54027000331502

INTELLIGENT DATA ANALYSIS IN MEDICINE AND PHARMACOLOGY

THE KLUWER INTERNATIONAL SERIES IN ENGINEERING AND COMPUTER SCIENCE

INTELLIGENT DATA ANALYSIS IN MEDICINE AND PHARMACOLOGY

edited by

Nada Lavrač
J. Stefan Institute
Ljubljana, Slovenia

Elpida T. Keravnou
University of Cyprus
Nicosia, Cyprus

Blaž Zupan
J. Stefan Institute
Ljubljana, Slovenia

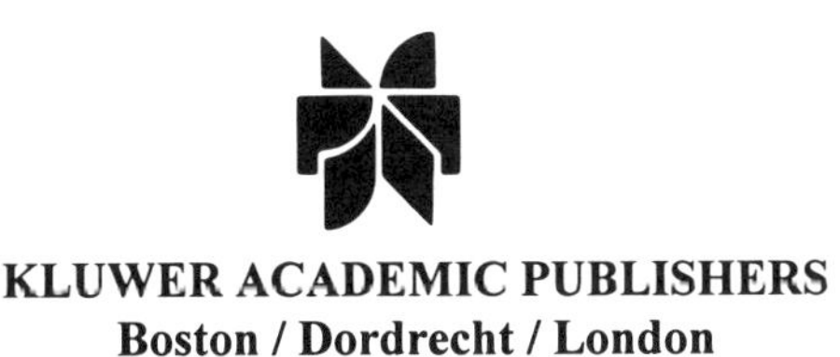

KLUWER ACADEMIC PUBLISHERS
Boston / Dordrecht / London

Distributors for North America:
Kluwer Academic Publishers
101 Philip Drive
Assinippi Park
Norwell, Massachusetts 02061 USA

Distributors for all other countries:
Kluwer Academic Publishers Group
Distribution Centre
Post Office Box 322
3300 AH Dordrecht, THE NETHERLANDS

Library of Congress Cataloging-in-Publication Data

A C.I.P. Catalogue record for this book is available
from the Library of Congress.

Illustration on front cover by Vjekoslav Vojo Radoičić

The publisher offers discounts on this book when ordered in bulk quantities. For more information contact: Sales Department, Kluwer Academic Publishers, 101 Philip Drive, Assinippi Park, Norwell, MA 02061

Printed on acid-free paper.

Printed in the United States of America

Contents

Preface

Intelligent data analysis, data mining and knowledge discovery in databases have recently gained the attention of a large number of researchers and practitioners. This is witnessed by the rapidly increasing number of submissions and participants at related conferences and workshops, by the emergence of new journals in this area (e.g., Data Mining and Knowledge Discovery, Intelligent Data Analysis, etc.) and by the increasing number of new applications in this field. In our view, the awareness of these challenging research fields and emerging technologies has been much larger in industry than in medicine and pharmacology. Hence, the main purpose of this book is to increase the awareness of the various techniques and methods that are available for intelligent data analysis in medicine and pharmacology, and to present case studies of their application.

The core of this book consists of selected (and thoroughly revised) papers presented at the First International Workshop on Intelligent Data Analysis in Medicine and Pharmacology (IDAMAP-96) held in Budapest in August 1996 as part of the 12th European Conference on Artificial Intelligence (ECAI-96). IDAMAP-96 was organized with the motivation to gather scientists and practitioners interested in computational data analysis methods applied to medicine and pharmacology, aimed at narrowing the increasing gap between extensive amounts of data stored in medical and pharmacological databases on the one hand, and the interpretation, understanding and effective use of stored data on the other hand. Besides the revised Workshop papers, the book contains a selection of contributions by invited authors aimed to broaden the scope of the book.

The expected readership of the book are researchers and practitioners interested in intelligent data analysis, data mining, and knowledge discovery in databases, particularly those that aim at using these technologies in medicine and pharmacology. Researchers and students in artificial intelligence and statistics should find this book of interest as well. Finally, much of the presented material will be interesting to physicians and pharmacologists challenged by new computational technologies, or simply in need of effectively utilizing the overwhelming volumes of data collected as a result of improved computer support in their daily professional practice. Further interest should be due to the need to solve problems emerging from automated data collection in modern hospitals, such as the analysis of electronic patient records, the analysis of data from patient-data management systems, intelligent alarming, as well as efficient and effective monitoring. Since the book is a collection of research papers it is primarily addressed at researchers and practitioners in the field. However, parts of it can be used as advanced readings for university courses in medical informatics (at the undergraduate and graduate level).

We wish to thank the authors of book chapters, the members of the IDAMAP-96 program committee (Pedro Barahona, Riccardo Bellazzi, Cristiana Larizza and Werner Horn) for their reviews, as well as the organizers of the ECAI-96 conference, in particular the workshop coordinator Elisabeth Andree. Our thanks goes also to Kluwer Academic Publishers, particularly Scott Delman, for their interest in this project. We are grateful to the J. Stefan Institute, Ljubljana, the Ministry of Science and Technology of Slovenia, and the University of Cyprus, Nicosia, for providing the research environment and funding enabling this work.

NADA LAVRAČ

ELPIDA T. KERAVNOU

BLAŽ ZUPAN

Ljubljana, Nicosia, March 1997

Contributing Authors

Marija Auersperg is a surgeon at the Institute of Oncology and a professor at the Medical Faculty in Ljubljana, Slovenia. For several years she had lead the thyroid carcinoma team at the Institute of Oncology.

J. Robert Beck (*jrbeck@bcm.tmc.edu*), M.D., is Vice President for Information Technology and Professor of Pathology at Baylor College of Medicine in Houston, Texas. His research encompasses the decision sciences in medicine, with particular interest in pharmacoeconomics, information technology applications, and diagnostic testing.

Riccardo Bellazzi (*ric@aim.unipv.it*), Ph.D., is an assistant professor at the Medical Informatics Laboratory of the Department of Computer and Systems Science, University of Pavia, Pavia, Italy. His research activity is mainly devoted to the application of AI-based techniques to the analysis and control of dynamic systems. He is currently involved in a telemedicine project called T-IDDM, for the intelligent management of diabetic patients.

Nikola Bešič (*nbesic@mail.onko-i.si*) is a surgeon at the Institute of Oncology in Ljubljana, Slovenia. He is a member of the thyroid carcinoma consortium. His research interests include the determination of prognostic factors and therapies for different types of thyroid carcinoma.

Marko Bohanec (*marko.bohanec@ijs.si*) is a research associate at the Department of Intelligent Systems, J. Stefan Institute, Ljubljana, Slovenia. His research and development interests are in decision support systems and machine learning. He has published in journals such as *Machine Learning*, *Acta Psychologica*, and *Information & Management.*

Makiko Daidoji (*daidoji@ia.noda.sut.ac.jp*) is a M.Sc. student of the Science University of Tokyo, Japan. She received a B.S. in 1996 from the Science University of Tokyo. She has been working in applied Inductive Logic Programming.

Andrej Dobnikar (*andrej.dobnikar@kri.fri.uni-lj.si*) is a professor at the Faculty of Computer and Information Science, University of Ljubljana, Slovenia. His research interests include neural networks, time-series prediction and pattern classification.

Sašo Džeroski (*Saso.Dzeroski@ijs.si*) has a Ph.D. degree in computer science and is a research associate at the Department of Intelligent Systems, J. Stefan Institute, Ljubljana, Slovenia. He is coauthor of *Inductive Logic Programming: Techniques and Applications*, Ellis Horwood 1994.

Dragan Gamberger (*gambi@lelhp1.irb.hr*) is a research associate at the Department of Physics, Rudjer Bošković Institute, Zagreb, Croatia. He developed the inductive learning system ILLM (Inductive Learning by Logic Minimization).

Josef Göppert (*goeppert@smst.de*) is a research assistant at the Department of Computer Engineering at the University of Tübingen, Germany. His research interests include applications and data analysis by artificial neural nets (ANN), especially the self-organizing map (SOM).

John Halter (*jah@bcm.tmc.edu*) is an assistant professor in the Department of Physical Medicine and Rehabilitation and the Division of Neuroscience at Baylor College of Medicine, Houston, Texas. He is also a member of the W.M. Keck Center for Computational Biology and on the executive committee for the Biomedical Computation and Visualization Laboratory. His research interests are in computational neuroscience, biomedical engineering and spinal cord injury.

Karsten R. Heidtke has a French diploma, a German Fachhochschuldiplom and a German university diploma, all in computer science. He is a Ph.D. student at the Max-Planck Institute for Molecular Genetics, Berlin, Germany with Steffen Schulze-Kremer.

Udo Heuser (*heuser@informatik.uni-tuebingen.de*) is a research assistant at the Department of Computer Engineering at the University of Tübingen, Germany. His diploma thesis discusses the classification of human brain waves using self-organizing maps (SOM).

Werner Horn (*werner@ai.univie.ac.at*), Ph.D., is Associate Professor of Artificial Intelligence at the Department of Medical Cybernetics and Artificial Intelligence of the University of Vienna, Austria. Since 1984 he has been Head of the Knowledge-Based Systems Group of the Austrian Research Institute for Artificial Intelligence. His main research interests include knowledge modeling, expert systems, knowledge acquisition, knowledge engineering, and specifically the embedding of knowledge-based modules into medical application systems.

Haku Ishida (*ishida@bcm.tmc.edu*), M.D., is Assistant Professor of Family Medicine and Laboratory Medicine at Kawasaki Medical School, Kurashiki, Japan. Dr. Ishida's research is applications of Information Technology to problems in laboratory medicine and primary care.

Michael W. Kattan (*MKattan@bcm.tmc.edu*), Ph.D., is Assistant Professor of Urology and Medical Informatics. He holds a primary appointment in the Scott Department of Urology and a secondary appointment in the Information Technology Program, both at Baylor College of Medicine, Houston, Texas. His research interests include medical decision making and machine learning.

Elpida T. Keravnou (*elpida@turing.cs.ucy.ac.cy*) is a professor at the Department of Computer Science of the University of Cyprus, and Chairperson of the Department. She is coauthor of *Competent Expert Systems: A Case Study in Fault Diagnosis*, Chapman and Hall, 1986, and *Expert Systems Architectures*, Chapman and Hall, 1988, and editor of *Deep Models for Medical Knowledge Engineering*, Elsevier Science Publishers, 1992. Her research interests are knowledge engineering, expert systems, temporal reasoning, diagnostic models, and artificial intelligence in medicine.

Ross D. King (*rdk@aber.ac.uk*) is a member of the Department of Computer Science at the University of Wales, Aberystwyth, U.K. Originally a member of the Inductive Logic Programming (ILP) groups at the Turing Institute, Scotland he was then at the Imperial Cancer Research Fund, London. He is the co-author of a number of important research papers examining the use of machine learning techniques in areas of biology.

Igor Kononenko (*igor.kononenko@fri.uni-lj.si*) is an associate professor at the Faculty of Computer and Information Science, University of Ljubljana, Slovenia. His research interests include artificial intelligence, machine learning and neural networks.

Igor Kranjec is a professor at the Department of Cardiology, University Medical Centre in Ljubljana, Slovenia.

Matjaž Kukar (*matjaz.kukar@fri.uni-lj.si*) is a research assistant at the Faculty of Computer and Information Science, University of Ljubljana, Slovenia. His research interests include machine learning and neural nets, applications in medicine and multimedia.

Cristiana Larizza (*cri@ipvlim1.unipv.it*), Ph.D., is an assistant professor at the Medical Informatics Laboratory of the Department of Computer and Systems Science, University of Pavia, Pavia, Italy. She has worked in the field of hospital information systems and decision support systems. Her current research activity includes temporal reasoning and intelligent data analysis.

Nada Lavrač (*nada.lavrac@ijs.si*) is a senior research associate at the Department of Intelligent Systems, J. Stefan Institute, Ljubljana, Slovenia. She is coauthor of *KARDIO: A Study in Deep and Qualitative Knowledge for Expert Systems*, The MIT Press 1989, and *Inductive Logic Programming: Techniques and Applications*, Ellis Horwood 1994. Her current research interests include machine learning, Inductive Logic Programming, and intelligent data analysis in medicine.

Subramani Mani (*mani@ics.uci.edu*) is a postgraduate researcher in the Department of Information and Computer Science, University of California at Irvine. He is interested in applications of machine learning, knowledge discovery and data mining, and Bayesian networks to medicine.

Silvia Miksch (*silvia@ifs.tuwien.ac.at*), Ph.D., is an assistant professor at the Institute of Software Technology, Vienna University of Technology, Austria. She was post-graduate fellow at Knowledge System Laboratory (KSL), Stanford University, California. Her general research interests are: temporal representation and reasoning, task-oriented design, protocol- and guideline-based care, planning, scheduling, time series analysis and filtering techniques, visualization, and evaluation of knowledge-based systems in real-world environments.

Fumio Mizoguchi (*mizo@ia.noda.sut.ac.jp*) is a professor and Director of Intelligent System Laboratory, the Science University of Tokyo, Japan. He received the B.Sc. degree in 1966, the M.Sc. degree in 1968 in Industrial Chemistry from the Science University of Tokyo, and Ph.D. in 1978 from the University of Tokyo. He has been working in Artificial Intelligence with various approaches. The most recent approaches are the use of Constraint Logic Programming and Inductive Logic Programming for real world problems.

Dunja Mladenić (*dunja.mladenic@ijs.si*) is a final year Ph.D. student in Computer Science at the Department of Intelligent Systems, J. Stefan Institute, Ljubljana, Slovenia. Her current research focuses on the use of machine learning in data analysis, with particular interests in learning from text applied on World Wide Web documents and intelligent agents.

Stephen H. Muggleton (*steve@comlab.ox.ac.uk*) is Research Fellow of Wolfson College, holder of a EPSRC Advanced Fellowship, and a member of the Sub-Faculty of Computation at the University of Oxford, U.K. Currently the Head of the Inductive Logic Programming (ILP) group at Oxford, he also coined the term "Inductive Logic Programming". He is the co-editor of the long-running series *Machine Intelligence*, editor of the book *Inductive Logic Programming*, and the author of a number of journal articles describing the theory, implementation, and application of ILP.

Hayato Ohwada (*ohwada@ia.noda.sut.ac.jp*) is Assistant Professor of Industrial Administration at the Science University of Tokyo, Japan. He received the B.Sc. degree in 1983, the M.Sc. degree in 1985 and the Ph.D. in 1988 from the Science University of Tokyo. He has been working in Inductive Logic Programming, Constraint Logic Programming and Intelligent Decision Support Systems.

Franz Paky (*franz.paky@magnet.at*), M.D., is Head of the Department of Pediatrics of the Hospital of Mödling, Austria. He is practicing pediatrician in Vienna. In 1984 he was member of the Respiratory Intensive Care Unit of the Hospital for Sick Children in London, U.K. His fields of interest include pedriatrics, neonatology, mechanical ventilation of infants, and applied computer science and medical expert systems.

Michael J. Pazzani (*pazzani@ics.uci.edu*) is Associate Professor and Chairman of the Department of Information and Computer Science, University of California at Irvine. His research interests include inductive learning, theory revision and information retrieval using machine learning.

Iztok A. Pilih is a trauma surgeon at the Department of Trauma Surgery, Celje General Hospital, Slovenia. He has completed his M.Sc. degree studying patients with severe head injury.

Christian Popow (*popow@vm.akh-wien.ac.at*), M.D., is Associate Professor of Pediatrics and Vice Head of the Department of Neonatology and Intensive Care of the Department of Pediatrics, University of Vienna, Austria. His special fields of interest include clinical neonatology, lung mechanics, mechanical ventilation of newborn infants, applied computer science, especially patient data management systems and medical expert systems.

Tine S. Prevec (*tine.prevec@uikn.mf.uni-lj.si*) is Professor of Neurology at the School of Medicine, University of Ljubljana, Slovenia. At the Department of Neurology in Innsbruck, Austria, he has studied the cognitive functions in patients recovering after a severe head injury.

Miran Rems, M.D., is a medical doctor at the Surgery Unit of General Hospital Jesenice, Slovenia. He is specially interested in computer-based analysis of medical data.

Alberto Riva (*alb@aim.unipv.it*) obtained a Ph.D. in Bioengineering at the University of Pavia, Italy, and is now a contract researcher with the Laboratory of Medical Informatics of the University Hospital of Pavia. He has worked in the fields of blackboard architectures and probabilistic reasoning under uncertainty. His current research interests are focused on the development of distributed artificial intelligence systems for medical applications.

Marko Robnik-Šikonja (*marko.robnik@fri.uni-lj.si*) is a research assistant at the Faculty of Computer and Information Science, University of Ljubljana, Slovenia. His research interests include machine learning, constructive induction and regression.

Wolfgang Rosenstiel (*rosenstiel@informatik.uni-tuebingen.de*) is Professor for Informatics (Computer Engineering) at the University of Tübingen and director of the Department "System Design in Microelectronics" at the research centre informatics (FZI), Karlsruhe, Germany. His research interests include high level synthesis, hardware software codesign, computer architecture, parallel computing and neural nets. He is TPC member of Eurodac, ICCAD, VLSI and others, member of the editorial board of DAES-Journal and member of IFIP 10.5.

Peter T. Scardino (*scardino@bcm.tmc.edu*), M.D., is a professor and Chairman of the Scott Department of Urology at Baylor College of Medicine, Houston, Texas. He is the primary investigator of a specialized program of research excellence (SPORE) grant in prostate cancer from the National Cancer Institute.

Steffen Schulze-Kremer (*steffen@chemie.fu-berlin.de*) has a Ph.D. in biochemistry and is a researcher at the Max-Planck Institute for Molecular Genetics in Berlin, Germany. He is author of the book *Molecular Bioinformatics: Algorithms and Applications*, Walter de Gruyter, 1996.

Yuval Shahar (*shahar@smi.stanford.edu*) M.D., Ph.D., is a senior research scientist since 1995 at the Section on Medical Informatics, School of Medicine, Stanford University, California, and Head of its planning and temporal reasoning group. His main research interests focus on planning and temporal reasoning for clinical applications. He is also interested in the representation, sharing, modification, recognition, and critiquing of clinical management plans, in representation and acquisition of general and task-specific medical knowledge, and in decision-theoretical aspects of clinical decision making.

William R. Shankle (*rshankle@uci.edu*) has joint appointments with the Departments of Neurology and Information and Computer Science, University of California at Irvine. His research interests include cognitive modeling and machine learning methods applied to developmental and degenerative conditions of the human brain.

Shiroaki Shirato is an associate professor and Vice-chairman at the Department of Ophthalmology, Faculty of Medicine, the University of Tokyo, Japan. He is the director of the glaucoma service at the Department of Ophthalmology, the University of Tokyo. He received the degree of M.D. in 1983 from the University of Tokyo.

Karsten Siems has a Ph.D. in chemistry and is project leader at Analyticon and Biotecon GmbH, Berlin, Germany.

Smiljana Slavec is General Manager of Infonet, Kranj, Slovenia, a company developing integrated medical information systems and decision support systems for medical treatment of patients.

Padhraic Smyth (*smyth@ics.uci.edu*) is an assistant professor in the Department of Information and Computer Science, University of California at Irvine. His research interests are knowledge discovery and data mining, statistical pattern recognition and machine learning.

Ashwin Srinivasan (*Ashwin.Srinivasan@comlab.ox.ac.uk*) is Research Officer, and a member of the Sub-Faculty of Computation at the University of Oxford, U.K. Since 1991, he has been part of the Inductive Logic Programming (ILP) groups at the Turing Institute, Scotland and at Oxford who have pioneered the application of ILP methods to biochemistry and molecular biology.

Michael J.E. Sternberg (*m_sternberg@icrf.icnet.uk*) is Head of the Biomolecular Modelling Laboratory, Imperial Cancer Research Fund, U.K. His main research interest has been in the area of computer modelling of biological molecules. In particular for the last eight years he has been a vital part of major research collaborations examining the application machine learning techniques to modeling problems.

Andreas Stevens (*stevens@uni-tuebingen.de*) is a lecturer and a senior physician at the University Clinic for Psychiatry and Psychotherapy at the University of Tübingen, Germany. His research interests are the neurobiology of cognitive processes and their alteration in psychiatric disease, quantitative EEG and infrared brain spectroscopy. He is member of the DGPPN and the "Neurowissenschaftliche Gesellschaft".

Branko Šter (*branko.ster@kri.fri.uni-lj.si*) is a junior researcher at the Faculty of Computer and Information Science, University of Ljubljana, Slovenia. His research interests include neural networks, pattern classification and time-series prediction.

Božo Urh is an information system developer in the medical-software development company Infonet, Kranj, Slovenia. He is particularly interested in the research and development of decision support and medical data analysis software.

Dietrich Wettschereck (*Dietrich.Wettschereck@gmd.de*) is a post-doctoral researcher at GMD, the German National Research Center for Information Technology, Sankt Augustin, Germany. He received his Ph.D. degree from Oregon State University.

Blaž Zupan (*blaz.zupan@ijs.si*) is a research assistant at the Department of Intelligent Systems, J. Stefan Institute, Ljubljana, Slovenia. His research interests include machine learning, computer-aided support for medical decision making, and medical informatics. Since 1993, he has also been involved in realistic neural modeling and medical data analysis projects at Baylor College of Medicine, Houston, Texas.

1 INTELLIGENT DATA ANALYSIS IN MEDICINE AND PHARMACOLOGY: AN OVERVIEW

Nada Lavrač,
Elpida T. Keravnou,
and Blaž Zupan

Abstract: Extensive amounts of data gathered in medical and pharmacological databases request the development of specialized tools for storing and accessing of data, data analysis, and effective use of stored data. Intelligent data analysis methods provide the means to overcome the resulting gap between data gathering and data comprehension. This chapter starts by presenting our view on the relation of intelligent data analysis to knowledge discovery in databases and data mining, and gives arguments why we have decided to use the term intelligent data analysis in the title of this book. It then discusses the needs and goals of intelligent data analysis in medicine and pharmacology. Next, it gives an overview of book chapters, characterizing them with respect to the intelligent data analysis methods used, as well as their application areas. Finally, it presents the overall purpose of this book.

1.1 INTRODUCTION

Now that we have gathered so much data, what do we do with it?
Usama Fayyad and Ramasamy Uthurusamy
editorial, *Communications of ACM*
Special issue on Data Mining, November 1996

Recently, many statements of this kind have appeared in journals, conference proceedings, and other materials that deal with data analysis, knowledge discovery, and machine learning. They all express a concern about how to "make sense" of large volumes of data being generated and stored in almost all fields of human activity.

Especially in the last few years, the digital revolution has provided relatively inexpensive and readily available means to collect and store the data. In the domain of medicine, in the mid-nineties one of the fathers of artificial intelligence in medicine, Edward H. Shortliffe, partially blamed the underdeveloped hospital infrastructure for the failure to fulfill the initial promise of the field [Shortliffe 1993]. Recently, however, the situation has changed rapidly: modern hospitals are well equipped with monitoring and other data collection devices, and data is gathered and shared in inter- and intra-hospital information systems. In fact, medical informatics has become a must and an integral part of every successful medical institution [Spackman et al., 1993].

The increase in data volume causes great difficulties in extracting useful information for decision support. Traditional manual data analysis has become insufficient, and methods for efficient computer-based analysis indispensable. From this need, a new interdisciplinary field, knowledge discovery in databases (KDD), was born [Frawley et al., 1991]. KDD encompasses statistical, pattern recognition, machine learning, and visualization tools to support the analysis of data and discovery of regularities that are encoded within the data.

The results of computer-based analysis have to be communicated to the users in an understandable way. In this respect, the analysis tools have to deliver transparent results and most often facilitate human intervention in the analysis process. A good example of such methods are symbolic machine learning algorithms that, as a result of data analysis, derive a symbolic model (e.g., a decision tree or a set of rules) of preferably low complexity but high transparency and accuracy.

1.2 INTELLIGENT DATA ANALYSIS AND ITS RELATION TO KNOWLEDGE DISCOVERY IN DATABASES

In order to argue for the selection of the term intelligent data analysis used in this book, we need to give a definition of what we understand under this term, and clarify its relation to the more established and more frequently used terms knowledge discovery in databases and data mining.

Knowledge discovery in databases (KDD) is frequently defined as a *process* [Fayyad et al., 1996] consisting of the following steps:

- understanding the domain,
- forming the dataset and cleaning the data,
- extracting of regularities hidden in the data thus formulating knowledge in the form of patterns, rules, etc.; this step in the overall KDD process is usually referred to as *data mining* (DM),
- postprocessing of discovered knowledge, and
- exploitation of the results.

KDD is an interactive and iterative process in which many steps need to be repeatedly applied in order to provide for an appropriate solution to the data analysis problem. In this process, *data visualization* plays an important role. The *data mining* step in KDD deals with the extraction of knowledge from (typically large masses of) data, thus describing the data in terms of the interesting regularities discovered.

Intelligent data analysis (IDA) is largely related to KDD. In our view, IDA also refers to the interactive and iterative process of data analysis, with the distinguishing feature that the architectures, methodologies and techniques used in this process are those of artificial intelligence. Figure 1.1 shows the relation of IDA to knowledge discovery in databases and data mining.

There is a large intersection between KDD and IDA. The two fields have in common the topic of investigation, which is data analysis, and they share many common methods. However, there are some differences in the characteristics of applied methods and domains under investigation. As stated above, the main difference is that IDA uses AI methods and tools, while KDD employs both AI and non-AI methods (e.g., machine learning data mining techniques are in the intersection of the two fields, whereas classical statistical methods belong to KDD but not to IDA). Another aspect involves the size of data: KDD is typically concerned with the extraction of knowledge from very large datasets, whereas in IDA the datasets are either large or moderately sized. This also affects the type of data mining tools used: in KDD the data mining tools are

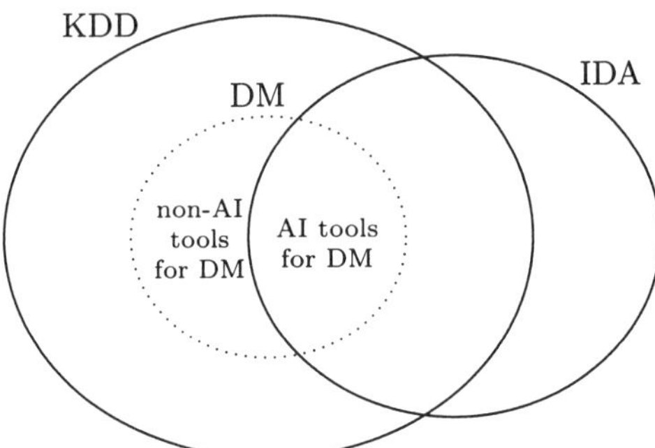

Figure 1.1 The relation between intelligent data analysis (IDA), knowledge discovery in databases (KDD), and data mining (DM).

executed mostly in batch mode (despite the fact that the entire KDD process is interactive), whereas in IDA the tools can either be batch or applied as interactive assistants.

1.3 INTELLIGENT DATA ANALYSIS IN MEDICINE AND PHARMACOLOGY

The gap between data generation and data comprehension is widening in all fields of human activity. In medicine and pharmacology, overcoming this gap is particularly crucial since medical decision making needs to be supported by arguments based on basic medical and pharmacological knowledge as well as knowledge, regularities and trends extracted from data.

1.3.1 The need for IDA in medicine and pharmacology

There are two main aspects that define the significance of and the need for intelligent data analysis in medicine and pharmacology:

- The first important aspect concerns the support of specific knowledge-based problem solving activities (diagnosis, prognosis, monitoring, etc.) through the intelligent analysis of given patient's raw data, e.g., a time series of data collected in monitoring. Data are mostly numeric and often quite noisy and incomplete. The aim is to glean out, in a dynamic fashion, useful abstractions (e.g., summaries) on the patient's (past, current, and hypothesized future) situation which can be matched against the relevant (diagnostic, prognostic, monitoring, etc.) knowledge for the purposes of the particular problem solving activity. Such data analysis methods are referred to as *data abstraction methods*, a term originally coined by Clancey in his now classical proposal on heuristic classification [Clancey 1985], where these methods form an integral part of the reasoning process. Recently, data abstraction methods have been concerned with the interpretation of temporal data (*temporal data abstraction*), where temporal trends and more complex temporal patterns constitute main types of such abstractions. Since the primary goal of (temporal) data abstraction methods is on-line decision support, their quality assessment is performance-based: for instance, does a method provide adequate support for diagnostic and prognostic reasoning, does it predict well a trend or a value to be expected at the next point of time? In this context, *visualization of data* is extremely important for supporting decision making and even invaluable for successfully performing a problem solving task.

- The second aspect concerns the discovery of new (medical, pharmacological) knowledge that can be extracted through data mining of representative collections of example cases, described by symbolic or numeric descriptors. The available datasets are often incomplete (missing data) and noisy (erroneous). The methods for extracting meaningful and understandable symbolic knowledge will be referred to as *data mining methods*. The quality assessment of these methods is based both on the performance (classification and prediction accuracy, misclassification cost, sensitivity, specificity, etc.), as well as the understandability and significance of the discovered knowledge.

Data abstraction, whose goal is to describe the data in more abstract terms, can also be used in the preprocessing of data for further analysis by data mining techniques and tools.

1.3.2 Goals of IDA research in medicine and pharmacology

Any research in medicine or pharmacology aims to directly or indirectly enhance the provision of health care. IDA research in these fields is no exception. The general goal of IDA in pharmacology is to enhance the knowledge and understanding of the structure and properties of therapeutic agents, or agents harmful to human health. Specific goals of IDA in medicine are:

- the intelligent interpretation of patient data in a context-sensitive manner and the presentation of such interpretations in a visual or symbolic form; the temporal dimension in the representation and intelligent interpretation of patient data is of primary importance,

- the extraction (discovery) of medical knowledge for diagnostic, screening, prognostic, monitoring, therapy support or overall patient management tasks.

IDA research in medicine and pharmacology is driven by a very pragmatic aim: the enhancement of health care. As such, the benchmark tests for these methods and techniques can only be real world problems. Viable IDA proposals for medicine or pharmacology must be accompanied by detailed requirements that delineate the spectrum of real applications addressed by such proposals; in-depth evaluation of resulting systems thus constitutes a critical aspect.

Another consideration is the role of IDA systems in a clinical or pharmacological setting. Their role is clearly that of an intelligent assistant that tries to bridge the gap between data gathering and data comprehension, in order to enable the physician or the pharmacologist to perform his task more efficiently and effectively. If the physician has at his disposal the right information at the right time then doubtless he will be in a better position to reach correct decisions or instigate correct actions within the given time constraints. The information revolution made it possible to collect and store large volumes of data from diverse sources on electronic media. These data can be on a single case (e.g., one patient) or on multiple cases. Raw data as such are of little value since their sheer volume and/or the very specific level at which they are expressed make its utilization (operationalization) in the context of problem solving impossible. However such data can be converted to a mine of information wealth if the real gems of information are gleaned out by computationally intelligent means. The useful, operational information/knowledge, which is expressed at the right level of abstraction, is then readily available to support the decision making of the physician in managing a patient or of a pharmacologist in analyzing a therapeutic agent.

Important issues that arise from the rapidly emerging globality of data and information are:

- the provision of standards in terminology, vocabularies and formats to support multi-linguality and sharing of data,
- standards for the abstraction and visualization of data,
- standards for interfaces between different sources of data,
- seamless integration of heterogeneous data; images and signals are important types of data,
- standards for electronic patient records, and
- reusability of data, knowledge, and tools.

Clinical and pharmacological data constitute an invaluable resource, the proper utilization of which impinges directly on the essential aim of health care which is "correct patient management". Investing in the development of appropriate IDA methods, techniques and tools for the analysis of clinical and pharmacological data is thoroughly justified and this research ought to form a main thrust of activity by the relevant research communities.

1.4 BOOK OVERVIEW

Based on the main aspects of the use of IDA methods in medicine and pharmacology, discussed in Section 1.3.1, we propose the classification of IDA methods into data abstraction methods and data mining methods. The top level organization of the book chapters is based on the areas: data abstraction (Part I) and data mining (Part II). Figure 1.2 shows the further division of chapters according to the methods used.

1.4.1 Data abstraction methods

Data abstraction methods are intended to support specific knowledge-based problem solving activities (data interpretation, diagnosis, prognosis, monitoring, etc.) by gleaning out the useful abstractions from the raw, mostly numeric patient data. *Temporal data abstraction methods* represent an important subgroup where the processed data are temporal. The derivation of abstractions is often done in a context sensitive and/or distributed manner and it applies to discrete and continuous supplies of data. Useful types of temporal abstractions are trends, periodic happenings, and other forms of temporal patterns. Temporal abstractions can also be discovered by visualization. The abstraction can be performed over a single case (e.g., a single patient) or over a collection of cases.

In this book, most of the contributions under temporal data abstraction are concerned with a single case, that is information on a single patient. Moreover the discussed approaches are knowledge-driven in the sense that aspects of the performed computations are driven by domain knowledge. Overall, the single case temporal data abstraction approaches included in this book are divided into context-sensitive (the chapters by Miksch et al. and Shahar), periodicity-based (the chapter by Keravnou) and distributed (the chapter by Bellazzi et al.).

For many medical domains the interpretation of patient data depends on relevant contexts. For example, the results of some laboratory examination can be interpreted differently under the two contexts "the patient is not receiving any treatment", and "the patient is receiving treatment X". Contexts are dynamic entities and hence they also need to be derived and revised, from lower

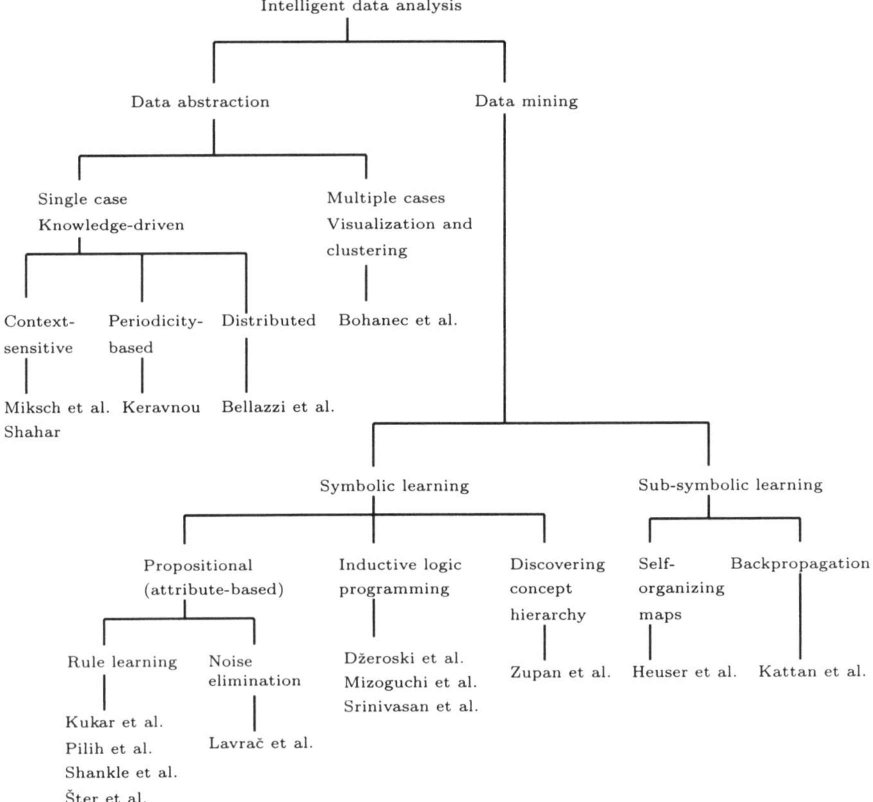

Figure 1.2 Organization of book chapters according to the IDA methods used.

level patient data, as a necessary step for the accurate derivation of temporal abstractions, such as significant temporal trends, on the status of the patient. Being dynamic entities, contexts have (finite) persistences and there can be multiple, overlapping contexts for a given patient. This is addressed by Miksch et al. and Shahar.

Periodic occurrences are intrinsically relevant to medical practice; symptoms can occur in repetitive patterns, disorders can be characterized with cyclic behavior, and cycles are inherent in treatment protocols. The expression of repetitive behavior, repetitive actions and repetitive phenomena as well as the derivation of such happenings (of any degree of complexity) from lower level information are necessary considerations for many medical domains. By nature periodic occurrences are composite occurrences, whereby the default assumption is that periods of dormancy exist between successive components. Overall, periodic occurrences constitute an important type of temporal abstractions. This problem is addressed in the chapter by Keravnou.

The advantages of distributed processing are well known and recently the advent of the Internet has given a new dimension and perspective to telematics tools and applications in a rapidly emerging Information Society. Hence it is not surprising that the field of telemedicine is acquiring more and more prominence in this new era of information technology with a view to bringing health care into the homes of the patients. The approach by Bellazzi et al. on distributed temporal data abstraction is therefore timely placed in the context of these developments. The processing of patient data is distributed between two components operating asynchronously, at different frequencies, and with different computational demands.

The temporal abstractions derived from some case, such as a patient, constitute an abstract (temporal) case. From multiple such abstract cases, new knowledge for the particular domain can be generated. However, the visualization and clustering of multiple concrete cases from a temporal perspective, as illustrated in the chapter by Bohanec et al., provides an effective, user-friendly, and computationally cheap way of gleaning out relevant temporal patterns within recently-past time windows which, when correlated across longer-past time windows, can lead to the discovery of more generic temporal patterns.

1.4.2 Data mining methods

Data mining methods are intended to extract knowledge preferably in a meaningful and understandable symbolic form. Most frequently applied methods in this context are supervised symbolic learning methods. For example, effective tools for inductive learning exist that can be used to generate understandable diagnostic and prognostic rules. Symbolic clustering, discovery of concept hierarchies, qualitative model discovery, and learning of probabilistic causal networks fit in this framework as well. Sub-symbolic learning and case-based reasoning methods can also be classified in the data mining category. Other frequently applied sub-symbolic methods are nearest neighbor, Bayesian classifier, and (non-symbolic) clustering.

In this book, the contributions to data mining are limited to symbolic and sub-symbolic learning approaches. Their common aim is the discovery of knowledge in symbolic or sub-symbolic forms, by generalizing from multiple cases.

The symbolic learning approaches included in this book are divided into propositional (attribute-based) approaches, inductive logic programming approaches (the chapters by Mizoguchi et al., and Srinivasan et al.), and a decomposition approach to discovering a concept hierarchy (the chapter by Zupan et al.). Propositional learning approaches form the largest subgroup of the symbolic learning approaches. This subgroup is further divided into the approaches for learning rules from the example cases (the chapters by Kukar et al., Pilih et al., Shankle et al., and Šter et al.) and an approach to noise elimination from example cases (the chapter by Lavrač et al.). The chapter by Džeroski et al. uses propositional and inductive logic programming approaches, as well as sub-symbolic learning.

Rules were proposed from the early days of knowledge-based systems, and expert systems in particular, as a prime formalism for expressing knowledge in a symbolic way. Propositional rules are simple, categorical rules, with no variables, which nonetheless are considered adequately expressive for many real applications. Predicate rules on the other hand are substantially more expressive and thus the techniques of inductive logic programming have been developed for domains where the additional expressiveness is required. Hierarchical structures provide a natural way for organizing a given body of knowledge at different levels of abstraction, thus combating the complexity of flat structures where one is "forced" to consider all the detail together. Effective, and thus successful, rule bases are not flat but they are hierarchically organized in terms of explicit concept hierarchies. The approach by Zupan et al. aims to convert a "flat" collection of propositional rules to a hierarchical collection of simpler rules by learning the underlying concept hierarchy.

The viability of rule learning approaches depends heavily on the quality of the processed case examples. Noise in data is an unavoidable phenomenon in many real domains, both in medicine and pharmacology, and thus its presence has to be acknowledged and managed by computational means. Basically there are two types of approaches to noise handling: either to eliminate the noise as a preprocessing step prior to the learning of rules, such as the approach proposed by Lavrač et al., or to handle the noise in the learning of rules.

The symbolic learning approaches constitute the bulk of the data mining contributions. However for the sake of providing a more balanced picture of the relevant state-of-the-art, the inclusion of some contributions from the sub-symbolic learning area was deemed necessary. This part of the book features two chapters on two sub-symbolic learning approaches, the self organizing maps (the chapter by Heuser et al.) and backpropagation neural networks (the chapter by Kattan et al.). It should be mentioned that the chapters by Džeroski et al., Kukar et al., and Šter et al. also describe experiments using neural networks.

1.4.3 Alternative classifications of book chapters

The contributions in this book can be classified in other ways to the one used as the basis for the organization of chapters in the book. Below we discuss two alternative classifications of the included material.

First, the contributions can be classified according to the development of new methods (the chapters by Keravnou, Lavrač et al., Miksch et al., Shahar, and Zupan et al.), the adaptation of methods (the chapters by Heuser et al. and Mizoguchi et al.), the comparative evaluation of methods in medical domains (the chapters by Kukar et al., Shankle et al., and Šter et al.), and applications (the chapters by Bellazzi et al., Bohanec et al., Džeroski et al., Heuser et al., Kattan et al., Kukar et al., Miksch et al., Mizoguchi et al., Pilih et al., and Srinivasan et al.).

Second, the contributions can be classified on the basis of which area they address, medicine or pharmacology. From this classification perspective, the content of the book is unbalanced since only two chapters (the ones by Džeroski et al. and Srinivasan et al.) address problems in biochemistry. Džeroski et al. present a study in structure elucidation of diterpenes, a class of organic compounds of substantial potential in the search for new pharmaceutical effectors. The study of Srinivasan et al. focuses on potentially harmful, rather than therapeutic, agents and, more specifically, it concerns the discovery of structure-activity relationships for a group of cancer related compounds. Enhancing the knowledge in such dangerous compounds is even more vital than discovering new therapeutic agents for combating their harmful effects and constitutes an effective basis for preventive care, at the same time resulting in the formulation of appropriate standards for industrial practices. The other fourteen chapters are concerned with problems from medicine. These chapters can be further classified in accordance with the problem solving tasks they address. Zupan et al. address concept refinement from a generic point of view and thus their approach is applicable in the context of different problem solving tasks. Keravnou and Shahar address data interpretation and again their approaches can be used in the context of different tasks, such as monitoring or diagnostic tasks. Heuser et al., Kattan et al., Lavrač et al., Mizoguchi et al., and Shankle et al. address diagnostic (or screening) tasks. Kukar et al., Pilih et al. and Šter et al. address prognostic tasks. Miksch et al. address a monitoring task. Bellazzi et al. address a patient management task and finally Bohanec et al. address a therapy support task.

1.5 THE PURPOSE OF THE BOOK

In our view, the awareness of the challenging new fields of intelligent data analysis, data mining and knowledge discovery in databases, and emerging new technologies has been much larger in industry, finance, and economy than in medicine and pharmacology. Hence, the purpose of this book is to increase the awareness of various techniques and methods that are available for intelligent data analysis in medicine and pharmacology, and to present some case studies of their application.

The principal aim of this book is to give a coverage of the state-of-the-art in intelligent data analysis in medicine and pharmacology and to illustrate the diversity of the field. Presently the field attracts attention from researchers with different motivations and backgrounds, such as (traditional) machine learning, case-based learning, knowledge-based problem solving, temporal reasoning, qualitative modeling etc. The outcome of this research can be roughly classified under the two areas, data abstraction and data mining. Consequently, the book is organized along these two axes.

Within the scope of the principal aim, subordinate aims are to present new theoretical achievements and to place these in the context of real-world medical and pharmacological applications. In other words, the overall aim is to give an accurate picture of the state-of-the-art in this field, both in theory and practice. Most of the chapters of amalgamate theory with practice.

We expect that researchers and practitioners interested in intelligent data analysis, data mining, and knowledge discovery in databases, particularly those that aim at using these technologies in the field of medicine or pharmacology, will constitute a main readership for the book. In addition, the book will be of broader interest to the researchers, practitioners and students in artificial intelligence, statistics, and knowledge discovery in databases. Finally, much of this reading should be interesting to physicians and pharmacologists who simply wish to get acquainted with the challenging new computational technologies, or because of the needs caused by the overwhelming existence of enormous amounts of data, stored as a result of improved computational support in their daily professional life. This interest is based on the increased needs to solve problems that result from the automated data collection in modern hospitals, such as the analysis of computer-based patient records (CPR), analysis of data from patient-data management systems (PDMS), intelligent alarming, as well as effective and efficient monitoring.

Since the book is a collection of research papers it is primarily addressed at the researchers in the field. However, parts of it may be utilized in the context of university courses (undergraduate and graduate) in medical informatics.

Acknowledgments

Nada Lavrač and Blaž Zupan are supported by research grants provided by the Ministry of Science and Technology of Slovenia. The support for Elpida T. Keravnou is provided by a research grant from the University of Cyprus.

References

Clancey, W. J. (1985). Heuristic classification. *Artificial Intelligence*, 27:289–350.

Fayyad, U. M., Piatetsky-Shapiro, G., and Smyth, P. (1996). The KDD process for extracting useful knowledge from volumes of data. *Communications of the ACM*, 39(11):27–41.

Frawley, W., Piatetsky-Shapiro, G., and Matheus, C. (1991). Knowledge discovery in databases: An overview. In Piatetsky-Shapiro, G. and Frawley, W., editors, *Knowledge Discovery in Databases*. The AAAI Press, Menlo Park, CA.

Shortliffe, E. H. (1993). The adolescence of AI in medicine: Will field come of age in the '90s? *Artificial Intelligence in Medicine*, 5(2):93–106.

Spackman, K., Elert, J. D., and Beck, J. R. (1993). The CIO and the medical informaticist: Alliance for progress. In *Proc. Annual Symposium on Computer Applications in Medical Care*, pages 525–528.

I Data Abstraction

2 TIME-ORIENTED ANALYSIS OF HIGH-FREQUENCY DATA IN ICU MONITORING

Silvia Miksch,
Werner Horn,
Christian Popow,
and Franz Paky

Abstract: Interpretation of high-frequency data (sampled every second) in Intensive Care Units (ICUs) requires a time-oriented analysis resulting in a high-level abstraction. This chapter presents analysis methods of such data to abstract qualitative descriptions over a period of time. The methods are sensitive to the context and the abstracted descriptions cover both the current situation and the time course of the monitored parameters. The aim of the time-oriented analysis is to arrive at unified qualitative values or patterns, comprehensible to health care providers and easy to use for decision support. The methods are guided by the expectation of skilled physicians about the physiological course of parameter development. They incorporate knowledge about data points, data intervals, and expected qualitative trend patterns. The applicability and usefulness are illustrated by examples from VIE-VENT, an open-loop knowledge-based monitoring and therapy planning system for artificially ventilated newborn infants.

2.1 THE NEED FOR DERIVING TEMPORAL PATTERNS

Monitoring and therapy planning in real-world environments involves numerous data analysis problems. First, long-term monitoring requires the processing of a huge volume of data generated from several (monitoring) devices and individuals. Second, the available data and information occur at various observation frequencies (e.g., high or low frequency data), at various regularities (e.g., continuously or discontinuously sampled data), and are of various types (e.g., qualitative or quantitative data). Third, the time-oriented analysis process has to cope with a combination of all these data sources. Fourth, the underlying domain knowledge about the interactions of parameters is vague and incomplete. Fifth, the interpretation context is shifting depending on observed data. Sixth, the underlying expectations regarding the development of parameters are different according to the interpretation context and to the degrees of parameters' abnormality. Seventh, the acquired data is more noisy than expected because of measurement errors, on-line transmission problems, or input from different people in different environments and in different experimental settings.

Interest in the problem of automating the data analysis has grown steadily under the label knowledge discovery in databases (KDD) and data mining [Fayyad et al., 1996]. Traditional theories of data analysis [Avent and Charlton, 1990, Kay, 1993] mostly deal with well-defined problems. However, in many real-world cases the underlying structure-function models or the domain knowledge and models are poorly understood or not applicable because of incomplete knowledge and complexity as well as the vague qualitative data involved (e.g., qualitative expected trend descriptions). Therefore statistical analysis, control theory, or other techniques are often unusable, inappropriate or at least only partially applicable.

To overcome the mentioned limitations, time-oriented analysis methods were proposed to derive qualitative values or patterns of the current and the past situation of a patient. An advantage of using qualitative descriptions is their unified usability in the system model, regardless of their origin. These derived qualitative values or patterns are used for different tasks within the monitoring and therapy planning process (e.g., to clarify data, to recommend therapeutic actions). Several different approaches have been introduced to perform such a temporal data abstraction (e.g., [Haimowitz et al., 1995, Shahar and Musen, 1996], see Section 2.2). However, dealing with high-frequency data, shifting contexts, and different expectations on the development of parameters require particular temporal abstraction methods to arrive at unified qualitative values or patterns.

We propose context-sensitive and expectation-guided temporal abstraction methods to perform the time-oriented data analysis. The methods incorporate knowledge about data points, data intervals, and expected qualitative trend patterns to arrive at unified qualitative descriptions of parameters (*temporal data abstraction*). Our methods are based on context-sensitive schemata for data-point transformation and curve fitting which express the dynamics of and the reactions to different degrees of parameters' abnormalities, as well as on smoothing and adjustment mechanisms to keep the qualitative descriptions stable in case of shifting contexts or data oscillating near thresholds. Our temporal abstraction methods combine AI techniques with time-series analysis, namely linear regression modeling. The stepwise linear regression model approximates vague medical knowledge, which could be determined only in verbal terms. The derived qualitative values or patterns are used for data validation, for recommending therapeutic actions, for assessing the effectiveness of these actions within a certain period, and for user- and time-oriented data visualization.

Our approach is oriented towards, but not limited to, our application domain of artificial ventilation of newborn infants in intensive care units. The temporal abstraction methods are integrated and implemented in VIE-VENT, an open-loop knowledge-based monitoring and therapy planning system for artificially ventilated newborn infants [Miksch et al., 1993, Miksch et al., 1996, Horn et al., 1997]. VIE-VENT had been tested and evaluated in real clinical scenarios. The applicability and usefulness of our approach are illustrated by an example from VIE-VENT.

The rest of the chapter is organized as follows: Section 2.2 explains why existing methods are not applicable and fail to meet our requirements. Section 2.3 presents the application domain by introducing the basic concepts and giving a sample case. Section 2.4 concentrates on the context-sensitive and expectation-guided temporal abstraction methods and illustrates them using the sample case. Finally, our experiences within a real-clinical setting are described, concluding with the strengths and limitations of the proposed approach.

2.2 OTHER APPROACHES TO DATA-ABSTRACTION AND THEIR LIMITATIONS

Several different approaches have been introduced to perform temporal abstraction tasks. The systems were implemented mainly for clinical domains. A pioneering work in the area of knowledge-based monitoring and therapy planning systems was the Ventilator Manager (VM, [Fagan et al., 1980]), which was designed to manage postsurgical mechanically ventilated patients. VM was developed in the late 1970s as one of a series of experiments studying the effectiveness of the MYCIN formalism. In recent years the most significant and encouraging approaches were the temporal utility package (TUP,

[Kohane, 1986]), the temporal control structure system (TCS, [Russ, 1989]), the TOPAZ system [Kahn, 1991], the temporal-abstraction module in the M-HTP project [Larizza et al., 1992], the temporal resource management in the Guardian project [Hayes-Roth et al., 1992], the trend detecting mechanism based on trend templates in the $TrenD_x$ project [Haimowitz et al., 1995], the RÉSUMÉ project [Shahar and Musen, 1993, Shahar and Musen, 1996], the T-IDDM project [Bellazzi et al., 1996, Larizza et al., 1997], the aggregation and forgetting mechanisms in the NéoGanesh project [Dojat and Sayettat, 1995], and the recognition of temporal scenarios [Ramaux et al., 1997]. A comprehensive review of various temporal-reasoning approaches and useful references are given in [Shahar and Musen, 1996]. In the following we concentrate only on the two approaches most closely related to our approach, pointing out their differences and limitations for our purpose.

Haimowitz and coworkers [Haimowitz et al., 1995] have developed the concept of trend templates ($TrenD_x$) to represent all the available information during an observation process. A trend template defines disorders as typical patterns of relevant parameters. These patterns consist of a partially ordered set of temporal intervals with uncertain endpoints. The trend templates are used to detect trends in series of time-stamped data. The drawbacks of this approach lie in the predefinition of the expected normal behavior of parameters during the whole observation process and the usage of absolute value thresholds matching a trend template. The absolute thresholds do not take into account the different degrees of parameters' abnormalities. In many domains it is impossible to define such static trajectories of the observed parameters in advance. Depending on the degrees of parameters' abnormalities and on the various contexts, different normal behaviors are possible. These normal expectations vary according to the patient's status in the past. Therefore these thresholds have to be derived dynamically during the observation period. For example, the decreasing of transcutaneous partial pressure of carbon dioxide ($P_{tc}CO_2$) from 94 $mmHg$ to 90 $mmHg$ during the last 25 minutes would be assessed as "decrease too slow" because the patient's respiratory status was extremely above the target range in the past. However, the same amount of change (4 units) from 54 $mmHg$ to 50 $mmHg$ during the same time interval (25 minutes) would be assessed as "normal decrease" if the patient's respiratory status was slightly above the target range.

RÉSUMÉ [Shahar and Musen, 1993, Shahar and Musen, 1996] performs temporal abstraction of time-stamped data without predefined trends. The system is based on a knowledge-based temporal-abstraction method (KBTA), which is decomposed into five subtasks: temporal context restriction, vertical temporal inference, horizontal temporal inference, temporal interpolation, and temporal pattern matching. They have applied RÉSUMÉ to different clinical domains (e.g., children's growth, AIDS, diabetes) and one engineering domain (traffic control). However, their approach is only applicable for a particular class of problem features: First, it concentrates on mechanisms to cope with low-frequency observations which cannot easily be adapted for high-frequency data due to their different properties. Second, RÉSUMÉ covers only limited domain dynamics (e.g., the classifiers for different degrees of parameters' abnormalities need to be derived dynamically during run-time). Third, it requires predefined domain knowledge to perform the temporal interpolation (e.g., gap functions), which is not available in some domains. Fourth, the high level abstraction mechanism (pattern matching based on external and internal knowledge) is superfluous for therapy planning in ICUs because the domain-specific heuristic knowledge needed is often not available in appropriate way.

Our approach benefits from using all the available information based on temporal ontologies (time points and intervals [Allen 1991, Dean and McDermott, 1987], different granularities (continuously and discontinuously sampled data) and various kinds of data (quantitative and qualitative data). Our temporal data-abstraction methods cover the different degrees of parameters' abnormalities caused by shifting contexts and their corresponding dynamics (e.g., "the higher the degree of a parameter's abnormality the bigger is the amount of positive parameter's change which is classified as normal") as well as expected qualitative trend descriptions (e.g., "the transcutaneous partial pressure of oxygen ($P_{tc}O_2$) value should reach the normal region within approximately 10 to 20 minutes") to arrive at unified qualitative descriptions of parameters. To keep our qualitative descriptions stable we apply smoothing and adjustment methods.

Additionally, we do not predefine absolute, time-dependent expected normal behavior of parameters during the whole observation process (as in [Haimowitz et al., 1995]), because the course of a parameter according to an absolute temporal dimension (axis) is not known in advance. We derive schemata for curve fitting in relation to the specific states of each parameter. The combination of different parameters' states reflects a particular context. Improving or worsening of these parameters are assumed to be best described as exponential functions. The costs to compare such exponential functions are reduced by stepwise linearization.

2.3 APPLICATION DOMAIN AND BASIC CONCEPTS

In this section we will explain the application domain, specify the input and the output of our temporal data-abstraction methods, introduce a sample case, and explain the basic notion of our concepts "context-sensitive" and "expectation-guided".

2.3.1 Application domain: Monitoring and therapy planning of artificially ventilated newborn infants in NICUs

Medical diagnosis and therapy planning at modern Intensive Care Units (ICUs) have been refined by the technical improvement of available equipment. We are particularly interested in the monitoring and therapy-planning tasks of artificially ventilated newborn infants in Neonatal ICUs (NICUs). These tasks can be improved by applying derived qualitative values or patterns (temporal data abstraction).

Our temporal abstraction methods are integrated, implemented, and evaluated in VIE-VENT. This is an open-loop knowledge-based monitoring and therapy planning system for artificially ventilated newborn infants [Miksch et al., 1993, Miksch et al., 1995]. It incorporates alarming, monitoring, and therapy planning tasks within one system. The data-driven architecture of VIE-VENT consists of five modules: data selection, data validation, temporal data abstraction, data interpretation and therapy planning. All these steps are involved in each cycle of data collection from monitors. VIE-VENT is especially designed for practical use under real-time constraints at NICUs. Its various components are built in analogy to the clinical reasoning process.

2.3.2 Input and output

VIE-VENT's input data set can be divided into continuously and discontinuously sampled data. Continuously sampled data (e.g., blood-gas measurements, like $P_{tc}O_2$, $P_{tc}CO_2$, S_aO_2, and ventilator settings, like PIP, F_iO_2) are taken from the output of the data selection module every 10 seconds. Discontinuously sampled data are entered into the system on request by the user depending on different conditions (e.g., critical ventilatory condition of the neonate, elapsed time intervals). The system output consists in primarily of therapeutic recommendations for changing the ventilator setting. Additionally, VIE-VENT gives warnings in critical situations, as well as comments and explanations about the health condition of the neonate.

The input to the temporal data-abstraction methods includes a set of time-stamped parameters (the continuously sampled data which are recorded every 10 seconds and the discontinuously sampled data at a particular time-stamp) and expected qualitative trend patterns (e.g., "the parameter $P_{tc}CO_2$ is moving one qualitative step towards the target range within 20 to 30 minutes.") The specific context of the observed parameters is automatically deduced from the input parameters, mainly the ventilator settings. The output of the data-abstraction methods is a set of time-point- and interval-based, context-specific, qualitative descriptions. These qualitative descriptions can be a separate abstraction at a particular time-stamp and/or a combination of different time-specific abstractions (a higher level of abstraction, e.g., a combination of different time-stamped qualitative data-point categories or a combination of time-point- and interval-based values called qualitative trend category).

2.3.3 A sample case

Figure 2.1 shows a sample case of VIE-VENT. In the following sections this sample case is used to illustrate our temporal data-abstraction methods. The left-hand region shows the blood-gas measurements (transcutaneous CO_2, CO_2, S_aO_2) and their corresponding qualitative temporal abstractions on the top. The actual ventilator settings (first column, e.g., F_iO_2 is 38%), and VIE-VENT's therapeutic recommendations at the current time (second column, e.g., decrease F_iO_2 to 30%) are given below. The upper right-hand region shows two status lines. First, the combination of different time-specific abstractions is labeled by "Status" (e.g., "hyperoxemia" is the combination of the qualitative data-point categories of S_aO_2 and $P_{tc}O_2$). Second, additional warnings are labeled by "Warnings". The right-hand region gives plots of the most important parameters over the last four hours. Scrolling to previous time periods in the plots is possible by pushing the buttons [<<] for a four-hour step backward, [<] for an one-hour step backward, [>>] and [>] for forward stepping. The therapeutic recommendations are displayed as black vertical lines in the corresponding curve of the ventilator setting (In the VIE-VENT application the user interface is colored, therefore the recommendations are displayed as red vertical lines).

2.3.4 Meaning of "context-sensitive"

The abstraction problem becomes more difficult when the behavior of a system involves interactions among components or interactions with people or with the environment. Under these conditions, correct abstractions become context-sensitive. It is possible to determine *a priori* a set of sensor parameters with their fixed plausible ranges. However, if the context is shifting, e.g., one component gets in a critical condition or a changing of specific phases or of protocols occurs, a capability for dynamic adjustment of threshold values is needed.

The context is automatically deduced from the set of input parameters. For example, we monitor the patient during the whole artificial ventilation process. The ventilation process can be divided into different phases, namely an initial phase, a phase of controlled ventilation (intermittent positive pressure ventilation, "ippv"), a phase of weaning (intermittent mandatory ventilation, "imv"), and a phase of returning to spontaneous breathing. All phases characterize a particular context and can be deduced from the current ventilator setting. In

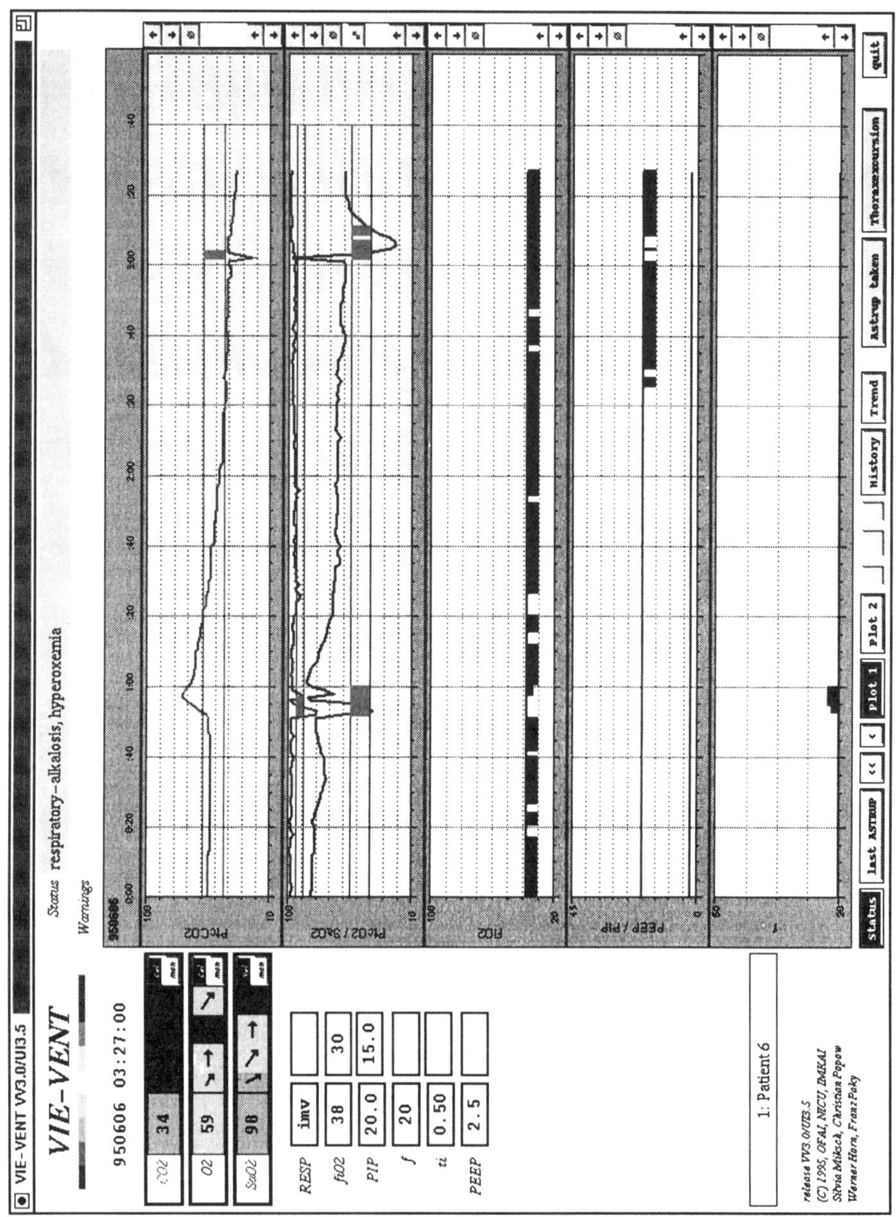

Figure 2.1 Sample case of VIE-VENT.

Figure 2.1 the context "imv" is shown in the first row of the ventilator settings labeled by "RESP".

2.3.5 Meaning of "expectation-guided"

Usually, the temporal abstraction is either exclusively based on the observed input parameters (see [Shahar and Musen, 1993, Shahar and Musen, 1996]) or predefined trajectories of observed parameters are used (see [Haimowitz et al., 1995]). The first neglects available knowledge; in many domains expectations of parameters' courses are obtainable. However, trajectories of observed parameters are often difficult to define in advance. The problem lies in the lack of an appropriate curve-fitting model to predict the development of parameters from actual measurements. Nevertheless, verbal descriptions about expectations of parameters' developments, which are obtained from domain experts. We improved our temporal data-abstraction process, including *expected qualitative trend descriptions*, which are derived from domain experts.

2.4 TEMPORAL DATA-ABSTRACTION METHODS

The aim of the temporal data-abstraction process is to arrive at unified, context-sensitive qualitative descriptions. The data abstraction is based on time points, time intervals and expected qualitative trend descriptions within a particular context. Dealing with high-frequency data, shifting contexts, and different expectations of the parameters' development requires particular temporal abstraction methods to arrive at unified qualitative values or patterns. Our temporal data-abstraction process consists of five different methods: (1) transformation of quantitative point data into qualitative values (context-sensitive schemata for data-point transformation), (2) smoothing of data oscillating near thresholds, (3) smoothing of schemata for data-point transformation, (4) context-sensitive adjustment of qualitative values, and (5) transformation of interval data (context-sensitive and expectation-guided schemata for trend-curve fitting).

The schemata for data-point transformation transform single observations into qualitative values. To keep the qualitative values stable in case of shifting contexts or data oscillating near thresholds, we apply different smoothing methods. In critical states of the patient we have to adjust the qualitative values avoiding severe lung damage (context-sensitive adjustment of qualitative values). The schemata for curve fitting represent the dynamically changing knowledge for classifying the observed parameters in combination with different expectations of the parameters' courses during time periods.

Table 2.1 The unified scheme for abstracting the seven qualitative data-point categories.

Code	*Category*	
s3	extremely	
s2	substantially	ABOVE
s1	slightly	
normal	target range	NORMAL
g1	slightly	
g2	substantially	BELOW
g3	extremely	

2.4.1 Context-sensitive schema for data-point transformation

The transformation of quantitative point data into qualitative values is usually performed by dividing the numerical value range of a parameter into regions of interest. Each region represents a qualitative value. The region defines the only common property of the numerical and qualitative values within a particular context and at a specific time-stamp. It is comparable to the *point temporal abstraction* task of Shahar and Musen [Shahar and Musen, 1993].

The basis of our transformation of the blood-gas measurements are context-sensitive *schemata for data-point transformation*, relating single values to seven qualitative categories of blood-gas abnormalities (qualitative *data-point* categories). The seven numerical regions of interest are not equal sized. The value range of an interval is smaller the nearer the target range. This is an important feature representing the dynamics related to the different degrees of parameters' abnormalities. It is extensively used in the schemata for trend-curve fitting. The schemata for data-point transformation (Table 2.1) are defined for all kinds of blood-gas measurements depending on the blood-gas sampling site (arterial, capillary, venous, transcutaneous) and all different contexts (e.g., "imv"). The different contexts require specific predefined target values depending on different attainable goals. Figure 2.2 shows the schema of $P_{tc}CO_2$ during "ippv". For example, the transformation of the transcutaneous $P_{tc}CO_2$ value of 34 $mmHg$ during "ippv" results in a qualitative $P_{tc}CO_2$ value of *g1* ("slightly below target range") whereas during "imv" it would represent *g2* ("substantially below target range"). The $w_{i,x}$ values divide the qualitative regions. The transformation of interval data is based on these qualitative data-point categories, which are described later.

In Figure 2.1 the temporal abstraction of the blood-gas measurements is displayed in the left upper corner. The qualitative data-point categories are expressed using a color chart with different gradation (e.g., deep pink repre-

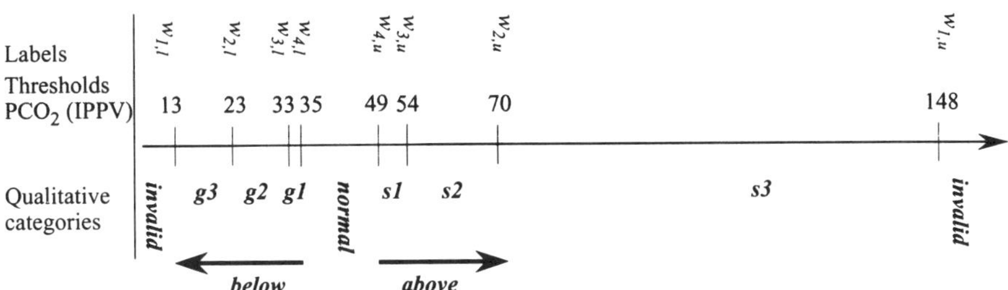

Figure 2.2 Schema for data-point transformation of $P_{tc}CO_2$ during context "ippv". The labels $w_{i,x}$ indicate the thresholds of the regions of interests. The corresponding numerical thresholds are recorded in the second row. The third row shows the abbreviations of the seven derived qualitative data-point categories.

sents values extremely above the target range (s3), lime green represents values extremely below the target range (g3); Figure 2.1 shows only the gray-scale gradation of VIE-VENT's user interface). The above example of the transcutaneous $P_{tc}CO_2$ value of 34 $mmHg$ during "imv" is displayed in color chartreuse.

2.4.2 Smoothing of data oscillating near thresholds

To avoid rapid changes of the qualitative categories triggered by data which oscillate near the thresholds of the schema for data-point transformation, we apply a smoothing method. The key idea is to keep the qualitative categories stable if the quantitative values cross the border to the next qualitative category just minimally for a few moments. Our smoothing method is based on the size of the regions of interests, predefined ε regions, and a maximum smoothing activation time period. Alternative smoothing approaches could use statistical measurements (e.g., interval of confidence) or fuzzy sets to classify the parameter values.

The smoothing method starts at time point t if the current qualitative data-point category $qual(a_t)$ is not equal to the previous qualitative data-point category $qual(a_{t-1})$ and a_t is in the ε region. The ε region defines the smoothing area around the quantitative border value w_i. Its size depends on the size of the qualitative region. During the smoothing time interval the new actual category $qual(a_{t+n})$ gets the value $qual(a_{t-1})$. Smoothing stops if the maximum smoothing activation time period (e.g., 5 minutes) has been elapsed, or if the a_{t+n} value leaves the ε region.

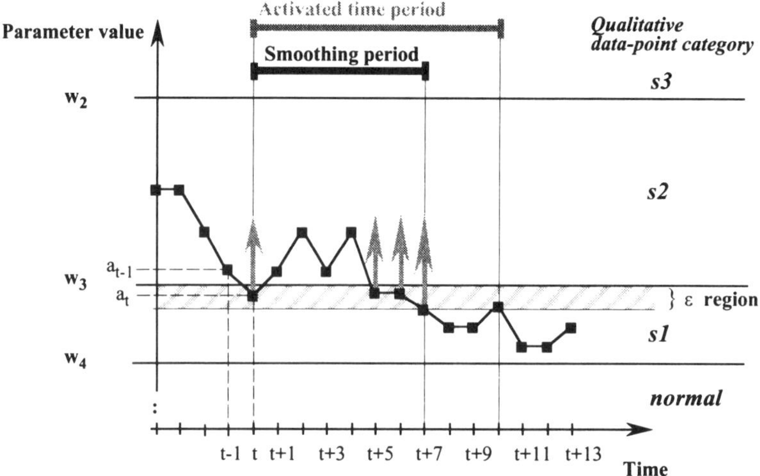

Figure 2.3 Example of smoothing of data oscillating near thresholds.

Figure 2.3 gives an example of our smoothing method. At time point t the smoothing method is activated, because $a_t \in [w_3, w_4]$ and $(a_{t-1} \in [w_2, w_3])$. This would result in $qual(a_t) \neq qual(a_{t-1})$. The condition $a_t \geq w_3 - \varepsilon$ is satisfied. We start smoothing at time point t. Shifting of the qualitative categories starts. The gray arrows illustrate the shifting of data values from the qualitative data-point category $s1$ to the qualitative category $s2$. At time points $t+1$ to $t+4$ no shifting is necessary because the qualitative category is the same as at the starting point of the smoothing. The data smoothing ends at time point $t+8$ because $a_{t+8} < w_3 - \varepsilon$. In this example, the predefined maximum time period of 10 time ticks has not been exhausted. Smoothing stops always after the predefined maximum activation time period.

2.4.3 Smoothing of data-point transformation schemata

The schemata for data-point transformation are defined for all contexts (i.e., modes of ventilation: "imv", "ippv") representing different target values. Changing the context would therefore result in an abrupt change of the schema for data-point transformation and by this in a sudden shift of the qualitative category. As a consequence, this could lead to recommendations for rather drastic changes of the ventilator settings. To avoid too-abrupt changes of the qualitative categories, we smooth the thresholds of the schemata for data-point transformation within a predefined time period (three to eight hours depending on the "aggressiveness" of the user).

For example, if the mode of ventilation is changed from "ippv" to "imv", the thresholds of the schemata for data-point transformation are changed stepwise during eight hours in the case of a conservative user. This results in a slow change of the target range in the next eight hours, and with respect to the therapeutic consequences, in a graceful start of the weaning process.

2.4.4 *Context-sensitive adjustment of qualitative values*

For extremely critical or life-threatening situations, the thresholds defined in the schemata for data-point transformation are too strict. In such cases we adjust the qualitative value of a parameter, which is equal to a shift of the numerical threshold values. The adjustment of qualitative values holds as long as the precondition of "life-threatening situation" is true.

For example, the degree of artificial ventilation determined by values of the ventilator settings can lead to the modification of the transformation process. If the peak inspiratory pressure (PIP, measured in cmH_2O) is very high, higher $P_{tc}CO_2$ values are tolerated as better ones in order to prevent extreme pressure settings. The following rule represents this kind of knowledge:

`if` $(30 < PIP \leq 35)$ `and` ($P_{tc}CO_2$ `is 'extremely below target range'`)
`then` ($P_{tc}CO_2$ `is changed to 'substantially below target range'`)

2.4.5 *Transformation of interval data*

Similar to the transformation of numerical data points to qualitative values, interval data are transformed to qualitative descriptions resulting in a verbal categorization of the change of parameters over time. Physicians expectations of how a blood-gas value has to change over time to reach the target range in a physiologically proper way are expressed in verbal terms. For example, "the parameter $P_{tc}O_2$ is moving one qualitative step towards the target range within 10 to 30 minutes." These qualitative statements are called *expected qualitative trend descriptions.* The qualitative classification of the abnormality of a blood-gas value resulted in different sized qualitative ranges ($s3$, $s2$, $s1$, *normal*, $g1$, $g2$, $g3$) shown in Figure 2.2. Combining these qualitative data-point categories with the expected qualitative trend descriptions we reach the *schemata for trend-curve fitting.* The schemata for trend-curve fitting express the dynamics of and the reactions to different degrees of parameter abnormalities. A physician classifies a higher degree of a parameter abnormality as more severe and classifies a faster positive change of this parameter as normal. The different sizes of the data-point categories express this circumstance. The corresponding dynamically derived trends depending on the expected qualitative trend descriptions represent different dynamic changes.

Based on physiological criteria, four kinds of trends of our 10-second data samples can be discerned:

- *very short-term* trend: sample of data points based on the *last* minute,
- *short-term* trend: sample of data points based on the *last 10* minutes,
- *medium-term* trend: sample of data points based on the *last 30* minutes,
- *long-term* trend: sample of data points based on the *last 3* hours.

Comparing different kinds of trends is a useful method of assessing the result of previous therapeutic actions, of detecting if oscillation is too rapid, and of isolating the occurrence of artifacts (see [Horn et al., 1997]).

The transformation of interval data into qualitative values is the last step of the temporal data-abstraction process. All necessary smoothing procedures have already been applied. Therefore only validated and reliable data are involved. In case of missing or invalid measurements certain criteria of validity to proceed with the trend-based data-abstraction process are needed.

In a time-oriented analysis process, the position of a measurement in the sequence of time-ordered data influences the reasoning process: namely, recent measurements are more important than past measurements. Hence, criteria dealing only with an average distribution of measurements are insufficient (e.g., compare [Larizza et al., 1997]). Due to this, we specified two criteria of validity to ensure that the used trend is actually meaningful: a certain minimum amount of valid measurements within the whole time interval, and a certain amount of valid measurements within the last 20 percent of the time interval. These limits are defined by experts based on their clinical experience. They may easily be adapted to a specific clinical situation based on the frequency at which data values arrive. An enhanced presentation of different kinds of data validation and repair methods is given in [Horn et al., 1997].

The guiding principle of our approach is illustrated in the left-hand side of Figure 2.4. The *schema for trend-curve fitting* represents the qualitative trend expectations acquired from the medical experts. This schema transforms the different quantitative trend values (e.g., short-term or medium-term trends) into ten qualitative categories guided by physiological criteria. The y axis shows the threshold levels and the corresponding qualitative data-point categories. The value space of a parameter is divided into an upper and a lower region by the normal range. The dark gray area represents the expected qualitative trend description for a normal change of a parameter in the upper and the lower region, respectively. The derived qualitative trend categories are

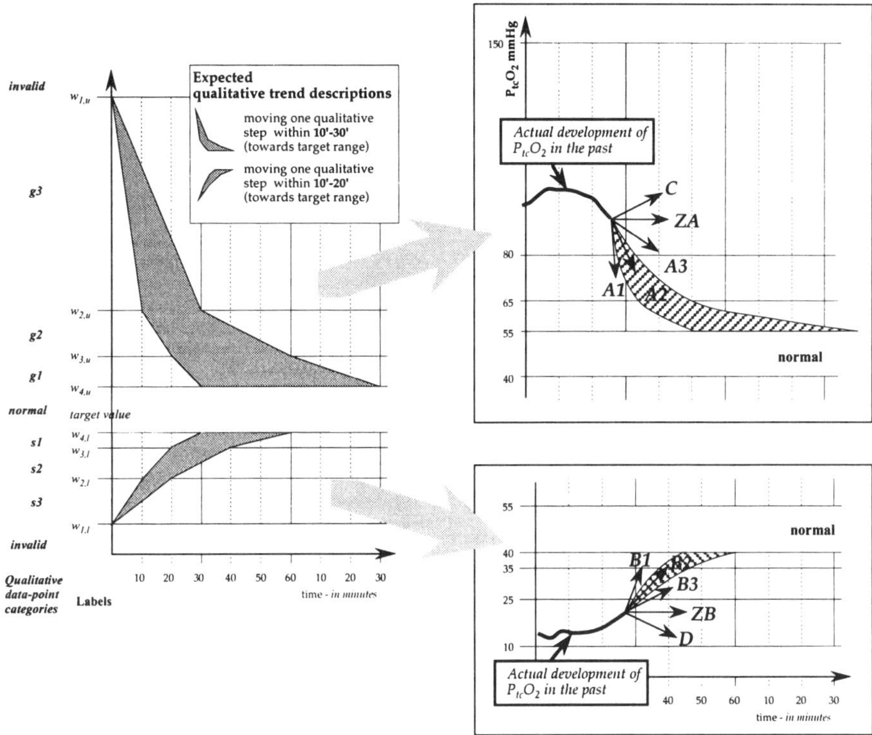

Figure 2.4 Schema for trend-curve fitting of $P_{tc}O_2$. On the left-hand side the light-gray rectangle indicates the qualitative point-categories. The dark gray area indicates the expected qualitative trend description of a normal change of a parameter in the upper and the lower region, respectively. The right-hand side illustrates the matching of trend-curve fitting in the upper and the lower regions and the corresponding ten qualitative trend-categories.

written in bold, capital letters listed in the right-hand side of Figure 2.4. The abbreviations are explained in Table 2.2.

Improving or worsening of parameters is fitted by exponential functions. An appropriate approach classifying trend data is to transform the curve (borders of the dark gray area) shown in Figure 2.4 into an exponential function and to compare it with the actual growth rate. To classify the trend parameters, we used a dynamic comparison algorithm which performs a stepwise linearization of the expected exponential function to overcome complexity. For example, if

Table 2.2 The unified context-sensitive and expectation-guided schema for trend-curve fitting.

Code	*Category UPPER*	*Code*	*Category LOWER*
A1	decrease too fast	B1	increase too fast
A2	normal decrease	B2	normal increase
A3	decrease too slow	B3	increase too slow
ZA	zero change	ZB	zero change
C	dangerous increase	D	dangerous decrease

a $P_{tc}O_2$ data point during the context "imv" is classified as $s1$, $s2$ or $s3$ ("... above target range") we would expect a therapeutic intervention to result in a decrease of type $A2$ (dark gray area) as "normal" trend.

The results of this algorithm are classifications of all parameters to one of the ten qualitative trend categories. The target range of a parameter divides the qualitative regions into an upper part ($A1$, $A2$, $A3$, ZA, C) and a lower part ($B1$, $B2$, $B3$, ZB, D) as explained in Table 2.2. The classification process results in instantiations of qualitative trend descriptions for each blood-gas measurement, for each kind of trend, and for each activated context.

In Figure 2.1 the qualitative trend categories are visualized by colored arrows next to the qualitative data-point categories (the three boxes CO_2, O_2, SaO_2 in the upper left corner). The four arrows of each box show the directions of the very-short, short, medium, and long-term trends. For example, all qualitative trend categories of transcutaneous CO_2 during the context "imv" are derived as D (their directions are down-going and the color is deep-pink represented as deep-gray in Figure 2.1). This expresses a dangerous decrease of the measurement. Consequently, our therapy planning module recommends a therapeutic action to decrease PIP from 20 to 15 cmH_2O (see ventilator parameters on left-hand side and the fourth plot on the right-hand side of Figure 2.1).

2.5 APPLICABILITY AND PRACTICAL USEFULNESS

We have tested the applicability of our approach both on generated data sets and on real data. The generated data sets were used to simulate extreme cases. The results obtained demonstrated the robustness of VIE-VENT. Real data were obtained from a NICU using on-line data acquisition. We collected sequences of 16-28 hours of continuous recording of transcutaneous blood-gas measurements and pulsoximetry. Discontinuously sampled data were taken from the computer-based patient records. The evaluation of these cases demonstrated the applicability of our approach in the clinical setting.

The usefulness of the qualitative categories and their visualizations have been manifested in different ways. First, they support the health care providers in getting a closer insight into their medical reasoning process. This has eased the fine-tuning of our therapy planning component. Second, the qualitative trend categories improved our data validation component. Third, applying the qualitative trend categories for formulating and assessing therapeutic actions resulted in a graceful weaning process avoiding too abrupt changes of therapeutic recommendations. In Figure 2.1 the therapeutic recommendations are displayed as black vertical impulses in the corresponding plot of the ventilator setting. The therapeutic recommendations show a very consistent and reasonable picture, except in cases where the measurements were set invalid (gray areas between the two horizontal lines in the two upper plots in Figure 2.1).

During our evaluation phase we discovered also limitations of our temporal data-abstraction methods. First, information about the frequency of temporal abstractions in the past (e.g., "three episodes of hyperoxemia during the last 3 hours occurred") would be very useful for future reasoning processes. Second, dealing with real data during longer time periods has to take into account that more recently observed data are more important for the reasoning process than data observed in older time periods. Therefore, the data-abstraction methods have to include a memory which weights the time-ordered data.

2.6 CONCLUSION

We demonstrated very powerful time-oriented analysis methods for the interpretation of data collected at the NICUs. The guiding principle is the temporal abstraction of quantitative data to qualitative values based on a unified scheme for all parameters. This scheme incorporates both an abstraction of the current value of a parameter and an abstraction of the current trend of the parameter. The abstraction scheme is easily comprehensible to health care providers and easy to use for decision support.

The data analysis methods combine all the available information to perform a context-sensitive and expectation-guided temporal abstraction process. In designing our abstraction, we concentrated on knowledge-based monitoring and therapy planning in real clinical environments. Dealing with high-frequency data, shifting contexts, and different expectations of the development of parameters requires particular temporal abstraction methods to arrive at unified qualitative values or patterns. Our temporal data-abstraction methods incorporate knowledge about data points, data intervals, and expected qualitative trend patterns. Additionally, the problem definitions are not as clear as expected, because the underlying structure-function models for predicting the time course of clinical parameters are poorly understood and incomplete knowledge is involved. Therefore theories of data analysis are only partially applicable. We overcome these limitations by applying qualitative statements (called *expected qualitative trend descriptions*), which are obtainable from domain experts. These qualitative statements are approximated using linear regression models. To keep the qualitative descriptions stable in case of shifting contexts or data oscillating near thresholds we apply smoothing and adjustment methods.

Integrating the time-oriented data analysis methods in VIE-VENT results in easily comprehensible and transparent definitions of the data-interpretation, therapy-planning, and data validation modules. Data interpretation can be performed on different levels using data-point and data-interval (trend) abstractions as well as a combination of different abstraction categories. The derived qualitative values and patterns are used for recommending therapeutic actions as well as for assessing the effectiveness of these actions within a certain period.

The clinical experience shows that our temporal data-abstraction methods provide the ground basis for improved therapy planning in neonatal ICUs. The physicians are able to recognize the patient's respiratory status immediately from VIE-VENT's graphical user interface. The therapeutic recommendations which are based on the abstracted data support a graceful weaning process, avoiding too abrupt changes of ventilator settings.

Acknowledgments

We greatly appreciate the support given to the Austrian Research Institute of Artificial Intelligence (ÖFAI) by the Austrian Federal Ministry of Science and Transport, Vienna.

References

Allen, J.F. (1991). Time and time again: The many ways to represent time. *International Journal of Intelligent Systems*, 6:341–355.

Avent, R.K. and Charlton, J.D. (1990). A critical review of trend-detection methologies for biomedical monitoring systems. *Critical Reviews in Biomedical Engineering*, 16(6):621–659.

Bellazzi, R., Larizza, C., Riva, A., Mira, A., Fiocchi, S. and Stefanelli, M. (1996). Distributed intelligent data analysis in diabetic patient management, In Cimino, J. J., editor, *Proceedings of the 1996 AMIA Annual Fall Symposium (formerly SCAMC)*, Washington, DC, pages 194–198. Philadelphia: Hanley-Belfus.

Dean, T.L. and McDermott, D.V. (1987). Temporal data base management. *Artificial Intelligence*, 32(1):1–55.

Dojat, M. and Sayettat, C. (1995). A realistic model for temporal reasoning in real-time patient monitoring. *Applied Artificial Intelligence*, 10(2):121–143.

Fagan, L.M., Shortliffe, E.H. and Buchanan, B.G. (1980). Computer-based medical decision making: from MYCIN to VM. *Automedica*, 3:97–106.

Fayyad, U., Piatetsky-Shapiro, G., and Smyth, P. (1996). The KDD process for extracting useful knowledge from volumes of data. *Communication of the ACM*, 39(11):27–34.

Haimowitz, I.J., Le, P.P., and Kohane, I.S. (1995). Clinical monitoring using regression-based trend templates. *Artificial Intelligence in Medicine*, 7(6):473–496.

Hayes-Roth, B., Washington, R., Ash, D., Hewett, R., Collinot, A., Vina, A., and Seiver, A. (1992). GUARDIAN: A prototype intelligent agent for intensive-care monitoring. *Artificial Intelligence in Medicine*, 4(2):165–185.

Horn, W., Miksch, S., Egghart, G., Popow, C., and Paky, F. (1997). Effective data validation of high-frequency data: time-point-, time-interval-, and trend-based methods. *Computer in Biology and Medicine, Special Issue: Time-Oriented Systems in Medicine*, forthcoming.

Kahn, M.G. (1991). Combining physiologic models and symbolic methods to interpret time-varying patient data. *Methods of Information in Medicine*, 30(3):167–178.

Kay, S.M. (1993). *Fundamentals of statistical signal processing.* Engelwood, New Jersey: Prentice Hall.

Kohane, I.S. (1986). Medical reasoning in medical expert systems. In Salamon, R., et al., editors, *Proceedings of the Fifth Conference on Medical Informatics (MEDINFO-86)*, pages 170–174, North-Holland.

Larizza, C., Moglia, A., and Stefanelli, M. (1992). M-HTP: A system for monitoring heart transplant patients. *Artificial Intelligence in Medicine*, 4(2):111–126.

Larizza, C., Bellazzi, R., and Riva, A.(1997). Temporal abstractions for diabetic patients management, In Keravnou, E., et al., editors, *Artificial Intelligence in Medicine (Proc. AIME-97)*, pages 319–330. Springer Verlag.

Miksch, S., Horn, W., Popow, C., and Paky, F. (1993). VIE-VENT: Knowledge-based monitoring and therapy planning of the artificial ventilation of newborn infants. In Andreassen, S., et al., editors, *Artificial Intelligence in Medicine (Proc. AIME-93)*, pages 218–229. Amsterdam: IOS Press.

Miksch, S., Horn, W., Popow, C., and Paky, F. (1995). Therapy planning using qualitative trend descriptions. In Barahona, P., et al., editors, *Artificial Intelligence in Medicine (Proc. AIME-95)*, pages 197–208. Springer Verlag.

Miksch, S., Horn, W., Popow, C., and Paky, F. (1996). Utilizing temporal data abstraction for data validation and therapy planning for artificially ventilated newborn infants. *Artificial Intelligence in Medicine*, 8(6):543–576.

Ramaux, N., Fontaine, D., and Dojat, M. (1997). Temporal scenario recognition for intelligent monitoring, In Keravnou, E., et al., editors, *Artificial Intelligence in Medicine (Proc. AIME-97)*, pages 335–342, Springer Verlag.

Russ, T.A. (1989). Using hindsight in medical decision making. In Kingsland, L.C., editor, *Proceedings of the Thirteenth Annual Symposium on Computer Applications in Medical Care (SCAMC-89)*, pages 38–44. Washington, DC: IEEE Computer Society Press.

Shahar, Y. and Musen, M.A. (1993). RÉSUMÉ: A temporal-abstraction system for patient monitoring. *Computers and Biomedical Research*, 26(3):255–273.

Shahar, Y. and Musen, M.A. (1996). Knowledge-based temporal abstraction in clinical domains. *Artificial Intelligence in Medicine, Special Issue on Temporal Reasoning in Medicine*, 8(3):267–298.

3 CONTEXT-SENSITIVE TEMPORAL ABSTRACTION OF CLINICAL DATA

Yuval Shahar

Abstract: Temporal abstraction in medical domains is the task of abstracting higher-level, interval-based concepts (e.g., 3 weeks of moderate anemia) from time-stamped clinical data (e.g., daily measurements of hemoglobin) in a context-sensitive manner. We have developed and implemented a formal knowledge-based framework for decomposing and solving that task that supports acquisition, maintenance, reuse of domain-independent temporal abstraction knowledge in different clinical domains, and sharing of domain-specific temporal abstraction properties among different applications in the same domain. In this chapter, we focus on the representation necessary for creation during runtime of appropriate contexts for interpretation of clinical data. Clinical interpretation contexts are temporally extended states of affairs (e.g., effect of insulin as part of the management of diabetes) that affect the interpretation of clinical data. Interpretation contexts are induced by measured patient data, concluded abstractions, external interventions such as therapy administration, and the goals of the interpretation process. We define four types of interpretation-contexts (basic, composite, generalized, and nonconvex), discuss the conceptual and computational advantages of separating interpretation contexts from both the propositions inducing them and the abstractions created within them, and provide an example within the domain of monitoring diabetes patients.

3.1 INTRODUCTION

Most clinical domains and tasks require the collection of substantial numbers of patient data over time and the abstraction of those data into higher-level concepts, meaningful for that domain and for the context in which the data were collected. Physicians who have to make decisions based on the original patient data may be overwhelmed by the number of data if their ability to reason with the data does not scale up to modern-day data-storage capabilities.

Typically, clinical data include a time stamp in which each particular datum was valid; an emerging pattern over a span of time, especially in a specific context (e.g., therapy with a particular drug), has much more significance than an isolated finding or even a set of findings. Thus, it is highly desirable for an automated knowledge-based decision-support tool that assists physicians who monitor patients over significant periods to provide short, informative, context-sensitive summaries of time-oriented clinical data stored on electronic media. Such a tool should be able to answer queries at various levels of abstraction about abstract concepts that summarize the data. Data summaries are valuable to the physician, support an automated system's diagnostic or therapeutic recommendations, and monitor plans suggested by the physician or by the decision-support system. A meaningful summary cannot use only time points, such as data-collection dates; it must be able to characterize significant features over *periods* of time, such as "2 weeks of grade-II bone-marrow toxicity in the context of therapy for potential complications of a bone-marrow transplantation event" (Figure 3.1) and more complex patterns. The **temporal abstraction (TA) task** is thus an interpretation task: given time-stamped data and external events, produce context-specific, intervalbased, relevant abstractions of the data (a more formal definition is stated in Section 3.3, where we present the formal ontology—terms and relations—of the TA task).

In Section 3.2 of this chapter we introduce the knowledge-based temporal abstraction (KBTA) method for solving the TA task. One of the important subtasks into which this method decomposes the TA task is that of creating appropriate time-oriented contexts for interpretation of clinical data. In Section 3.3, we define briefly the formal ontology used by the TA mechanisms (the computational modules that can solve the tasks created by the KBTA method). In Section 3.4, we present the context-forming mechanism, which uses that ontology, when mapped to the matching clinical-domain knowledge, to create temporal contexts for interpretation of clinical data in a context-sensitive manner. We also explain the meaning of the distinctions made by the context-forming mechanism among four types of interpretation contexts (basic, composite, generalized, and nonconvex) and the conceptual and computational advantages of the separation of interpretation-context propositions from both the propositions inducing them and the abstractions created within them. These advantages are especially pertinent in clinical domains, which are typically knowledge intensive. In Section 3.5, we present an application of the KBTA method and its interpretation-context model to a clinical domain (diabetes therapy) in which the RÉSUMÉ system was evaluated. Section 3.6 concludes with a brief summary and discussion.

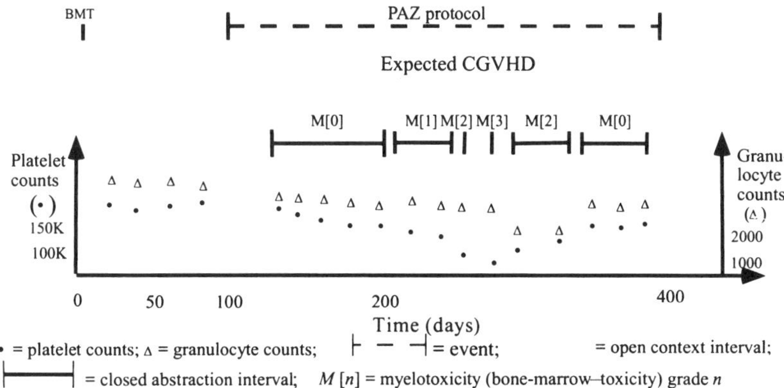

Figure 3.1 Abstraction of platelet and granulocyte values during administration of the predisone/azathioprine (PAZ) clinical protocol for treating patients who have chronic graft-versus-host disease (CGVHD). The time line starts with a bone-marrow transplantation (BMT) event.

3.2 KNOWLEDGE-BASED TEMPORAL ABSTRACTION

A method solving the TA task, especially in medical domains, encounters several conceptual and computational problems: (1) both the input data and the required output abstractions might include several data types (e.g., numeric values of blood gases, symbolic values of physical signs) and various abstraction levels (e.g., physicians might perform some of the abstraction process before entering the result); (2) input data might arrive out of temporal order (e.g., arrival of last week's laboratory report), and existing interpretations must be revised nonmonotonically; (3) several alternate clinical interpretations might need to be maintained and followed over time; (4) clinical parameters have context-specific temporal properties, such as expected persistence of measured values and classification functions (e.g., the meaning of the value low of the hemoglobin-state abstraction depends on the context); (5) acquisition of knowledge from expert physicians and maintenance of that knowledge should be facilitated. The method should enable reusing its domain-independent knowledge for solving the TA task in other clinical domains, and enable sharing of domain-specific knowledge with other tasks in the same domain.

The framework that we are using for solving the TA task is based on our work on temporal abstraction mechanisms [Shahar et al., 1992, Shahar and Musen, 1993, Shahar, 1994, Shahar and Musen, 1996, Shahar, 1997]. We have defined a general problem-solving method [Eriksson et al., 1995] for interpreting data in time-oriented domains, with clear semantics for both the method and its domain-specific knowledge requirements: the **knowledge-based temporal abstraction (KBTA) method**. The KBTA method comprises a knowledge-level representation of the TA task and of the knowledge required to solve that task. The KBTA method has a formal model of input and output entities, their relations, and their properties—the **KBTA ontology** [Shahar, 1994, Shahar, 1997].

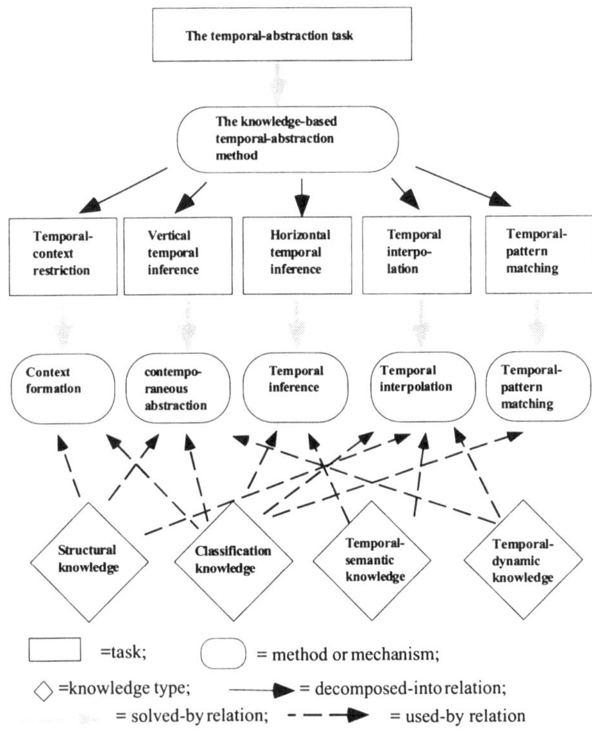

Figure 3.2 The knowledge-based temporal abstraction method and its mechanisms.

The KBTA method decomposes the TA task into five parallel subtasks (Figure 3.2):

Temporal context restriction. Creation of contexts relevant for data interpretation (e.g., effect of a drug), to focus and limit the scope of the inference (we elaborate on this task in Section 3.4).

Vertical temporal inference. Inference from values of contemporaneous input data or abstractions (e.g., results of several different blood tests conducted during the same day) into values of higher-level concepts (e.g., classification into bone-marrow toxicity Grade II). Note that classification functions are often context sensitive (e.g., different clinical guidelines define differently MODERATE ANEMIA, a state abstraction of the hemoglobin-level clinical parameter).

Horizontal temporal inference. Inference from similar-type propositions that hold over different time intervals (e.g., joining different-value abstractions of the same parameter that hold over two meeting time intervals and computing the new abstraction's value). In fact, two subtasks are involved in horizontal temporal inference. *Temporal semantic inference* infers specific types of interval-based logical conclusions, given interval-based propositions, using a deductive extension of Shoham's temporal semantic properties [Shoham, 1987]. For instance, unlike two anemia periods, two episodes of 9-month pregnancies can never be summarized as an episode of an 18-month pregnancy—even if they followed each other—since they are not *concatenable*, a temporal semantic property. Similarly, a week-long episode of coma implies an abstraction of coma during each day (i.e., it has the *downward-hereditary* temporal semantic property); that is not necessarily true for the abstraction "a week of oscillating blood pressure." *Temporal horizontal inference* determines the domain value of an abstraction created from two joined abstractions (e.g., for most parameters and interpretation contexts, decreasing and same might be concatenated into NONINCREASING). Although more stable than classification functions, temporal semantic properties might be sensitive to the context.

Temporal interpolation. Bridging of gaps between similar-type but temporally disjoint point- or interval-based propositions to create longer intervals (e.g., joining two disjoint episodes of anemia, occurring during different days, into a longer episode, bridging the gap between them). We use *local* (forward and backward from an abstraction interval) and *global* (between two abstraction intervals) *truth-persistence functions* to model a belief in the value of an abstraction [Shahar, 1994]. Global truth-persistence (Δ) functions return the maximal temporal gap threshold that can be bridged (with a high-enough probability) between two temporally disjoint abstractions, given the parameter involved, its value(s), the length of each abstraction, and the interpretation context of the abstractions. Both local and global truth-persistence functions are highly dependent on context.

Temporal pattern matching. Creation of intervals by matching patterns over disjoint intervals over which propositions of various types hold. Temporal patterns might be meaningful only for certain contexts and should not be created (and their creation should not be attempted) in others.

The five subtasks of the KBTA method are solved by **five temporal abstraction mechanisms** (nondecomposable computational modules) that we have defined (see Figure 3.2). The temporal abstraction mechanisms depend on four well-defined domain-specific **knowledge types**: *structural* knowledge (e.g., IS-A, PART-OF and ABSTRACTED-INTO relations), *classification* (functional) knowledge (e.g., mapping of hemoglobin values into hemoglobin states), *temporal semantic* (logical) knowledge (e.g., the CONCATENABLE property [Shoham, 1987]), and *temporal dynamic* (probabilistic) knowledge (e.g., temporal persistence functions that bridge gaps between temporally disjoint intervals [Shahar, 1994]). Values for the four knowledge types are specified as the domain's **temporal abstraction ontology** when developing a temporal abstraction system for a particular domain and task.

We have implemented the KBTA method as the **RÉSUMÉ** system [Shahar and Musen, 1993] and applied it with encouraging results to several clinical domains such as chronic graft-versus-host disease [Shahar and Musen, 1993], monitoring of children's growth [Kuilboer et al., 1993], therapy of AIDS patients [Shahar, 1994], and therapy of patients who have diabetes [Shahar and Musen, 1996]. The RÉSUMÉ system is currently used within the **Tzolkin** temporal mediator server, a part of the **EON** architecture for support of clinical-guideline-based therapy [Musen et al., 1996].

3.3 THE TEMPORAL ABSTRACTION ONTOLOGY

Informally, the KBTA temporal model includes both time intervals and time points. *Time points* are the basic temporal primitives, but propositions, such as occurrence of events and existence of parameter values, can be interpreted only over *time intervals*. Therefore, all propositions are *fluents* [McCarthy and Hayes, 1969] and, in our model, must be interpreted over a particular time *period* (e.g., the value of the temperature parameter during time interval $[\tau_1, \tau_2)$. The knowledge-based TA ontology contains the following entities.

Time stamps $\tau_i \in T$ comprise the basic primitives of time. A time-standardization function, $f_S(\tau_i)$, can map a time stamp into an integer amount of any pre-defined temporal granularity unit $G_i \in \Gamma$ (e.g., hour). Time stamps are measured in G_i units with respect to a zero-point time stamp. There is a time unit G_0 of the lowest granularity. A finite positive or negative amount of G_i units is a *time measure.* There is a total order on time stamps. Subtraction of any time stamp from another must be defined and should return a time measure. Addition or subtraction of a time measure to or from a time stamp must return a time stamp.

Time interval is an ordered pair of time stamps that denote the endpoints, $[I.start, I.end]$, of the interval. A zero length interval in which $I.start = I.end$ is a time point.

Interpretation context $\xi \in \Xi$ is a proposition representing a state of affairs relevant to interpretation (e.g., "the drug insulin exerts its effect during this interval"). When an interpretation context exists during a particular time interval, parameters may be interpreted differently within that time interval. IS-A and SUBCONTEXT relations are defined over the set of interpretation contexts. *Basic* interpretation contexts are atomic propositions. *Composite interpretation contexts* are created by the conjunction of a basic or a composite interpretation context and one of its subcontexts. Intuitively, composite interpretation contexts permit the definition of a hierarchy of increasingly specific contexts. *Generalized* and *nonconvex interpretation contexts* are special types of interpretation contexts (see Sections 3.4.2 and 3.4.3). Unlike the propositions creating them, interpretation contexts have the *concatenable* [Shoham, 1987] temporal semantic property as a default. Thus, two almost-consecutive nine-month *pregnancy* abstractions should not be joined into an 18-month pregnancy, but the two respective *being-pregnant* nine-month context intervals might be concatenated into an 18-month context.

Context interval is a structure $\langle \xi, I \rangle$ containing an interpretation context ξ and a time interval I (i.e., an interpretation context during an interval).

Event, or event proposition, $e \in E$ is the occurrence of an external willful act or process, such as the administration of a drug. Events are instantiated event schemata; an event schema has a series a_i of event attributes (e.g., drug dose) that must be mapped to attribute values ν_i. A PART-OF (or *subevent*) relation is defined over event schemata.

Event interval is a structure $\langle e, I \rangle$, consisting of an event proposition e and a time interval I that represents the duration of the event.

Parameter, or parameter schema, $\pi \in \Pi$ is a measurable or describable state of the world. Parameters may represent raw input data (e.g., a hemoglobin level) or abstractions from the raw data (e.g., a state of anemia). Parameter schemata have various *properties*, such as a domain V_π of possible symbolic or numeric values, measurement units, temporal semantic properties, or temporal persistence. An *extended parameter* is a combination $\langle \pi, \xi \rangle$ of a parameter π and an interpretation context ξ. An extended parameter is also a parameter and can have properties. Extended parameters have a special property, a value $\nu \in V_\pi$, which is typically known only at runtime (i.e., parameter values require a context). A *parameter proposition* is the combination of a parameter, a parameter value, and an interpretation context, $\langle \pi, \nu, \xi \rangle$ (e.g., "the state of hemoglobin is low in the context of chemotherapy").

Parameter interval $\langle \pi, \nu, \xi, I \rangle$ is a parameter proposition and a time interval, representing the value of a parameter in a specific context during a particular time interval.

Abstraction function $\theta \in \Theta$ is a unary or multiple-argument function from one or more parameters to an abstract parameter. The abstract parameter has one of three abstraction types: *state*, *gradient*, and *rate*. An additional type of abstraction is *pattern* which defines a temporal pattern of several other parameters. An abstraction of a parameter is a parameter (thus, both hemoglobin and the state of hemoglobin are parameters, with distinct properties).

Abstraction is a parameter interval $\langle \pi, \nu, \xi, I \rangle$ where π is an abstract parameter. Abstractions may be abstraction points or abstraction intervals.

Abstraction goal $\psi \in \Psi$ is a proposition that indicates a goal or intention that is relevant to the TA task (e.g., the intention to control a diabetes patient's blood-glucose values).

Abstraction-goal interval is a structure $\langle \psi, I \rangle$, where ψ is a temporal abstraction goal that is posted during the interval I. An abstraction-goal interval induces interpretation contexts.

Interpretation contexts are induced by (or inferred dynamically from) event, parameter, or abstraction-goal propositions. The time intervals over which the inducing propositions exist impose temporal constraints on the interval in which the inferred context will be valid. For example, the interpretation context of insulin's effect on blood-glucose values might begin at least 30 minutes following the event of insulin administration and end up to 8 hours after terminating the administration. These constraints are represented formally in a *dynamic induction relation of a context interval* (**DIRC**). A DIRC is a relation over propositions and time measures, in which each member is a structure of the form $\langle \xi, \varphi, ss, se, es, ee \rangle$. Intuitively, the inducing proposition is assumed, at runtime, to be interpreted over some time interval I with known end points. The symbol ξ is the induced interpretation context. The symbol $\varphi \in P$ represents the inducing proposition, an event, an abstraction-goal, or a parameter proposition. Each of the other four symbols is either the "wild card" symbol *, or a time measure, which denote, respectively, the temporal distance between the start point of I and the start point of the induced context interval, the distance between the start point of I and the end point of the induced context interval, the distance between the end point of I and the start point of the context interval, and the distance between the end point of I and the end point of the induced context interval (Figure 3.3). Note that the resultant context interval need not span the same temporal scope as the inducing proposition, but can have any of Allen's 13 relations to it [Allen, 1984] (see Figure 3.3b). A *context-forming proposition* is an inducing proposition in at least one DIRC.

A TA ontology of a clinical domain is an event ontology, a context ontology, a parameter ontology, a set of abstraction-goal propositions, and the set of all DIRCs for a particular domain. The event ontology of a domain consists of the set of all the relevant event schemata and propositions. The context ontology defines the set of all the relevant contexts and subcontexts. The parameter ontology is composed of the set of all the relevant parameter propositions and their properties. The TA task also assumes the existence of a set of temporal queries, expressed in a predefined temporal abstraction language. A *temporal query* is a set of temporal and value constraints over the components of a set of parameter and context intervals [Shahar, 1994].

The TA task solved by the KBTA method in a clinical domain is thus the following: Given a set of event and abstraction-goal intervals, a set of parameter intervals, and the clinical domain's TA ontology, produce an interpretation—that is, a set of context intervals and a set of new abstractions such that the interpretation can answer any temporal query about all the abstractions derivable from the transitive closure of the input data and the domain's TA ontology.

The four types of domain-specific knowledge required by the TA mechanisms, apart from the event and context ontologies, are represented in the RÉSUMÉ system in the **parameter-properties ontology**, a representation of the parameter ontology [Shahar and Musen, 1993]. The parameter-properties ontology is a frame hierarchy that represents knowledge about parameter propo-

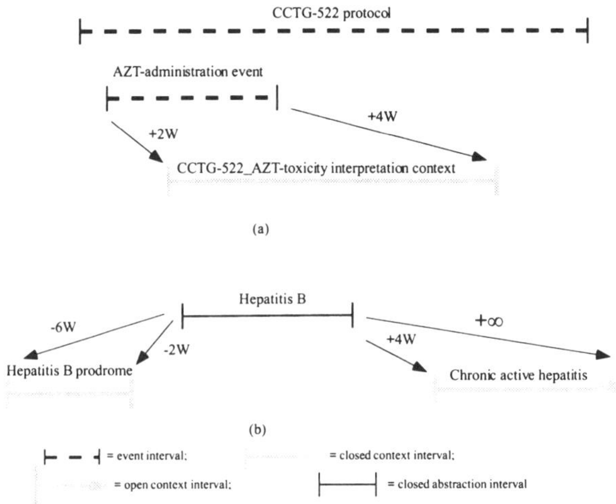

Figure 3.3 Dynamic induction relations of context intervals (DIRCs).
(a) An AZT-toxicity interpretation context induced by an AZT-administration event in the context of the CCTG-522 experimental protocol for AIDS therapy. The interpretation context starts 2 weeks after the start of the inducing event, and ends 4 weeks after its end.
(b) Prospective (chronic active hepatitis) and retrospective (hepatitis B prodrome) interpretation contexts induced by the hepatitis B parameter proposition.

sitions (e.g., classification knowledge about various values of the hemoglobin-value state abstraction) and specializes that knowledge within different interpretation contexts (e.g., therapy by different drugs). Figure 3.4 shows a part of the RÉSUMÉ parameter-properties ontology in the domain of protocol-based care.

Note that the knowledge regarding the granulocyte-count state abstract parameter is specialized in the context of the CCTG-522 experimental protocol for therapy of patients who have AIDS, in the context of the prednisone/azathioprine (PAZ) experimental protocol for treating chronic graft-versus-host disease, and in the subcontext of each part of the PAZ protocol.

3.4 DYNAMIC INDUCTION OF CONTEXT INTERVALS

Abstractions are meaningful only within the span of a context interval, such as administration of the drug AZT as part of a particular protocol for therapy of AIDS. Context intervals create a *frame of reference* for interpretation, and thus enable a TA mechanism to conclude abstractions for—and only for—that

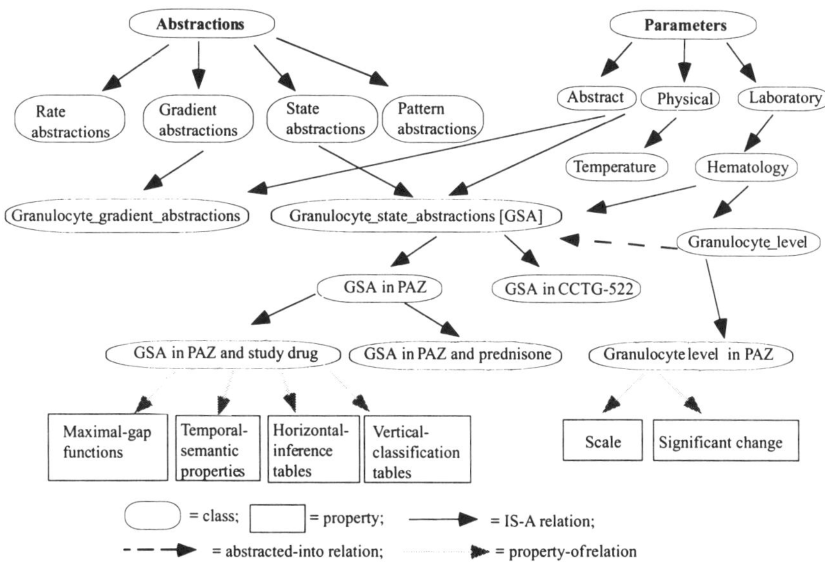

Figure 3.4 A portion of the RÉSUMÉ parameter-properties ontology in the domain of protocol-based care, showing a specialization of the temporal abstraction properties for the granulocyte_state_abstraction (GSA) abstract parameter in the context of the prednisone/azathioprine (PAZ) experimental protocol for treating chronic graft-versus-host disease, and in the context of each part of that protocol.

context. Thus, specificity is increased and the computational burden is reduced. Context intervals are created by the **context-forming mechanism**.

As explained in Section 3.3, DIRCs represent relationships between context intervals and several types of propositions that can induce them. Context intervals might be induced by the existence of an *abstraction-goal* interval, such as "therapy of insulin-dependent diabetes," or by the existence of an *event interval*, that is, an external process or action, such as treatment in accordance with a particular clinical protocol. A context interval can also be induced by the existence of a *parameter interval* that includes a *context-forming* (see Section 3.3) parameter proposition $\langle \pi, \nu, \xi \rangle$—namely, the value ν of the parameter π, in the context ξ, is sufficiently important to change the frame of reference for one or more other parameters (e.g., the low value of the hemoglobin-state abstract parameter in the context of protocol CCTG-522 might affect the interpretation of values of the platelet-value parameter).

A *composite interpretation context* (see Section 3.3) can be composed by the context-forming mechanism at runtime from a conjunction of two or more concluded basic interpretation contexts that hold contemporaneously, such that basic context ξ_{i+1} has a SUBCONTEXT relation to basic context ξ_i. The composite interpretation context would be interpreted over a context interval formed from a *temporal intersection* of the two or more corresponding context intervals. For example, components of a composite interpretation context are often induced by an *event chain*—a connected series of events $\langle e_1, e_2, \ldots, e_n \rangle$, where e_{i+1} is a subevent of e_i. In that case, the composite interpretation context would denote an interpretation context induced by the most specific subevent, such as administration of a particular drug as part of a certain protocol. (Subevents of an event typically induce interpretation contexts that have a SUBCONTEXT relation to the interpretation context induced by the event.) This knowledge is used as a default in the context ontology, and can also be exploited during a manual or automated process of acquisition of knowledge, either for knowledge elicitation or for knowledge verification and cross-validation. Interpretation contexts can be extended by concatenating two *meeting* [Allen, 1984] equal-context intervals.

Dynamic induction of context intervals by parameter propositions might lead to new interpretations of existing parameter intervals, thus potentially inducing new context intervals within which another or even the original parameter value (the input datum) might have new interpretations. However, we can prove [Shahar, 1994] that no contradictions or infinite loops can be generated by the context-forming process.

Observation 1. The context-forming process has no "oscillation cycles" among different interpretations of the same parameter (i.e., the same parameter proposition can never be retracted and eventually reasserted).
Justification. Parameter propositions are not retracted by the addition of a new interpretation context. Rather, a new interpretation is added to the set of true parameter propositions. (Retractions *can* occur due to the nonmonotonic nature of temporal abstraction, but in different circumstances, such as arrival of additional data with a present transaction time but with an old valid time, forcing a *view update* [Shahar, 1994].) Therefore, if a parameter proposition $\langle \pi, \nu_1, \xi_1 \rangle$ induces a new interpretation context ξ_2 over some interval, and within the scope of that interval the parameter π is interpreted to have another value, a new parameter proposition $\langle \pi, \nu_2, \xi_2 \rangle$ would simply be inferred and added to the set of true propositions. This, of course, creates no contradictions since the parameter π—or some abstraction of π, say, state(π)—is interpreted within two different contexts and can thus have two different values at the same time.

Observation 2. The context-forming process is finite.
Justification. The total number of different interpretation contexts that, potentially, can be inferred (including composite ones) is bounded by the size of the context ontology and the number of potential *subcontext chains* (which can

form composite contexts) of interpretation contexts that have SUBCONTEXT relations. Furthermore, for each parameter π, the number of possible induced context intervals is bound by the number of DIRCs in which a parameter proposition including π is an inducing proposition. Since observation 1 ascertained that there are no loops either, the process must end for any finite number of input (interval-based) propositions.

3.4.1 *Advantages of explicit contexts and DIRCs*

Explicit interpretation contexts, separate from the propositions inducing them and from abstractions using them, have significant conceptual and computational advantages for context-specific interpretation of time-stamped data.

First, since the four temporal measures of a DIRC, representing temporal constraints over an induced context interval with respect to the start time and the end time of the inducing proposition, can be positive, negative, or infinite time measures, the context interval induced by a context-forming proposition can have any one of [Allen, 1984] 13 binary temporal relations (e.g., BEFORE, AFTER, or OVERLAPS) to the time interval over which the inducing proposition is interpreted (see Figure 3.3). Thus, a context-forming proposition interval can create, in addition to a **direct** (concurrent) context interval, **retrospective** context intervals (e.g., potential preceding symptoms of a disease), **prospective** context intervals (e.g., potential complications of a disease), or both (see Figure 3.3). Intuitively, retrospective interpretation contexts represent a form of **abductive** reasoning (e.g., from effects to causes, such as preceding events), while prospective interpretation contexts represent a form of **deductive** reasoning (e.g., from an event to potential complications), or **foresight**. (Note, however, that we infer only a potential interpretation context, not an abstraction.) The context-forming mechanism creates retrospective and prospective contexts mainly to enable the use of context-specific TA functions, such as the correct mapping functions related to ABSTRACTED-INTO relations and the relevant temporal persistence functions [Shahar, 1994], that should not be considered in other contexts. Creation of explicit contexts enables the TA mechanisms to focus on the abstractions appropriate for particular contexts, such as potential consequences of a certain event, and to avoid unnecessary computations in other contexts. In addition, the ability to create dynamically retrospective contexts enables a form of **hindsight** [Russ, 1989], since the interpretation of *present* data can induce new interpretation contexts for the past and thus shed new light on *old* data. Note that the representations of both hindsight and foresight are outside of the scope of formalisms such as the event calculus [Kowalski and Sergot, 1986], in which, in effect, events must directly and instantaneously create state transitions. No delay is permitted for future effects, and past effects are impossible. In our formalism, a proposition cannot create directly another proposition, but can induce, over any other temporal interval relative to the proposition's temporal scope, an environment (a context) which enables a TA mechanism, *potentially*, to infer another proposition.

Second, since a context-forming proposition can be an inducing proposition in more than one DIRC, the *same proposition* can *induce* dynamically *several interpretation contexts*, either in the past, the present, or the future, relative to the temporal scope of the interval over which it is interpreted. Thus, we can model, for instance, several potential effects of the same action, each of which creates a different interpretation context, or several inferences from the same temporal pattern, once detected.

Third, the *same interpretation* context (e.g., potential bone-marrow toxicity) might be induced by *different propositions*, possibly even of different types and occurring over different periods (e.g., different types of chemotherapy and radiotherapy events). The domain's TA ontology would then be representing the fact that, within the particular interpretation context induced by any of these propositions (perhaps with different temporal constraints for each proposition), certain parameters would be interpreted in the same way (e.g., we can represent the properties of the hemoglobin-state parameter within the scope of a bone-marrowtoxicity context interval, without the need to list all the events that can lead to the creation of such a context interval). Thus, the separation of interpretation contexts from their inducing propositions also facilitates maintenance and reusability of the TA knowledge base.

Finally, since several context intervals, during which different interpretation contexts hold, can exist contemporaneously, it is possible to represent several abstraction intervals in which the *same abstract parameter* (e.g., the state of the hemoglobin level) has *different values* at the *same time*—one for each valid and relevant context (e.g., "LOW hemoglobin state" in the context of having AIDS without complications, and "NORMAL hemoglobin state" in the context of being treated by the drug AZT, which has expected side effects). Thus, the context-forming mechanism supports maintenance of several *concurrent* **views** of the abstractions in the abstraction database, denoting several possible interpretations of the same data. This is one of the reasons that parameter propositions (including temporal pattern queries to the abstraction database) must include an interpretation context: The parameter value alone might otherwise be meaningless.

3.4.2 Generalized interpretation contexts

Additional distinctions important for the TA task are enabled by the explicit use of interpretation contexts and DIRCs. A **simple interpretation context** is a *basic* or a *composite* interpretation context. Our discussion till now concerned simple interpretation contexts. Usually, abstractions are specific to a particular simple interpretation context, and *cannot* be joined (by the temporal inference or temporal interpolation mechanisms) to abstractions in other interpretation contexts (e.g., two "LOW hemoglobin state" abstractions might denote different ranges in two different subcontexts of the same interpretation context induced by a chemotherapy-protocol event). This restriction is reasonable, since the primary reason for having contexts is to *limit* the scope of reasoning and of the applicability of certain types of knowledge.

However, it is both desirable and possible to denote that, for certain classes of parameters, contexts, and subcontexts, the abstractions are *sharable* among two meeting different context intervals (i.e., with different interpretation contexts). Such abstractions denote the same state, with respect to the task-related implications of the state, in all sharing contexts. For instance, two meeting "LOW hemoglobin state" abstractions in two different contexts might indeed denote different ranges in the two contexts, and the hemoglobin-state parameter might even have only two possible values in one context, and three in the other, but an expert hematologist still might want to express the fact that the LOW value of the hemoglobin-state abstraction can be joined meaningfully to summarize a particular hematological state of the patient during the joined time period. The sharable abstraction values would then be defined within a new **generalized interpretation context** that is equivalent to neither of the two shared subcontexts (e.g., those induced by two different parts of the same clinical protocol), nor to their parent context (e.g., the one induced by the clinical protocol itself, within which the hemoglobin-state parameter might have yet another, default, LOW hemoglobin-state range). This generalized context can be viewed as a generalization of two or more subcontexts of the parent interpretation context. The proposition "LOW hemoglobin-state (within the generalized context)" would then have the logical *concatenable* [Shoham, 1987] property and can thus be joined across the temporal scope of two different subcontexts.

3.4.3 Nonconvex interpretation contexts

Sometimes, we might want to abstract the state of a parameter such as glucose in the preprandial (before meals) interpretation context, over two or more temporally *disjoint*, but semantically equivalent, preprandial interpretation contexts (e.g., the PRELUNCH and PRESUPPER interpretation contexts are both PREPRANDIAL interpretation contexts) (see Section 3.5.1). We might even want to create such an abstraction within only a particular preprandial context (e.g., several PRESUPPER interpretation contexts) skipping intermediate preprandial contexts (e.g., PREBREAKFAST and PRELUNCH interpretation contexts). This interpolation is different from sharing abstractions in a generalized interpretation context, since the abstractions in this case were created within the *same* interpretation contexts, but the interpolation operation joining them needs to skip temporal gaps, including possibly context intervals over which different interpretation contexts hold. The output is a new type of a parameter interval, with respect to temporal scope—a *nonconvex interval*, as defined by [Ladkin, 1986]. A "LOW glucose state" abstraction would be defined, therefore, within the **nonconvex interpretation context** of "prebreakfast episodes." Note that parameter propositions including such a nonconvex context will have different temporal semantic inference properties [Shahar, 1994] from the same parameter propositions except for a simple, convex, context. For instance, propositions will usually not be *downward hereditary* ([Shoham, 1987] in the usual sense of that property (i.e., the proposition holds within any subinterval of the original interval) unless subintervals are confined to only the convex or nonconvex intervals that the nonconvex superinterval comprises (e.g., only morning times).

Thus, the interpretation context of a parameter proposition is a combination of simple, generalized, and nonconvex interpretation contexts. Assume that a **Gen** (generalize) operator returns the generalizing-context parent (if it exists) of a parameter proposition in the parameter-properties ontology. Assume that a **Gen*** operator, that generalizes the Gen operator, returns the least common generalizing-context ancestor (if it exists) $\langle \pi, \nu, \xi_g \rangle$ of two parameter propositions $\langle \pi, \nu, \xi_1 \rangle$, $\langle \pi, \nu, \xi_2 \rangle$, in which the parameter π and the value ν are the same, but the interpretation context is different. Assume that an **NC** (nonconvex) operator returns the nonconvex-context extension (if it exists) of a parameter proposition. Then, the parameter proposition that represents the nonconvex join (over disjoint temporal spans) of two parameter propositions in which only the interpretation context is different can be represented as

$$NC(\text{Gen}^*(\langle \pi, \nu, \xi_1 \rangle, \langle \pi, \nu, \xi_2 \rangle))$$

Thus, we first look for a generalizing interpretation context for glucose-state abstractions in the PRELUNCH and PRESUPPER interpretation contexts, in this case the PREPRANDIAL one. Then we represent the parameter proposition "LOW preprandial glucose-state values" as the LOW value of the glucose-state parameter in the nonconvex extension of the PREPRANDIAL interpretation context. This proposition would be interpreted over some time interval to form a (nonconvex) parameter interval.

Generalized and nonconvex interpretation contexts are represented in the context ontology; the corresponding extended-parameter propositions are represented in the parameter ontology.

3.5 APPLICATION OF INTERPRETATION CONTEXTS IN THE DIABETES DOMAIN

As mentioned in Section 3.2, the RÉSUMÉ system was tested in several different clinical domains, such as chronic graft-versus-host disease [Shahar and Musen, 1993], monitoring of children's growth [Kuilboer et al., 1993], and therapy of AIDS patients [Shahar, 1994]. In this section, we demonstrate the use of interpretation contexts in a clinical domain in which we have evaluated the RÉSUMÉ system more formally: monitoring the therapy of patients who have insulin-dependent diabetes mellitus (DM) [Shahar and Musen, 1996].

We collaborated with two endocrinologists, acquiring within several meetings a TA ontology from one of the expert physicians. We created a parameter-properties ontology for the domain of insulin-dependent diabetes (Figure 3.5), an event ontology (which includes three types of insulin therapy, four types of meals, and physical exercise), and a context ontology (e.g., preprandial [measured at fasting time, before a meal] and postprandial [after a meal] contexts and subcontexts, and postexercise contexts) (Figure 3.6).

In the diabetes-therapy ontology, administrations of regular insulin, isophane insulin suspension (NPH), or Ultralente insulin are *events* inducing different insulin-action *interpretation contexts* that are *subcontexts* of the dm *interpretation context* (see Figure 3.7a) which represents the context of treating diabetes. Meals (breakfast, lunch, supper, and a bedtime snack) are events that induce preprandial and postprandial contexts (see Figure 3.7b). Thus, values for the Glucuse_state_DM_prebreakfast (the state of glucose in the context of DM and measurement before breakfast) parameter (see Figure 3.5) can be created, when relevant, regardless of absolute time.

To control the computational process, the overall DM context itself (which, as a top-level context for the diabetes domain, is necessary for activation of all of the domain-specific temporal abstraction inferences) is induced at runtime when the user asserts into the RÉSUMÉ system's runtime temporal fact base a DM-therapy abstraction-goal interval (Figure 3.8). This abstraction goal induces retrospectively the DM interpretation context (usually, during the two preceding weeks; the desired context-interval length is part of the corresponding DIRC in the knowledge base). All other contexts are induced automatically by events in the patient's record.

The Glucose_state parameter is a new parameter with six values defined from corresponding Glucose ranges used by the domain expert (HYPOGLYCEMIA, LOW, NORMAL, HIGH, VERY HIGH, EXTREMELY HIGH). These values are sensitive to the context in which they are generated; for instance, the postprandial context classification functions define a higher range of the NORMAL value. Glucose_state propositions (for all allowed values) have the value TRUE for the tem-

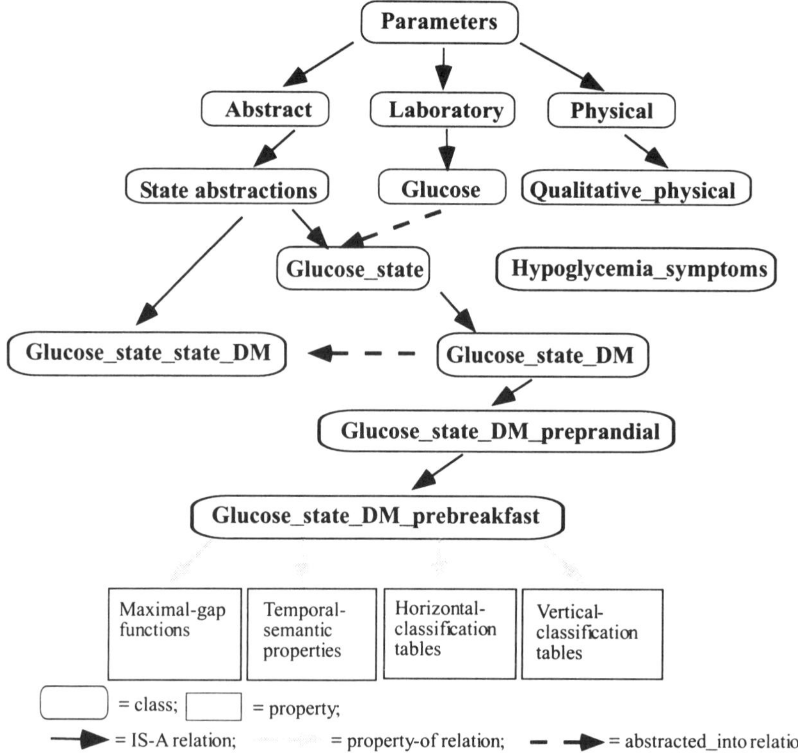

Figure 3.5 Part of the diabetes mellitus (DM) parameter-properties ontology. The Glucose parameter is abstracted into the Glucose_state parameter. This abstract parameter has a specialized subclass in the DM context, and is abstracted in that context into the Glucose_state_state parameter. The Glucose_state_DM class is further specialized in the preprandial and postprandial contexts, each of which has several subclasses corresponding to the different relevant premeal contexts.

poral semantic property *concatenable* (see Section 3.2) in the same meal-phase context. The Glucose_state_state parameter is a higher-level abstraction of the Glucose_state parameter, which maps its six values into three (LOW, NORMAL, HIGH, or L, N, H for short). It has different semantic properties, and allows creation of daily horizontal-inference patterns within a *nonconvex* preprandial context (see Section 3.4.3) representing abstraction over several meal phases, such as LLH (LOW, LOW and HIGH Glucose_state_state values over breakfast, lunch, and supper, respectively).

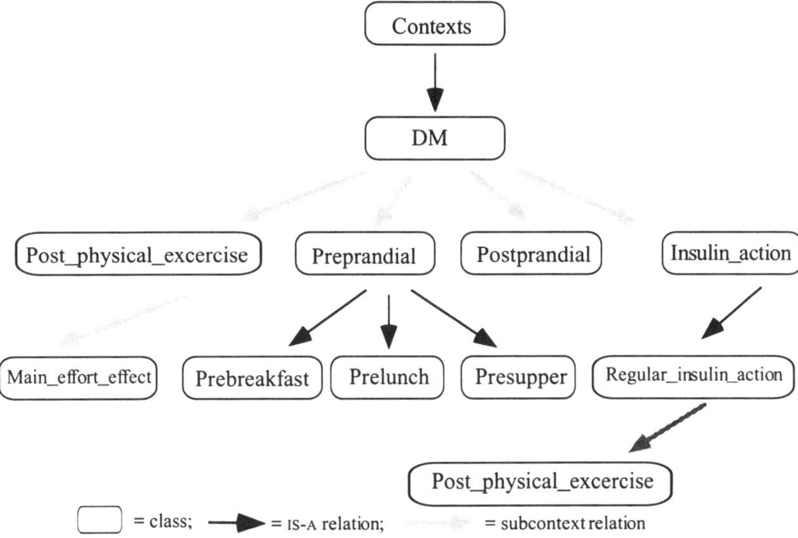

Figure 3.6 Part of the context ontology in the diabetes-mellitus (DM) therapy domain. Preprandial and postprandial contexts are induced before and after meal events, respectively.

Patterns such as LLH values for the Glucose_state_state parameter, especially in the preprandial subcontext, are extremely useful when a physician must decide how to modify a patient's insulin regimen. Furthermore, once created, the prevalence of such patterns can be calculated—an important step in determining whether the pattern is a common one for the patient.

Glucose_state_state values that are measured within *different phases* (e.g., prelunch and presupper), but within the *same day*, can be joined by interpolation within the same *generalized* (see Section 3.4.2) interpretation context (a nonconvex version of the generalized PREPRANDIAL context interval; see Section 3.4.3) creating an abstraction comprising several preprandial abstractions, up to 6 to 8 hours apart. The maximal gap is defined by a interphase Δ (global-persistence) function. Diurnal state abstractions that are measured in the *same phase* but over *different* (usually consecutive) *days*, such as several values of the Glucuse_state_DM_prebreakfast parameter, can be joined by interpolation within the same interpretation context (e.g., a nonconvex PREBREAKFAST context interval, that comprises all breakfasts within a given interval), up 24 to 28 hours apart, using another interphase Δ function. The two expert physicians formed (independently) temporal abstractions from more than 800 points of

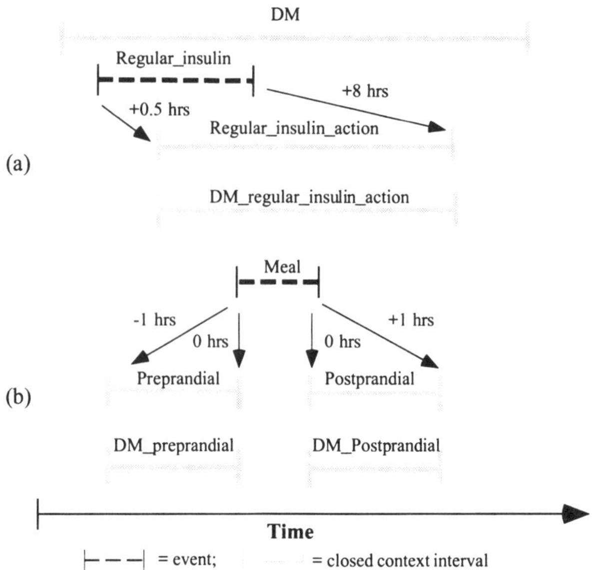

Figure 3.7 Formation of contexts in the diabetes-mellitus (dm)domain.
(a) Creation of a Regular_insulin_action context, induced by a Regular_insulin administration event, and of the corresponding DM subcontext.
(b) Creation of the Postprandial and Preprandial (prospective and retrospective, respectively) context intervals, induced by a Meal event, and formation of the corresponding DM subcontexts.

data, representing two weeks of glucose and insulin data from each of eight patients.

The RÉSUMÉ system created 132 (80.4%) of the 164 temporal abstractions that were noted by both experts [Shahar and Musen, 1996]. An example of the output is shown in Figure 3.8. In the particular time window shown, two significant abstractions are demonstrated: (1) A period of 5 days of HIGH presupper blood-glucose values in the presupper [nonconvex] context; (2) A set of three Glucose_state_state abstractions representing a repeating diurnal pattern, consisting of NORMAL or LOW blood-glucose levels during the morning and lunch measurements, and high glucose levels during the presupper measurements. The combined pattern suggests an adjustment of the intermediate-acting insulin and was noted in the data by both experts.

Examination of the output for the first three cases by one of the experts showed that the expert agreed with almost all (97%) of the produced abstractions—a result similar to the one we found in the domain of growth monitoring

[Kuilboer et al., 1993, Shahar, 1994]. We expected this high predictive value, since the domain's TA ontology directly reflected that expert's knowledge about these low- and intermediate-level abstractions.

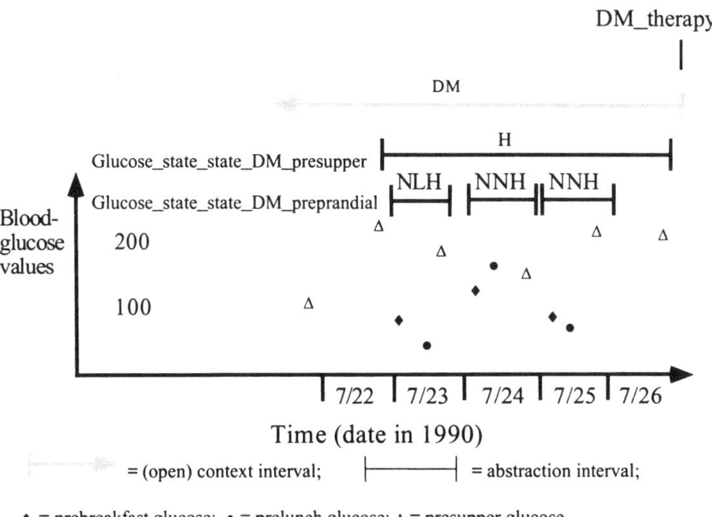

Figure 3.8 Abstraction of data by the RÉSUMÉ system in one of the diabetes-patients' cases. The DM_therapy abstraction goal induces a retrospective DM interpretation context. DM_therapy = diabetes-mellitustherapy abstraction goal; dm = diabetes-mellitustherapy interpretation context; Glucose_state_state_DM_presupper = Glucose_state_state abstraction in the dm and presupper composite context; Glucose_state_state_DM_preprandial = Glucose_state_state abstraction in the dm and preprandial composite context. L = LOW; N = NORMAL; H = HIGH.

3.6 DISCUSSION

Large amounts of time-oriented clinical data often need to be abstracted or queried, either for direct human purposes or as part of automated medical decision-support applications. On one hand, the data need to be interpreted in a context-sensitive manner, using all available knowledge about past and future data to make inferences as specific as possible. On the other hand, inference computations should be kept to a minimum, and thus should be evoked only when (potentially) clinically relevant. The interpretation-context framework supports both goals.

The TA mechanisms (except for context formation) operate within the temporal span of context intervals and *do not depend on the event and context ontologies.* These mechanisms assume the existence of context intervals and of interpretation contexts as part of the input parameter propositions. The context-forming mechanism is thus the only interface to the domain's event, context, and abstraction-goal ontologies, and shields the rest of the mechanisms from any need to know about external events and their structure, or how interpretation contexts are induced.

The introduction of explicit clinical interpretation contexts as independent mediating entities, separate from the propositions inducing them and from abstractions using them, has significant conceptual and computational advantages for context-specific interpretation of time-stamped data. Advantages include (1) Any temporal relation can hold between a context interval and its inducing proposition; interpretation contexts might be induced concurrently, in the future, and in the past, enabling a form of foresight and hindsight. Both past and delayed effects are outside of the scope of formalisms such as the event calculus [Kowalski and Sergot, 1986], in which events directly and instantaneously create state transitions; (2) the *same context-forming proposition* can *induce* one or more context intervals; (3) the *same interpretation context* might be induced by *different* propositions. The separation of interpretation contexts from their inducing propositions facilitates maintenance and reusability of temporal abstraction knowledge; and (4) parameter propositions include an explicit interpretation context, thus enabling a representation of several abstractions in which the *same abstract parameter* (e.g., the "state of hemoglobin-level" parameter) has *different values* at the same *time*—one for each of the context intervals that hold during the relevant period. Thus, interpretation contexts support maintenance of several *concurrent* interpretations of the same clinical data.

Acknowledgments

This work has been supported by grants LM05708 and LM06245 from the National Library of Medicine, and IRI-9528444 from the National Science Foundation. Computing resources were provided by the Stanford CAMIS project, funded under Grant No. LM05305 from the National Library of Medicine.

References

Allen, J.F. (1984). Towards a general theory of action and time. *Artificial Intelligence*, 23(2): 123–154.

Eriksson, H., Shahar, Y., Tu, S.W., Puerta, A.R., and Musen, M.A. (1995). Task modeling with reusable problem-solving methods. *Artificial Intelligence*, 79 (2): 293–326.

Kowalski, R.A. and Sergot, M.J. (1986). A logic-based calculus of events. *New Generation Computing*, 4: 67–95.

Kuilboer, M.M., Shahar, Y., Wilson, D.M., and Musen, M.A. (1993). Knowledge reuse: Temporal-abstraction mechanisms for the assessment of children's growth. In *Proc. of the Seventeenth Annual Symposium on Computer Applications in Medicine*, Washington, D.C., pages 449–453.

Ladkin, P. (1986). Time representation: A taxonomy of interval relations. In *Proc. of the Sixth National Conference on Artificial Intelligence*, Philadelphia, PA, pages 360–366.

McCarthy, J. and Hayes, P. (1969). Some philosophical problems from the standpoint of artificial intelligence. In Meltzer, B., Michie, D., and Swann, M., editors, *Machine Intelligence IV*, pages 463–502, Edinburgh University Press.

Musen, M.A., Tu, S.W., Das, A.K., and Shahar, Y. (1996). EON: A component-based approach to automation of protocol-directed therapy. *Journal of the American Medical Association*, 3(6): 367-388.

Russ, T.A. (1989). Using hindsight in medical decision making, In Kingsland, L. C., editor, *Proc. of the Thirteenth Annual Symposium on Computer Applications in Medical Care*, pages 38–44. IEEE Computing Society Press, Washington.

Shahar, Y., Tu, S.W., and Musen, M.A. (1992). Knowledge acquisition for temporal-abstraction mechanisms. *Knowledge Acquisition*, 4(2): 217–236.

Shahar, Y. and Musen, M.A. (1993). RÉSUMÉ: A temporal-abstraction system for patient monitoring. *Computers and Biomedical Research*, 26(3): 255273. Reprinted in van Bemmel, J.H. and McRay, T., editors, *Yearbook of Medical Informatics 1994* (F.K. Schattauer and The International Medical Informatics Association, Stuttgart, 1994), pages 443–461.

Shahar, Y. (1994). A knowledge-based method for temporal abstraction of clinical data. Ph.D. dissertation, Program in Medical Information Sciences, Knowledge Systems Laboratory Report No. KSL-94-64, Department of Computer Science report No. STAN-CS-TR-94-1529, Stanford University, Stanford, CA.

Shahar, Y., and Musen, M.A. (1996). Knowledge-based temporal abstraction in clinical domains. *Artificial Intelligence in Medicine*, 8(3): 267–298.

Shahar, Y. (1997). A framework for knowledge-based temporal abstraction. *Artificial Intelligence*, 90(1-2): 79–133.

Shoham, Y. (1987). Temporal logics in AI: Semantical and ontological considerations. *Artificial Intelligence*, 33(1): 89–104.

4 TEMPORAL ABSTRACTION OF MEDICAL DATA: DERIVING PERIODICITY

Elpida T. Keravnou

Abstract: Temporal abstraction, the derivation of abstractions from time-stamped data, is one of the central processes in medical knowledge-based systems. Important types of temporal abstractions include periodic occurrences, trends, and other temporal patterns. This chapter discusses the derivation of periodic abstractions at a theoretical, domain-independent level, and in the context of a specific temporal ontology.

4.1 TEMPORAL DATA ABSTRACTION

The focus of the chapter is the derivation of periodic occurrences from lower level information directly obtained from the record of some patient; the raw patient data so to speak. A patient record is viewed as a *historical database* consisting of a collection of time-stamped assertions of the form $< p, t >$, where p is a property and t is an interval of *valid-time*, meaning that at the current point in time it is believed that during time period t property p is valid (holds) with respect to the particular patient. A fair proportion of the assertions comprising the patient record would denote observations made at discrete points in time. The temporal assertions are divided into *abnormality observations* and *contextual information*. The latter could assert normal situations or happenings, things like age or sex, therapeutic interventions, or other contextual information of relevance to the particular domain.

The essence of the temporal data abstraction task is the derivation of temporal abstractions from a collection of temporally discrete assertions. The task operates with respect to a specific period of valid time and a specific patient record. Converting numeric values to qualitative values is a simple, but important type of data abstraction but no temporal reasoning is involved here. For some data abstraction to qualify as a *temporal* abstraction, temporal reasoning must play a central part in its derivation. We distinguish the following types of temporal data abstraction:

- persistence derivation,
- derivation of temporal trends,
- derivation of periodic occurrences, and
- derivation of general temporal patterns, i.e., clusters of related occurrences.

Each type can be further classified into subtypes.

Deriving maximal temporal extents of some concatenable [Shoham, 1987] property by *merging* together the temporal extents of overlapping assertions sharing that property may also be considered a simple form of temporal data abstraction. Merging of temporal assertions is discussed in [Keravnou, 1996b].

Persistence derivation is explained through an example. Suppose the record of some patient includes the two assertions "kyphoscoliosis at the age of 2 years" and "kyphoscoliosis at the age of 4 years". The problem is how to see beyond these two discrete sightings, both forwards and backwards in time, e.g., what can be inferred about the existence of this condition with regard to the particular patient before the age of 2 years, between the ages of 2 and 4 years, and after the age of 4 years? Persistence derivation is also discussed in [Keravnou, 1996b].

Merging and persistence derivation are necessary functionalities for obtaining maximal temporal extents of properties; the assertions derived this way subsume a number of the original assertions. We assume that the operations of merging and persistence derivation are applied to the raw patient data prior to attempting to derive potential trends and/or periodic occurrences. The derivation of trends is discussed in [Keravnou, 1996a]. The motivation for the research presented here is that the representation and derivation of periodicity and trends constitutes an important problem in the area of temporal reasoning that has significant practical consequences for many domains, e.g., the interpretation of clinical data [Haimowitz et al., 1995, Larizza et al., 1995, Miksch et al., 1996, Russ, 1995, Shahar and Musen, 1996, Wade, 1994].

The chapter is organized as follows. Section 4.2 overviews the adopted temporal ontology from the perspective of this research. Section 4.3 discusses the notions of periodicity, trends and patterns. Section 4.4 outlines the algorithms for the derivation of periodic occurrences. Finally, section 4.5 concludes the discussion.

4.2 TEMPORAL ONTOLOGY

For the natural modeling of many medical problems, multiplicity of temporal granularities is required for providing the relevant time abstractions. We believe that the adopted ontology [Keravnou, 1996a, Keravnou, 1996b] models multiple granularities in an appropriate way by introducing the notion of a conceptual time-axis and supporting the presence of multiple time-axes. A *time-axis*, α, is a conceptual temporal context defined in a discrete way as a sequence of time-values, Times(α) $= \{t_1, t_2, ..., t_n\}$, expressed with respect to an *origin* and a specific time-unit (granularity). The origin of a concrete time-axis is bound to a real time-point.

The other central primitive of the ontology is the *time-object*. A time-object, τ, is a dynamic entity for which time constitutes an integral aspect. It is viewed as a tight coupling between a *property* and an *existence*, where its existence can be expressed with respect to different time-axes. Thus $\tau \equiv < \varrho, \epsilon_\tau >$ where ϱ is the property of τ, and ϵ_τ : Axes $\rightarrow$ Eexps is the existence function of τ. The domain of ϵ_τ is the set of time-axes and its range is the set of absolute existence expressions. An absolute existence expression gives the (earliest) initiation and (latest) termination of some existence. If time-object, τ, has a valid existence on some time-axis, α, then $\epsilon_\tau(\alpha) = < t_s, t_f, \varsigma >$; $t_s, t_f \in Times(\alpha)$; $t_s \leq t_f$; and the status $\varsigma \in$ {closed, open, open-from-left, open-from-right, moving}. If there is openness in some valid existence of a time-object then its actual initiation and/or termination is not known. A special moving time-object is *now* which exists as a point-object on any relevant, concrete, time-axis and functions to partition time-objects into past, future, or ongoing. Three types of relations are defined for time-objects, temporal, structural, and causal relations. Structural relations enable the definition of compound occurrences.

Properties that constitute the other half of time-objects are atomic or compound (negations, disjunctions, or conjunctions), passive or active, and some are time-invariant. Examples of properties are “sex male”, “sore throat”, “severe coughing”, etc. We assume that an atomic property has the format $(< subject > [, < attribute_1 >, < value_1 >, ..., < attribute_n >, < value_n >])$. A property is associated with relevant granularities, e.g., “headache present” is associated with hours and days, but not months or years. This way the time-axes meaningful to a property can be defined. A property, ϱ, either has an infinite persistence, *infper*(ϱ), or a finite persistence, *finper*(ϱ). In the latter case it is also specified whether the property can *reoccur* (multiple instantiations of the given property in the same context are possible). Properties that describe normal situations are assumed to persist indefinitely. Property relations include causality, exclusion, necessitation, etc.

The adopted temporal ontology is discussed in detail in [Keravnou, 1996a]. Each temporal assertion included in the patient record defines a concrete time-object. Thus a patient record is viewed as a collection of concrete time-objects whose existences are specified with respect to a collection of concrete time-axes.

4.3 PERIODICITY, TRENDS AND PATTERNS

Periodic occurrences, trends, and patterns are types of compound occurrences. Repeated instantiations of some type of occurrence, in a regular fashion, forms a *periodic occurrence*. An abstract periodic occurrence is qualified through an occurrence type and the “algorithm” governing the repetition. A specific periodic occurrence is the collation of the relevant, individual, occurrences. A *temporal trend*, or simply trend, is an important kind of interval occurrence. An atomic trend describes a change, the direction of change, and the rate of change that takes place in the given interval of time, which can be translated into “something is normal, or moving away or towards normality (worsening or improving) and at what rate”. An example of a trend could be “low pressure, increasing, slowly”. The derivation of trends from patient data or the matching of patient data against prespecified generic trends (trend templates) is a topic of active research in medical temporal reasoning, where the issues of multiple granularities (different sampling frequencies between parameters) and default persistencies of properties arise [Haimowitz et al., 1995, Miksch et al., 1996, Russ, 1995, Shahar and Musen, 1996, Wade, 1994]. There are different kinds of *temporal patterns*. A sequence of meeting trends is a commonly used kind of pattern [Larizza et al., 1995]. A periodic occurrence is another example of patterns. A set of relative occurrences, or a set of causally related occurrences, could form patterns.

The notion of periodicity is very relevant to medical problem solving. It applies to disease processes, therapeutic interventions, and patient data. For example consider the following statements of periodic occurrences: s_1: this ailment causes morning nausea for about two weeks; s_2: expect headache every morning for about two hours over a period of one week which worsens each day; s_3: administer drug every four hours until the pain stops but not for more than two days; s_4: I experienced nausea for about an hour followed by headache after each meal. A periodic occurrence can be characterised as follows:

Repetition element. The occurrence that is repeating itself. This could be a compound occurrence. The repetition elements in the above statements are: s_1: nausea; s_2: two hours of headache; s_3: administration of drug x; s_4: an hour of nausea followed by headache. The temporal extent of the repetition element could be fixed or variable amongst its succession of instantiations but this extent may be incompletely specified, e.g., in statements s_1 and s_4 above where the durations of nausea and headache are, respectively, unspecified.

Repetition pattern. This defines a pattern of the particular repetition, which, if completely specified, would imply the initiation and termination of the temporal extent of the periodic occurrence in absolute, relative, or conditional terms, which in turn would imply the number of times that the repetition element materialises and the respective existences of these instantiations. Thus the repetition is either counted or indefinite. The repetition patterns for the above statements are: s_1: every morning for two weeks; s_2: every morning for one week; s_3: every four hours until either the pain stops or a two day period has elapsed; s_4: after each meal. In s_1, s_2, and s_3 the initiations of the instantiations of the repetition element are fixed and predetermined but these are variable for s_4.

Progression pattern. This specifies any constraints that define some sort of progression over the sequence of instantiations of the repetition element; usually such constraints would refer to attributes of the property involved. The progression pattern enables the specification of a trend in the context of periodicity. Of the above statements only s_2 includes a progression pattern which is "a worsening situation".

By default the existences of periodic time-objects are characterised with 'discontinuities' [Ladkin, 1986].

4.4 DERIVING PERIODICITY

A patient record can be organised in terms of a number of abstraction layers. Starting from the least abstract layer, the one that contains the raw (quantitative) patient data, the most abstract layer, the one that includes trends, periodic occurrences and other temporal patterns, can be obtained by successively applying the operations "qualitative abstraction", "merging and persistence abstraction" and "periodicity, trend and causality abstraction". The latter operation can be repeatedly applied to the top layer in order to obtain more and more complex trends and periodic occurrences, thus yielding a higher abstraction. For example, the repetition element of a periodic occurrence could be a trend or another periodic occurrence, or a sequence of related periodic occurrences could form a trend, etc.

In this section we discuss how to derive periodic occurrences in a nondirected fashion. The aim is to derive any periodic occurrence that is derivable from the patient information, rather than to determine whether the patient record entails some periodic occurrence(s) which is(are) matchable against a prespecified template for a given type of periodic occurrence.

Recall that the raw patient data comprise a collection of discrete (initially unrelated) time-objects, where the property of a time-object has the format $(< subject > [, < attribute_1 >, < value_1 >, ..., < attribute_n >, < value_n >])$. To start with, time-objects whose existences are not covered by the span of valid time that defines the temporal focus (time window) of the overall data abstraction process are screened out. The following time-objects are additionally screened out: (a) time-objects with infinitely persistent, or finitely persistent but not reoccurrying properties; and (b) time-objects that do not share the subject of their property with any other time-object. In either case there is just a single time-object with the same property/subject and since we need at least two time-objects to even potentially derive a periodic occurrence, none of these time-objects can possibly be involved in a periodic occurrence. Finally, time-objects that denote neither abnormalities nor actions are screened out. All the remaining time-objects participate in the processing. These are classified into *passive* time-objects, those whose property subject denotes an abnormality, and *active* time-objects, those whose property subject denotes an action, e.g., some therapeutic action or any other action.

The selected time-objects are then organised into the bottom layer of the relevant *periodicity map* (see Figure 4.1). A periodicity map is a 3-dimensional structure where the first dimension is defined by the discrete time-axis that constitutes the temporal context (window) of the whole processing (it is assumed that the granularity of this time-axis is meaningful to the properties of all selected time-objects – the processing can be repeated with different

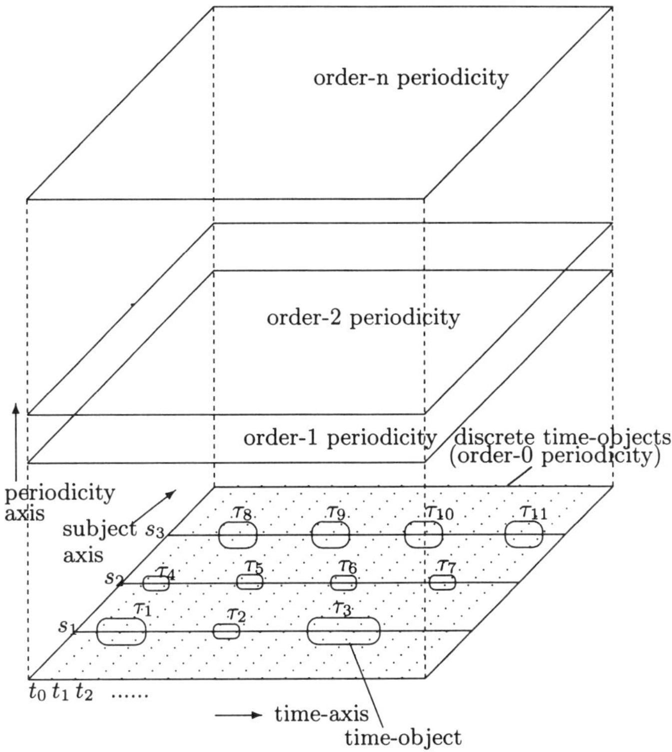

Figure 4.1 Multi-layer periodicity map.

time-axes and granularities), the second dimension is defined by the subjects of the properties involved, and the third dimension is defined by the orders of periodicity required (see below). Thus initially only the bottom layer of the periodicity map is filled, while higher layers are gradually filled by the results of the periodicity derivator. The bottom layer is referred to as order-0 periodicity layer because no periodic relations are depicted between the different time-objects on this layer; each time-object is seen as an 'independent' entity that represents a distinct occurrence in the lifetime of the particular patient and hence all subjects involved are mutually distinct. Furthermore no exclusivity relation holds between the properties of any pair of time-objects within the same subject.

Occurrences of order-0 periodicity are treated as non-decomposable occurrences in the context of the particular reasoning, i.e., they are not treated as periodic occurrences, even if they are. Since periodic occurrences could be of any degree of complexity, the periodicity derivator is repeatedly applied to the raw patient data augmented with the various derived abstractions. Thus different periodicity maps are constructed during the different phases of the processing, both in a horizontal and a vertical fashion; horizontally refers to different time-windows and granularities (and hence subjects), while vertically is when the results of some application of the derivator (the compound occurrences recorded on the higher layers of the relevant periodicity map) are fed as the input to a subsequent application of the derivator (they become the elements of the bottom layer of the new periodicity map). The latter enables the derivation of new periodic occurrences of even higher complexity, e.g. nested periodicity – the repetition element is itself a periodic occurrence. Thus, if for some periodicity map its order-0 time-objects are really periodic time-objects, an order-1 (see below) periodic time-object represents nested periodicity. Elements at the bottom layer of a periodicity map could be trends (output from the trend derivator) to enable the derivation of periodic (repeated) trends. This is different from the progression pattern of a periodic occurence, since the latter represents the threading of a trend over some periodic occurrence.

Thus, within the context of some periodicity map, 'true' periodic occurrences have an order of periodicity of at least 1. An order-1 periodic time-object consists of a sequence of order-0 time-objects, of the same subject; in other words, order-1 periodicity is periodicity within a single subject. For example, the sequence of time-objects (see Figure 4.1) τ_4, τ_5, τ_6, and τ_7, appear to form an order-1 periodic occurrence, where there is a correspondence between successive pairs of time-objects, i.e., τ_4 with τ_5, τ_5 with τ_6, etc. Similarly the sequence of time-objects τ_8, τ_9, τ_{10}, and τ_{11}, appears to compose an order-1 periodic occurrence. An order-2 periodicity is periodicity across two subjects. For example, the two sequences of time-objects discussed above that constitute order-1 periodic occurrences could form an order-2 periodic occurrence where the pairwise correspondences would be τ_4 with τ_8, τ_5 with τ_9, τ_6 with τ_{10}, and τ_7 with τ_{11}. In general, a periodic occurrence of order-n comprises, at the bottom layer, n distinct subject sequences of time-objects; each sequence has the same length. An order-n periodic occurrence is therefore periodicity across n distinct subjects, and it can be composed out of any combination of lower order periodic occurrences that yields n distinct subjects at the bottom layer. The aim is to achieve as much abstraction as possible, which in this context means deriving periodic occurrences of the highest possible order. In the rest of this section we sketch the algorithms for the following: (a) derivation of order-1 periodic occurences, i.e., periodicity within an individual subject; and (b) derivation of order-n periodic occurrences, where $n > 1$, i.e., periodicity across subjects. To be plausible, a derived periodic occurrence of any order must exhibit some form of *regularity*.

4.4.1 An algorithm for order-1 periodicity

The minimum number of order-0 time-objects of the same subject required to derive an order-1 periodic occurrence is 3. The aim is to derive periodic occurrences of maximal temporal extents by implicating the longest possible chains of order-0 time-objects.

A tree structure, referred to as *periodicity tree*, is grown such that it gives all potential periodic occurences of order-1; each branch of the tree represents an order-1 periodic occurrence, where each node gives the pair of order-0 time-objects that constitute a correspondence under the particular periodic occurrence. Each branch must thus include at least two nodes to ensure the participation of at least 3 order-0 time-objects. The operation of the algorithm is illustrated in Figure 4.2 for a specific sequence of order-0 time-objects. All branches except one include just 2 nodes which means that only in one branch all four of the specified order-0 time-objects participate. The excluded time-objects are circled at the bottom of the relevant branches. Thus the leftmost branch of the tree represents the potential periodic occurrence consisting of the sequence of time-objects τ_1, τ_2 and τ_3 with the relevant pairwise correspondences; time-object τ_4 does not participate in this periodic occurrence.

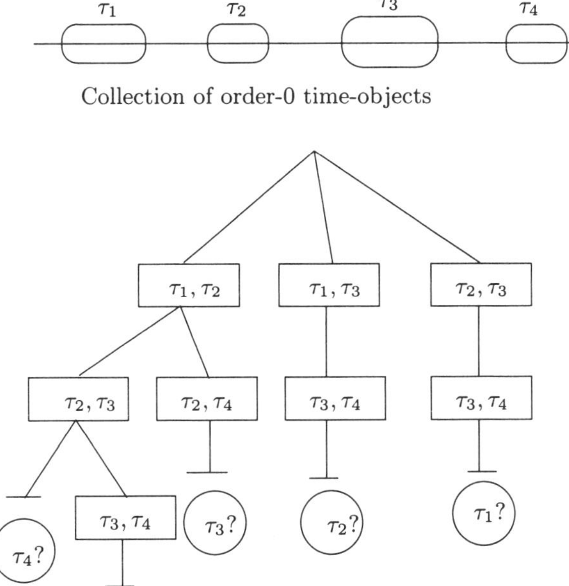

Figure 4.2 Illustrating a result of an algorithm for the derivation of order-1 periodicity.

The construction of the periodicity tree is the first step of the algorithm. The second step is the evaluation of the potential periodic occurrences to determine the plausible ones. The essence of the evaluation is the induction of the regularity that needs to underlie the presence of a plausible periodic occurrence. In other words, it tries to induce a single relation that defines the pairwise correspondences between successive elements composing the periodic occurrence. The objective is to prune all but one of the branches of the tree. The unpruned branch gives the order-1 periodic occurrence(s). If all the branches are pruned, then it is not possible to establish a credible periodic occurrence within the given sequence.

Let $\{R_1, R_2, .., R_n, f_1, f_2, .., f_m\}$ be the set of acceptable (temporal) correspondence relations (R) and functions (f) under order-1 periodicity, i.e., they denote the acceptable regularity patterns. Each relation is a binary temporal relation between time-objects, e.g., relation "immediately-succeeds" [Keravnou, 1996a]; similarly, each function has two arguments which are time-objects, e.g., the function that computes the temporal distance between the initiations of two time-objects. The correspondence relations and functions are sorted in the order of preference. Starting with the most preferred relation (function), each relation (function) is successively applied to all nodes of the tree to obtain labels for the arcs of the tree. For example, let us assume that relation R_k is applied to each node of the tree. When applied to some node that contains the pair of time-objects (τ_i, τ_j), the arc above the given node is given the label T (F) if $R_k(\tau_i, \tau_j)$ holds (does not hold). Once all the arcs are labeled, a branch of the tree that does not include at least two consecutive T's is prunable under R_k. If all the branches are prunable under R_k then R_k does not represent a viable correspondence relation (regularity pattern) for the given sequence. Functions are used in the same way (after all, the relations are predicate functions). A branch is prunable under a given function if it does not include at least two consecutive labels which are the same.

If some branch of a tree which is unprunable under $R_k(f_k)$ contains more than one sequence of at least two consecutive T (same) labels (e.g., a branch with labels T, T, T, F, F, T, T, T), then it may represent an instance of nested periodicity, i.e., regular repetition of an order-1 periodic occurrence (each sequence of T's corresponds to a separate order-1 periodic occurrence). The discovery of such higher complexity periodicity can be done by the repeated application of the discussed algorithm in the context of a new periodicity map, where the discovered order-1 periodic occurrences become order-0 periodic occurrences. It should be noted that the algorithm exhibits the following limitation. Suppose that under some relation, R_k, a branch of the given tree has the sequence of labels T, F, T, F, T. Such a branch is prunable under R_k because it does not contain two consecutive T's. However this pattern does exhibit some regularity, namely a sequencing of three pairings of time-objects. If a regularity can be established between the three pairs then a periodic occurrence may well exist. To overcome this limitation, the pruning part of the algorithm would need to be appropriately enhanced in order to avoid the missing of potential regularities of this form.

If an unpruned branch of a labeled tree is associated with some exclusions, then they would need to be justified if the excluded time-objects occur within the temporal extent of the plausible periodic occurrence. For example, if the periodic occurrence $\{\tau_1, \tau_3, \tau_4\}$ depicted in Figure 4.2 is decided as plausible under some relation R_k, i.e., both $R_k(\tau_1, \tau_3)$ and $R_k(\tau_3, \tau_4)$ hold, then the exclusion of time-object τ_2 needs to be justified. Justifications of exclusions are discussed below. If some exclusion that needs justification cannot be justified then the relevant (part of the) branch is again prunable under the given relation (function).

Each distinct plausible periodic occurrence under some relation (function) is saved. The relation (function) denotes the underlying regularity. As mentioned above the correspondence relations (functions) are successively applied in order of preference to yield the potential labels for the arcs of the tree. Therefore, the processing can stop as soon as a given labeling generates a plausible periodic occurrence covering all or a sufficient proportion of the time-objects involved.

The third step of the algorithm is to resolve the conflicts between the plausible periodic occurrences, and thus to retain the best plausible periodic occurrences. A conflict arises if periodic occurrences share elements. Different conflict resolution heuristics may be used. For example, if a periodic occurrence includes another periodic occurrence, the former is retained provided that it is associated with a more preferred correspondence relation; otherwise if the shorter occurrence has a much preferred correspondence relation (function) then it may be retained at the expense of the other.

The final step of the algorithm is to qualify, at a more abstract level, the retained plausible periodic occurrences, i.e., to specify their repetition elements, repetition patterns, and progression patterns (if any). Each retained periodic occurrence is represented as a compound time-object whose components are the relevant order-0 time-objects. The repetition element of a periodic occurrence consists of the given subject and a margin for the temporal extents of the included time-objects. If the extents of the component time-objects are more or less the same, or if they differ but in a regular way, e.g., progressively increasing or decreasing, then the credibility of the given periodic occurrence is enhanced even more since this provides additional regularity. The opposite happens if the temporal extents of the component time-objects are markedly and irregularly different. The repetition pattern of a periodic occurrence is the algorithm that, when given some instantiation of the repetition element, it determines the next appearance of the repetition element. This algorithm is directly obtained from the induced correspondence relation (function). Finally, the progression pattern (if any) is induced on the basis of the attribute-values of the properties of the component time-objects. E.g., if the subject denotes an abnormality (therapeutic action) a possible progression pattern could be "increased severity" ("reduced dosage"). The algorithm is summarized below.

Algorithm for order-1 periodicity

Input:
(a) Sequence of at least three order-0 time-objects with same subject.
(b) Acceptable regularity patterns in order of preference.

Output: Collection of credible order-1 periodic occurrences.

Step 1: Construct periodicity tree, giving potential periodic occurrences.

Step 2: Derive plausible periodic occurrences by labeling the arcs of the periodicity tree on the basis of the acceptable regularity patterns (and the justification of any exclusions, if this is necessary).

Step 3: Resolve conflicts between plausible periodic occurrences by retaining the best ones on the basis of various heuristics.

Step 4: Qualify each retained occurrence through a repetition element, a repetition pattern, and a progression pattern.

4.4.2 An algorithm for order-n periodicity

In this section we sketch an algorithm for deriving periodic occurrences of order-n, where $n > 1$, by discussing the central operation of this algorithm, which is the derivation of some regularity pattern across two distinct sequences of time-objects, each sequence having a different subject. A sequence of time-objects used in this context either defines some periodic occurrence or is a sequence of unrelated, order-0, time-objects. Furthermore, a sequence must consist of at least two time-objects.

This part of the algorithm is quite similar to the algorithm for order-1 periodicity. Again, a periodicity tree is constructed, labeled, and pruned under various regularity patterns. The operation is illustrated using the time-object sequences for subjects S_1 and S_2 given at the bottom layer of the periodicity map of Figure 4.1. The constructed periodicity tree is given in Figure 4.3. The essence is to establish matches between pairs of time-objects across the two sequences. The *potential matches* for some time-object are the time-objects

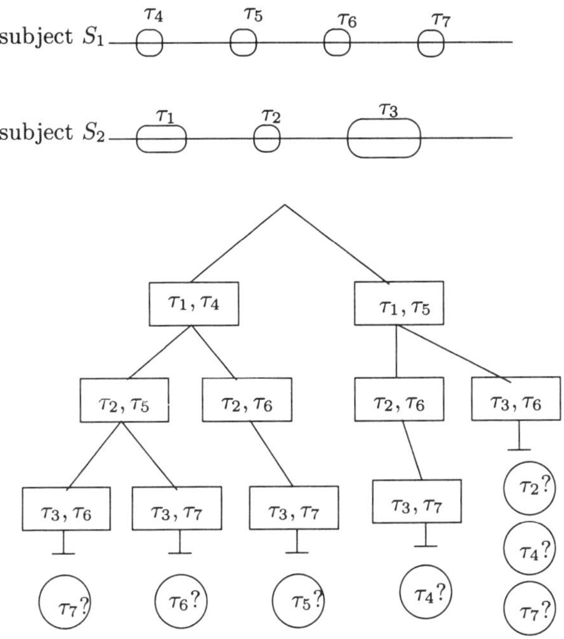

Figure 4.3 Illustrating the results of an algorithm for periodicity across two sequences.

from the other sequence whose temporal extent is covered (possibly partly) by the *temporal vicinity* of the given time-object. The temporal vicinity of a time-object is the temporal region between the termination of its predecessor time-object (or the beginning of the time-window if there is no predecessor) and the initiation of its successor (or the ending of the time-window if there is no successor). For example, the potential matches for τ_1 are τ_4 and τ_5, the potential match for τ_4 is τ_1, the potential matches for τ_3 are τ_6 and τ_7, etc. The periodicity tree is constructed on the basis of potential matches by using one of the time-object sequences, say the sequence with the fewer members, as the 'driver'. The same tree results irrespective of which sequence is used as the driver. The tree given in Figure 4.3 is constructed using the S_2 subject sequence as the driver. Under this specific construction the first choice point is given by the potential matches for τ_1; thus one possibility is to match τ_1 with τ_4 and the other possibility is to match τ_1 with τ_5. The next choice point is given by the potential matches for τ_2, which are τ_5 and τ_6. Finally, the construction of the specific tree is completed when the potential matches for τ_3 are incorporated in the tree.

The *depth* of an order-n periodicity tree is equal to the length of the shorter length sequence provided that the following conditions are satisfied:

- Each time-object belonging to the shorter length sequence has a non empty set of potential matches.

- If a time-object has a single potential match, this is not also the single potential match for another time-object on that sequence.

Time-objects with null potential matches are effectively deleted from the relevant sequence. If, due to such deletions, the length of some sequence drops below 2 then the processing is no longer viable and it should be terminated.

The depth of an order-n periodicity tree is given by

$$LS_1 - \mid C_1 \mid - \mid C_2 \mid - \ldots - \mid C_n \mid + n$$

where LS_1 is the length of the shorter length sequence, C_i, $i = 1,..,n$, are clusters of time-objects, on the shorter length sequence sharing their single potential match; out of each cluster at most one time-object can appear on any branch of the periodicity tree. Hence, if the depth of the tree is below 2, the processing must be abandoned. Thus, before the periodicity tree is constructed and evaluated, its depth is computed as a necessary validity check.

A branch of an order-n periodicity tree can be associated with a number of exclusions; this is so for every branch if the two sequences of time-objects are unequal in length. The total number of exclusions for a given branch is $LS_1 + LS_2 - 2DB$ where LS_1 and LS_2 are the respective lengths of the two sequences and DB is the depth of the particular branch.

Once a periodicity tree of a depth of at least 2 is constructed, the next step is to decide which branches of the tree represent plausible periodic occurrences across the given subjects. As for the algorithm for order-1 periodicity, this is determined on the basis of correspondence relations (functions) defining acceptable regularity patterns in order of preference. A high preference correspondence relation is "causality-link" [Keravnou, 1996a]. A branch labeled under some relation R_k is prunable if it does not contain at least 2, not necessarily consecutive, T labels. The nodes whose corresponding arcs are labeled with F's are pruned and the given branches are coalesced to include only nodes with T-labeled arcs. Similarly, a branch labeled under some correspondence function f_k is prunable if it does not contain at least two, not necessarily consecutive, same labels. The pruned nodes represent additional exclusions for the relevant branches. Distinct, plausible periodic occurrences (across two sequences) are saved in association with their underlying regularity patterns. The processing can stop as soon as a given correspondence relation (function) yields a plausible periodic occurrence corresponding to the entire branch or to a sufficient portion of it for some maximal depth branch of the periodicity tree.

A periodic occurrence across subjects is a sequence of pairs of (possibly compound) time-objects, each pair satisfying the same correspondence relation. Hence, the repetition element is a compound entity consisting of a pair of simpler entities. It is therefore denoted through the given pair of subjects, a margin for the temporal extent of the abstracted compound occurrence, as well as margins for the temporal extents of the two components individually, and the induced correspondence relation between the two components. The repetition pattern is the algorithm that determines the succession of instantiations of the repetition element. This algorithm may well be implicit in the induced correspondence relation. Also, if at least one of the original sequences is itself a periodic occurrence, then the repetition pattern could be dictated by the already established repetition pattern of the given, single subject, periodic occurrence. It can also be the amalgamation of the two individual repetition patterns (if both of the original sequences constitute periodic occurrences). Consider the following cases regarding the types of the two subjects S_1 and S_2 involved:

(a) One of the subjects, say S_1, is an action, e.g., a therapeutic action like taking some medication, or an ordinary action, like consuming a meal, and the other subject, S_2, is an abnormality subject. Suppose that the regularity across the two subjects is induced to be a causality-link from the S_1 time-object to the S_2 time-object. Here we have a case of a *dominant* correspondence where S_1 is the dominant 'partner' and S_2 is the subordinate partner. In this example, the S_2 time-objects represent side-effects of the S_1 time-objects. The overall repetition pattern is dictated by the dominant subject, i.e., by S_1 component of the repetition element (dominant component in the association). If this pattern is not already known, then the relevant sequence of S_1 time-objects can be fed to the order-1 periodicity algorithm to induce the repetition pattern. An alternative scenario to the above could be that the abnormality subject, S_2, is the dominant partner, i.e., the correspondence relation would be that the abnormality strongly suggests the undertaking of the therapeutic action. Under this scenario the overall repetition pattern is determined by the repetition pattern of the S_2 sequence.

(b) Both S_1 and S_2 are abnormality subjects. The same reasoning as for the above case applies if the induced correspondence relation ascribes the role of dominator to one of the subjects.

(c) Both S_1 and S_2 are actions. A strongly dominant correspondence such as causality cannot be directly established between pairs of actions; an action does not cause another action, rather an action causes something which suggests/enables the undertaking of the other action. The intermediate missing link, if any, can be subsequently discovered by attempting to increase the order of the given periodic occurrence by 1 through the incorporation of a new sequence of time-objects from a third distinct subject, S_3. However, a sort of dominance can be established between pairs of actions, e.g., if one action is a (necessary) precondition for the other action, the latter action requires the former action and hence dictates its undertaking. Thus the dominant partner is taken to be the latter action.

If no dominance relation between the two subjects can be established, the sequence of compound occurrences (matched pairs) is fed to the order-1 periodicity algorithm to derive the repetition pattern. The algorithm for order-n periodicity, $n > 1$, is sketched next.

Algorithm for order-n periodicity

Input:

(a) The order n of periodicity which is sought.
(b) Bottom two layers of relevant periodicity map, i.e., all sequences of order-0 time-objects and all periodic occurrences of order-1.
(c) Acceptable regularity patterns in order of preference. It is assumed that these are independent of the order of periodicity, i.e., the same regularity patterns are used for $n = 2, 3, ...$; if this assumption is incorrect then different sets of patterns are specified.

Output: Collection of credible order-n periodic occurrences.

Case for $n = 2$:

Invoke algorithm for periodicity across two sequences for each pair of sequences under the following combinations:

- Both sequences are order-1 periodic occurrences.
- One sequence is an order-1 periodic occurrence and the other is a sequence of order-0 time-objects.
- Both sequences consist of unrelated order-0 time-objects.

Case for $n > 2$:

1. Apply algorithm recursively to obtain periodic occurrences of order $(n-1)$.
2. For each derived periodic occurrence of order $(n-1)$, invoke algorithm for periodicity across two sequences, with every sequence of order-1 or order-0 periodicity.

4.4.3 Justification of exclusions

First we discuss the justification of exclusions with respect to order-1 periodic occurrences. In this context, a time-object is excluded in order to achieve the required regularity. In trying to justify the exclusion we aim to see whether the given time-object is definitely not a part of the particular periodic occurrence, but rather its materialization is due to some other factors independent of the periodic occurrence. If such a justification cannot be established then the excluded time-object may well be part of the given periodicity, the presence of which, however, marks some irregularity in the unfolding of the particular periodic occurrence. Suppose that the subject of the periodic occurrence is a therapeutic action, and hence the extra time-object denotes an additional application of the given action. For example, the periodic occurrence denotes the administration of some anti-fever medicine every six hours; if the 'extra' time-object is to be included in it, then we have that twice the given action was applied at three hour intervals. Should this irregularity be permitted, or can the exclusion of the particular time-object be justified? An action, especially a therapeutic action, is associated with some abnormality. So the extra instantiation of the action could be justified by establishing an accentuation of the associated abnormality at the particular time; the issue is therefore resolved by referring to other patient information which in this example impinges directly on the given periodic occurrence. If an accentuation of the abnormality is established, then the action instantiation is part of the periodic occurrence and the irregularity is noted and accepted. If, however, no accentuation of the abnormality is established, and provided the action is a multi-purpose one, then its extraneous instantiation may be attributed to a purpose other than the one assigned to the periodic occurrence; periodic instantiations of an action should have a common purpose. Thus if the extraneous action is attributed to an independent purpose then it does not belong to the periodic occurrence and its exclusion has been properly justified.

Now suppose that the subject of the order-1 periodic occurrence is an abnormality. If it is possible to establish that the extraneous appearances of the given abnormality are attributed to a cause independent to the one shared by the regular appearances of the abnormality, then again the exclusions are justified. Alternatively, it may be (subsequently discovered) that the extraneous appearances also happen in a regular fashion, thus having another, overlapping, order-1 periodic occurrence with the same subject. If the latter periodic occurrence had already been discovered, then its member time-objects would not have been considered extraneous with respect to another order-1 periodic occurrence with the same subject; an extraneous time-object is one that does not participate in any periodic occurrence and exists within the temporal span of some periodic occurrence. Thus if the extraneous time-objects are shown to compose a new order-1 periodic occurrence, then an attempt to merge the two, overlapping, order-1 periodic occurrences into a single periodic occurrence with a more complex repetition pattern is made. The same can happen for order-1 periodic occurrences that have actions as subjects.

Next we discuss the justification of exclusions in the context of periodicity across two sequences (i.e., subjects). The excluded time-object belongs to the one of the two sequences, and it was excluded because it could not be paired with some time-object on the other sequence. If the regularity of the periodic occurrence is not affected by the given omission, or, more strongly, if the regularity were to be disturbed by including the particular time-object, then most likely the time-object denotes a happening that does not belong to the scope of the periodic occurrence. Still it would be better to offer a more solid justification to its exclusion by explaining its presence along the lines discussed above for therapeutic actions and abnormalities.

A different picture, however, emerges if the exclusion of the given time-object affects adversely the regularity of the periodic occurrence, i.e., its inclusion results in establishing an acceptable, or of a higher preference, regularity (especially if the time-object belongs to the dominant subject, if any). In such a case it would appear that the exclusion of the time-object is erroneous and the reasoning reverts from trying to justify its exclusion to trying to justify the absence of a partner for it. Since incompleteness in medical data (patient records) is not an uncommon phenomenon, the simplest reason for the given absence is "unknown information". Thus, before looking for another explanation, the simplest explanation should be explored through a suitable enquiry. First suppose that the missing partner is an action. If it is established that the sought instantiation of the action definitely had not taken place, then the alternative would be to look for an instantiation of some other action that could have served the same purpose. Next suppose that the missing partner is an abnormality. Again, if it is established that the patient definitely had not exhibited the particular instantiation of the abnormality then it may be that the abnormality had been 'masked' in some way, or in the case where the unmatched partner is the dominant one, then it may be that for some reason it had not succeeded in yielding its subordinate partner.

4.5 CONCLUSIONS

Temporal data abstraction is an important process in medical problem solving which may also play a significant role in the discovery of new medical knowledge. This chapter has focused on one aspect of temporal data abstraction, namely the heuristic derivation of periodic occurrences of various orders of complexity, in the context of a specific temporal ontology. Periodicity, trends, as well as other patterns can be derived by statistical methods. Heuristic methods constitute effective alternatives.

What we have presented here are some preliminary results of an aspect of a larger, ongoing research effort that aims to define and implement an efficient, effective and reusable temporal kernel for medical knowledge-based problem solving in general.

References

Haimowitz, I.J., Phuc Le, P., and Kohane, I.S. (1995). Clinical monitoring using regression-based trend templates. *Artificial Intelligence in Medicine*, 7:473–496.

Keravnou, E.T. (1996a). An ontology of time using time-axes and time-objects as primitives. *Technical Report TR-96-9*, Dept. of Computer Science, University of Cyprus.

Keravnou, E.T. (1996b). Engineering time in medical knowledge-based systems through time-axes and time-objects. In *Proc. Third Int. Workshop on Temporal Representation and Reasoning (TIME-96)*, pages 160–167. IEEE Computer Society Press.

Ladkin, P. (1986). Primitives and units for time specification. In *Proc. AAAI-86*, pages 354–359.

Larizza, C., Bernuzzi, G., and Stefanelli, M. (1995). A General framework for building patient monitoring systems. In *Proc. Artificial Intelligence in Medicine Europe '95*, pages 91–102. Springer Verlag (LNAI, Vol. 935).

Miksch, S., Horn, W., Popow, C., and Paky, F. (1996). Utilizing temporal data abstraction for data validation and therapy planning for artificially ventilated newborn infants. *Artificial Intelligence in Medicine*, 8:543–576.

Russ, T.A. (1995). Use of data abstraction methods to simplify monitoring. *Artificial Intelligence in Medicine*, 7:497–514.

Shahar, Y., and Musen, M.A. (1996). Knowledge-based temporal abstraction in clinical domains. *Artificial Intelligence in Medicine*, 8:267–298.

Shoham, Y. (1987). Temporal logics in AI: semantical and ontological considerations. *Artificial Intelligence*, 33:89–104.

Wade, T.D., Byrns, P.J., Steiner, J.F., and Bondy, J. (1994). Finding temporal patterns - A set-based approach. *Artificial Intelligence in Medicine*, 6(3):263–271.

5 COOPERATIVE INTELLIGENT DATA ANALYSIS: AN APPLICATION TO DIABETIC PATIENTS MANAGEMENT

Riccardo Bellazzi,
Cristiana Larizza,
and Alberto Riva

Abstract: This chapter outlines the methodologies that can be used to perform distributed intelligent data analysis in a telemedicine system for diabetic patients management. We present a decision-support system architecture based on two modules, a Patient Unit and a Medical Unit, connected by telecommunication services. We outline how the two modules can cooperatively interpret patient data by resorting to temporal abstraction techniques combined with time series analysis.

5.1 INTRODUCTION

The widespread use of telecommunication networks pushes towards the definition of new AI methodologies and architectures, able to cope with the distributed nature of several application contexts. In particular, Intelligent Data Analysis (IDA) may be efficiently and effectively performed through the co-operation of a set of distributed software programs able to solve specialized tasks [Zhong and Ohsuga, 1995]. Distributed IDA (D-IDA) can be defined as the analysis of data realized by a decentralized and loosely coupled collection of Knowledge Sources, located in a number of distinct processor nodes [Smith and Davis, 1981].

D-IDA may have a crucial role in medicine, where several agents (physicians, nurses, patients) interact to achieve effective patient care. For example, in a networked distributed environment the therapeutic management task can be subdivided among a number of modules, in which D-IDA software tools and decision-support tools are integrated to assist the physical agents involved in the decision-making process. D-IDA seems particularly important in medical monitoring of chronic patients: in this context, out-patients follow a therapeutic protocol that is assessed by physicians on the basis of periodical visits, and are usually allowed to slightly modify the treatment in dependence of their health status and of occasional life-style modifications.

A Distributed Decision Support System for chronic patients can be realized through a simple hierarchical architecture that relies on the interaction between two decision-support units: a medical unit (MU) and a patient unit (PU). The MU is designed to assist the physician in defining the *treatment protocol* by periodically evaluating the patient's data. The treatment protocol is then communicated to the PU in order to bind the space of its admissible actions. The PU assists the patients in their self-monitoring activity, by giving proper therapeutic advice. Moreover, the PU deals with automatic data collection and transmission from the patient's house to the clinic, by communicating the therapeutic actions and the current patient state. The MU should also guide the PU functionalities, by selecting the knowledge sources to be exploited at the patient level: for instance, the PU rules that generate the alarms and suggestions can depend on the patient's life-style. Of course, the two modules may have different computational capabilities. While the PU must perform limited but efficient computations, the MU could resort to more complex techniques in order to properly assist physicians. It is also important to notice that, in a real clinical setting, the two units should usually work asynchronously; in fact, although periodical communications are required, it is not a-priori known when the two modules will be connected.

In this chapter we will concentrate on D-IDA software tools and cooperation modes needed to accomplish the different tasks of the two modules. In the following we will hence address the problem of performing home monitoring of pharmacodynamical parameters in diabetic patients, by using a distributed architecture in which a collection of different data analysis methods are exploited to assess and revise a therapeutic protocol.

5.2 MONITORING DIABETIC PATIENTS

An application domain in which D-IDA techniques may play a crucial role is home monitoring of Insulin-Dependent Diabetes Mellitus (IDDM) patients. IDDM is a major chronic disease in developed countries, caused by the destruction of the pancreatic cells producing insulin, the main hormone that regulates glucose metabolism. IDDM causes short-term complications, such as hyperglycemia, polyuria, glycosuria and ketonuria, as well as long-term complications, such as retinopathy, nephropathy, neuropathy and cardiovascular diseases. IDDM patients control their glucose metabolism through the delivery of exogenous insulin several times a day. The patients perform self-monitoring of Blood Glucose Levels (BGL) at home, usually before meals, and report the monitoring results in a diary. The accuracy of the patients' self-care is very important, since the onset and development of diabetic complications is strictly related to the degree of metabolic control that can thus be achieved. Recent studies [DCCT, 1993] show that a good metabolic control can significantly delay or prevent the development of long-term complications. Unfortunately, tight metabolic control involves 3 to 4 insulin injections per day or continuous sub-cutaneous injections, accurate home BGL monitoring, and an increase in the probability of hypoglycemic events.

Current information technologies may be exploited to improve the quality of patients monitoring by a) optimizing the rate of information exchange between patients and physicians, b) providing patients and physicians with support tools for taking proper decisions. The above mentioned motivations and previous experiences [Gomez et al., 1992] led to the definition of the Telematic Management of Insulin-Dependent Diabetes Mellitus (T-IDDM) project [Bellazzi et al., 1995a]. In the T-IDDM architecture, the IDDM patient management is realized through the cooperation of the two basic components described in the introduction: a *Patient Unit* (PU) and a *Medical Unit* (MU), interconnected by a telecommunication system. In the following section we will provide a more accurate description of the module interaction and functionalities. Further details on the architecture can be found in [Bellazzi et al., 1995b, Riva and Bellazzi, 1995].

5.3 A DISTRIBUTED ARCHITECTURE

In order to precisely define the architecture of our system, it is essential to understand the structure of the decisions involved in IDDM management: *who* usually takes decisions, *what decisions* are to be taken, and *what control rules* are employed.

The two "natural" decision-makers in the IDDM management problem are the *physician* and the *patient*. These two control agents are hierarchically interrelated. The physician determines the insulin therapy, the diet and also the *decision rules* for insulin adjustment that the patient must follow during self-monitoring. Thus, the physician establishes a *policy* for the patient's self-management, that is summarized in a *protocol*. The tasks of the physician are very complex, and the knowledge that is used to accomplish them must be as deep as possible. On the contrary, the task of the patient usually reduces to consulting a set of predefined decision tables and the required medical knowledge could be limited to an understanding of the basic action-reaction processes related to diabetes control.

The system we propose reflects the decision architecture outlined in the above analysis, and is therefore based on the cooperation between the two distinct agents previously introduced: the (PU) and a the (MU). The two modules are arranged in a hierarchical networked architecture that is distributed between the patient's house and the clinic, and is primarily aimed at increasing the frequency and quality of the information interchange between the patient and the physician. In other words, the patient will view the PU and the MU as means to obtain quicker and more accurate assistance by the physician, and the physician will consider the system as the key for controlling the metabolic behavior of a large number of patients. While the MU assists the physician in the definition of the basal insulin regimen and diet through a periodic evaluation of the patient's data, the PU allows for automatic data collection and transmission from the patient's house to the clinic, and assists the patients in their self-monitoring activity, suggesting the insulin dosage adjustments.

5.3.1 Distributed intelligent data analysis

The self-monitoring data of IDDM patients often contain only a portion of the information really needed to perform a proper control. For example, patients' diaries usually report only BGL, glycosuria and insulin values, while meals and physical exercise are not precisely described. Moreover, the monitoring data consist of highly unstable time series that are not easily interpreted through causal models. In our approach we propose to discover the real meaning of the data through D-IDA techniques.

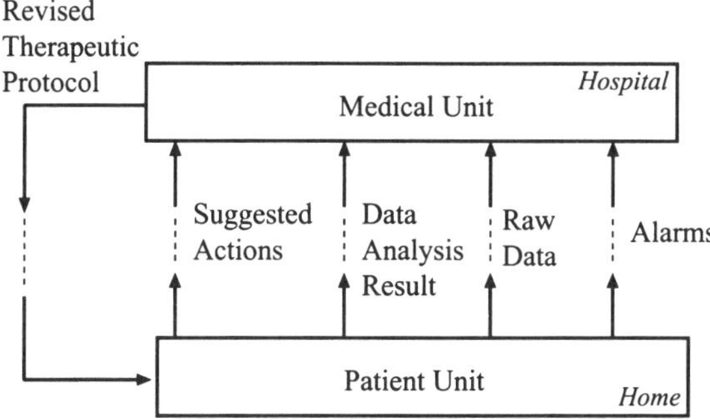

Figure 5.1 The Distributed Intelligent Data Analysis Architecture.

The basic philosophy of the D-IDA architecture is shown in Figure 5.1. Patient's data are collected by the PU, that should be able to *react* in real-time to critical situations that require an immediate therapeutic adjustment. The PU must also perform a preliminary data analysis, in order to detect in advance deviations from the expected metabolic control target. In this way, alarms and advice could be communicated to the patients, and an immediate connection to the MU could be required. The PU is constrained in its decision support activity by two important factors: a) the PU data processing is usually performed on devices with *limited memory and computational capabilities*, so, it is often not possible to implement routines able to analyze the overall patient behavior; b) some decisions, like protocol revisions, must be taken under the physician's responsibility. This means that the PU is allowed to suggest only slight insulin dose modifications and life-style checking (increasing or decreasing meals and physical exercise), while waiting for the MU decisions on the insulin type, on the injections timing and on the targets of the therapy. During each connection, the PU transmits to the MU the raw data, the results of the preliminary data processing and the suggestions given to the patient.

Starting from the PU outputs, the MU analyzes the data in a more complete and sophisticate way, in order to revise the current therapeutic protocol and to communicate it back to the PU. The pre-processing performed at the PU level is exploited by the MU in order to properly focus its data analysis only on the potential current problems. It is important to notice that the two modules exchange data as well as inference results: such cooperating activity represents a D-IDA in which the two modules interact in a bidirectional way to identify and solve metabolic instability problems.

5.4 THE MEDICAL UNIT

In current medical practice, the patient diary is revised and a new therapeutic protocol is assessed only when a patient undergoes the periodic control visit. On the contrary, by using the architecture described above, the MU is able to dynamically suggest to the physicians a protocol updating, by combining the home monitoring data coming from the PU with the historical information stored in the patients' data base. The MU knowledge-based system relies on an ontology of IDDM and on a number of inference mechanisms [Riva and Bellazzi, 1995, Riva and Bellazzi, 1996] to perform a three-steps procedure: an *intelligent data analysis* task extracts high-level metabolic and statistical parameters from the individual measurements; a *reasoning* task applies a set of statistical analyses in order to evaluate the state of the patient and a *decision making* task exploits the results of the first two tasks to choose or to adjust a protocol using heuristic or model-based techniques.

5.4.1 Intelligent data analysis

In order to allow a proper interpretation of the data, the MU subdivides the 24-hour daily period into a set of consecutive non-overlapping time slices. These time slices are generated on the basis of the information about the patient's life-style, in particular the meal times. The possible adjustments are then selected using the concept of *competent time slice*: an action in a certain time slice will be competent for the BGL measurements in the time slices that it directly affects. For example, an intake of regular insulin will be competent for the time slices that cover the subsequent six hours. Therefore, when a problem is detected in a particular time slice *t*, the possible adjustments will be the ones affecting the actions in the time slices that are competent over *t*. This information is used by the MU to suggest a new therapeutic protocol, that is passed to the PU. The protocol is composed of suggested actions (insulin intakes, diet, exercise) with their competent time slices, and of the PU control tables, that specify the strategies for coping with dangerous situations in the different time slices [Riva and Bellazzi, 1995]. The degree of competence of an insulin injection for a certain time slice is calculated on the basis of a pharmacodynamic model of the insulin action [Hovorka et al., 1990].

Whenever a dangerous condition, such as an episode of non-stationarity, is detected, the PU may suggest a protocol revision: the modified protocol must nevertheless be checked and confirmed by the MU. As mentioned in the previous section, when a new connection is established, the PU sends the data analysis results to the MU, together with the monitoring data and the suggested actions. The MU will check the adequacy of the actions by applying a number of available *data abstraction* methods.

In particular, temporal abstractions (TAs) have been recognized to be of fundamental importance in order to help data interpretation [Shahar and Musen, 1996, Keravnou, 1995]. TAs refer to an intelligent data analysis task: they are used to transform the fragmentary representation of the patient's history into a more compact one. The advantage of this kind of abstractions stands in the capability of representing a large set of raw data with only a few meaningful abstract entities which can provide a complete synthesis of the patient clinical condition. TAs performed by our system are based on a specific temporal model, based on *time-point* and *interval* primitives. In this model we assume that all the biological processes under monitoring generate time-stamped data representing single events, and that the relevant patterns of the observations (trends, levels, etc.), detected by TA mechanisms, may be represented as intervals. Defining proper mechanisms of temporal abstraction involves several well known problems. First, temporal abstractions should be sufficiently flexible in recognizing the most wide variety of patterns in a time series. They should, in fact, represent all the clinical situations potentially relevant to the domain. Second, the monitoring activity can, in general, focus on different kinds of clinical parameters, so the abstraction could be performed on both numerical and qualitative data drawn on irregular time grids. The temporal abstractions carried out by the system were chosen in order to satisfy the requirements of flexibility and generality mentioned above.

Following an explicit description of the *data abstractions ontology* [Larizza et al., 1995], two temporal abstraction types have been defined: BASIC and COMPLEX. BASIC TAs include STATE, TREND abstractions, which are used to perform analysis of longitudinal data, derived from the observation of symbolic or numerical parameters. Example of TREND TAs are "BGL increase" or "BGL stationarity". COMPLEX abstractions detect more complex patterns in the data through the search of temporal relationships between intervals, like "increase of BGL" AFTER "decrease of the insulin level".

Complex abstractions are particularly useful in our application domain, to detect critical situations. For example, IDDM patients may present hyperglycemia at breakfast, due to two different and opposite phenomena: the BGL may be high due to an insufficient insulin dose (Dawn Effect), or may be high because of a reaction after a nightly asymptomatic hypoglycemia, caused by an excessive insulin dosage (Somogy effect). The two effects are discriminated on the basis of the glycosuria values, that express the mean BGL values over the last eight hours. A high glycosuria value (*present*) combined with hyperglycemia can be related to a Dawn effect, while low glycosuria (*absent*) combined with hyperglycemia can be related to a Somogy effect. According to the domain medical knowledge, we defined a set of relevant critical situations that may be

Table 5.1 The set of TAs defined for the Before Breakfast time-slice.

BASIC TAS		
TA type	Finding	Temporal Abstractions
STATE	BGL	Hypoglycemia, Hyperglycemia, Normal BGL
	NPH Insulin	High NPH Insulin, Low NPH Insulin, Medium NPH Insulin
	Glycosuria	Glycosuria Absent/Traces, Glycosuria Present
	Physical Exercise	Extra Physical Exercise, No Extra Physical Exercise
TREND	BGL	BGL Increase, BGL Decrease, BGL Stationarity
	NPH Insulin	NPH Insulin Increase, NPH Insulin Decrease, NPH Insulin Stationarity

COMPLEX TAS	
Definition	TA
Hyperglycemia OVERLAPS Glycosuria Absent	Suspected Somogy Effect
Hyperglycemia OVERLAPS Glycosuria Present	Suspected Dawn Effect
Hypoglycemia OVERLAPS High Evening NPH Insulin	Induced Hypoglycemia
BGL Increase MEETS BGL Decrease	Metabolic Instability

efficiently recognized through TAs. A subset of the TAs defined for the before breakfast time-slice is shown in Table 5.1.

During patient monitoring, the MU searches for the episodes that are related to the simple analysis performed at the PU level. In this way, the PU results are used to select the TAs that are relevant to the current problem.

For example, if the PU marks out a persistent hyperglycemia at breakfast, the MU will search for the *Suspected Somogy* or *Suspected Dawn effect* episodes, without considering problems in other time slices. On the contrary, if the PU detects a hypoglycemia, the MU will search for an episode of *Induced Hypoglycemia*, without considering hyperglycemia-related episodes.

The derived TAs are exploited by the reasoning module of the MU to confirm or reject the protocol adjustments suggested by the PU. After being approved and possibly modified by physicians, the inference result is transmitted back to the PU in the form of a revised protocol.

5.4.2 Reasoning and decision making

The reasoning module exploits the TAs to extract from the data a set of high-level descriptors that characterize the current patient situation.

The simplest descriptor is derived by counting the most relevant episodes detected during the monitoring period and by measuring their total and mean temporal extent. A more informative descriptor is the patient's MODAL DAY that summarizes the patient situation during the monitoring period from different viewpoints. In this context interesting modal days are, for example, the BGL modal day (BG-MD), which represents the "mean" patient response to the therapy, and the control actions modal day (CA-MD), which summarizes the typical insulin regimen followed by the patient. Several approaches for deriving the BG-MD have been presented in the literature, from time series analysis to belief maintenance systems [Deutsch et al., 1995, Riva and Bellazzi, 1995]. We propose an approach to derive the patient MODAL DAY based on TAs. In our approach the BG-MD is extracted by calculating the probability distribution of the STATE abstractions defined for the BGL finding [Riva and Bellazzi, 1995]. This operation is simply performed by counting the number of occurrences of the STATE episodes, weighted by their time span. By using the same procedure we can extract also the CA-MD; in this case the analysis is performed on the NPH and regular insulin STATE abstractions (see Table 5.1). Furthermore, modal days can be derived on every episode that can be detected using a single measurement. We can therefore define the Somogy effect modal day, the Dawn effect modal day, and so on. In such a way it is possible to characterize the patient's behavior with a collection of modal days, that describe it from different perspectives. Typical patient behaviors can be found also by counting the occurrence of COMPLEX episodes, having a minimum time span greater than one day. For example, the counts of metabolic instability episodes, defined on a minimum time span of three days, can be summarized by calculating the percentage of time spent in the episode with respect to the total monitoring time. Other interesting results can be obtained through the time span distribution of the episodes; for example it could be of interest to know the number of increasing BGL episodes lasting for more than three days. It is clear that a great number of patient behaviors can be defined through TAs, and that the relevant ones have to be selected according to the physician's preferences and the data availability.

The decision process starts with an evaluation of the high-level descriptors calculated from the available data by the reasoning module. In particular, the modal day profiles are interpreted according to heuristic rules that reduce the set of the admissible protocol adjustments according to various kinds of "context" constraints (e.g. the total number of injections cannot be too high, some injection times are preferable over others). Such context constraints are exploited to perform a first screening on the possible protocol adjustments. Each of the remaining adjustments can be interpreted as a movement in the protocol space characterized by a direction and a distance from the current one.

In order to minimize the differences between the current protocol and the new one, we will prefer the adjustments that lead to protocols closest to the current one, according to the above defined metric.

If the amount of information is sufficiently high, the technique here described can be replaced by purely quantitative ones that rely on the ability to correctly identify a predictive model of the glucose metabolism. In this case the selection of the adequate adjustment can be performed by directly simulating the effect of each one of the protocols under consideration and choosing the one that yields the best BGL profile (optimal control). In general, different decision tools will be available, ranging from the most qualitative to the most quantitative ones, and the one to be used will be selected according to the number of missing data to be dealt with.

5.5 THE PATIENT UNIT

In dependence of the kind and amount of data, the PU may exploit different data analysis algorithms. If the data contain reliable information on the meal intakes and on the physical activity, it is possible to define suitable control strategies based on adaptive controllers [Bellazzi et al., 1995b].

Unfortunately, home monitoring data usually contain information only on BGL and glycosuria values. In this case, the PU data analysis is mainly related to the detection of *State* and *Trend* abstractions. In particular, we are now considering a number of simple and efficient techniques derived from the analysis of stock market prices time series, that exploits the *Running Average* calculation to detect stable trends in BGL time series. Given a generic unidimensional time series, the basic Running or Moving Average Estimate (RAE) for an observation is computed by calculating the average over the k preceding values; k is called the running average length. Modifications of the basic technique able to take into account linear trends in time can be found in [Frees, 1996]. Although the RA approach may seem naive, it can be proved that its predictions can be expressed as Weighted Least Squares estimates. A prediction obtained with the RAE technique is useful to detect local trend components in the BGL time series. Starting from this consideration, the econometricians derived a technique to predict increasing or decreasing trends based on two different RAEs. The first RAE (short-time RAE, ST-RAE) has a small RA length, and is hence sensitive to the latest BGL values, while the second RAE (long-time, LT-RAE) has a larger length, and is hence a smoother estimate of the local trend.

The relationships between the two curves can be classified into three significant patterns, that reflect the following typical situations (see Figure 5.2): pattern a) shows ST-RAE moving around LT-RAE; this situation reveals a stationary behavior, also when the original time series has a large variance; pattern

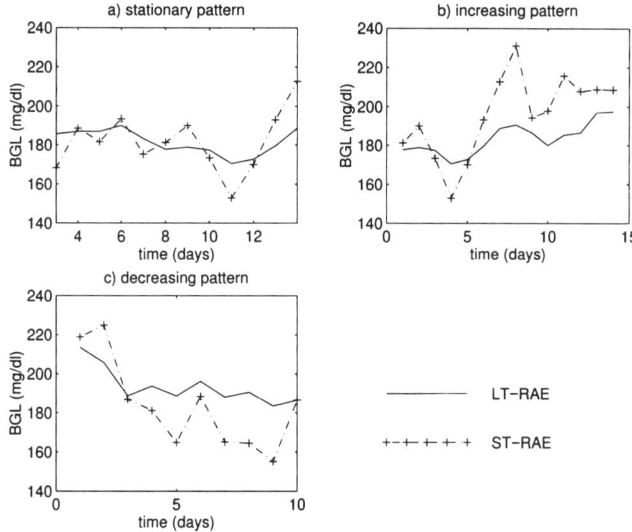

Figure 5.2 The three patterns derived from RAE analysis: a) stationary behavior; b) increasing behavior; c) decreasing behavior.

b) presents an abrupt change in the ST-RAE derivative, and a crossing point after which the ST-RAE is persistently higher than the LT-RAE; this situation clearly shows an increasing trend in the time series; pattern c) is the complement of pattern b), revealing a decreasing trend in the time series.

When applied to BGL time series, this kind of analysis can be used to detect in advance potentially dangerous trends. Pattern recognition may be effectively carried out by means of temporal abstraction mechanisms able to reveal persistent situations. In our architecture this task is performed at the PU level by using a minimum persistence time span and appropriate LT-RAE and ST-RAE lengths whose values are determined by the MU. We are evaluating the sensitivity of the analysis on the two last parameters.

The RAE analysis is particularly useful if measurements coming from different time slices are considered as separate time series. As a matter of fact, if the patient's metabolism is stable, the overall BGL values must show a cyclostationary behavior, with oscillations around a daily trajectory. By considering separate time series the daily periodical component of the measurements is filtered out, and it is hence easier to detect local trends in a particular time slice and to suggest the appropriate control actions.

The PU suggestions are related to two different therapy adjustments. The first one is based on the present BGL value and attempts to react against dangerous instantaneous situations (e.g., by modifying a single regular insulin dose or delaying a meal). The second therapy adjustment is based on the above described detection of local BGL trends and on a set of control tables. Each table is based on three inputs: the ST-RAE, the current ST- and LT-RAE patterns and the glycosuria level. The table output is a control action that deals with non-stationary behaviors by suggesting a modification to the most competent protocol action for the identified problem (for example, changing an NPH insulin dose). Such output always generates a connection request to submit the data analysis results to the MU for a more accurate investigation. A different control table is generated by the MU for each time slice, according to the constraints imposed by the patient's life-style.

The RAE technique, used for retrospective analysis of 6 patients monitored over 6 months, detected 98 instances of non-stationary patterns, 95 of which were judged to be clinically significant. The relevant episodes were detected in advance with respect to visual inspection by the physician, and the results obtained were often easier to interpret than the ones derived with more sophisticated techniques [Bellazzi et al., 1995b]. We are now evaluating the RAE technique in comparison with other low-computational-cost methods, such as piecewise linear autoregressive models.

5.6 AN EXAMPLE

The analysis of IDDM patients' data is a very complex task. Let us consider for example Figure 5.3, that shows the Blood Glucose Level (BGL) time series coming from home monitoring over 77 days of a 20 years old male IDDM patient. The patient underwent three insulin injections per day, at breakfast, lunch and dinner time, respectively. The insulin injections at breakfast and dinner were a mixture of regular and NPH (intermediate) insulin. BGL measurements were performed before meals. The mean of the BGL measurements over the 77 days period was 150.66 mg/dl, while the standard deviation was 69.3 mg/dl. Only a nominal diet plan was known, and there is no assurance that it was actually followed on each day. The patient gave only qualitative information on the physical exercise performed. The time series is highly unstable and our attempts to derive significant causal models from the data or to obtain significant estimates of mathematical or probabilistic model parameters were not successful. Figure 5.4 shows an example of the application of the RAE method to the time series of Before Breakfast BGL (BB-BGL) measurements of the data displayed in Figure 5.3.

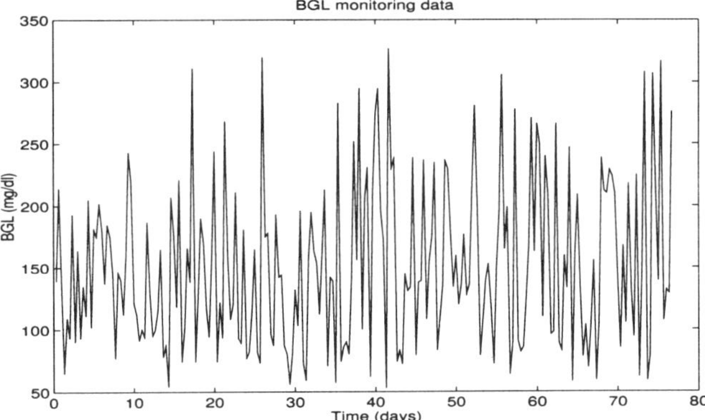

Figure 5.3 BGL monitoring data over 77 days (see text).

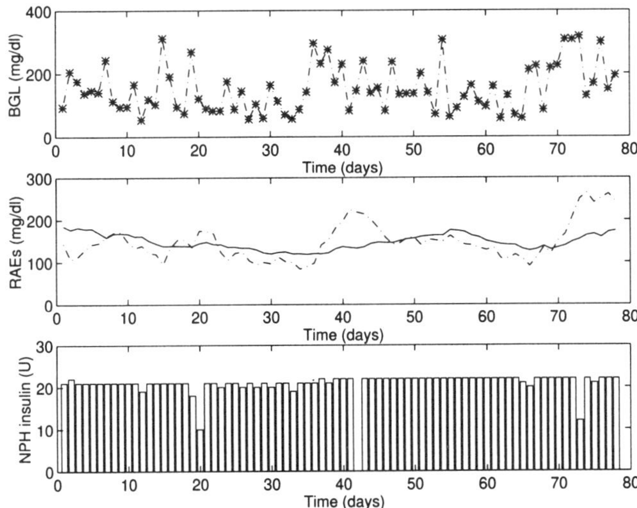

Figure 5.4 BB-BGL values over 77 days (top) the corresponding RAE (middle) and the NPH dosages (bottom). Five different trends are identifiable by considering the intersection between LT-RAE (solid line) and ST-RAE (dash-dotted line).

The ST-RAE is calculated with an RA length of 7 days, and the LT-RAE is calculated with an RA length of 21 days; the two curves allow for a straightforward interpretation of the different local patterns in the 77 days follow-up period. If patterns b) and c) are identified with a persistence of at least 4 days without

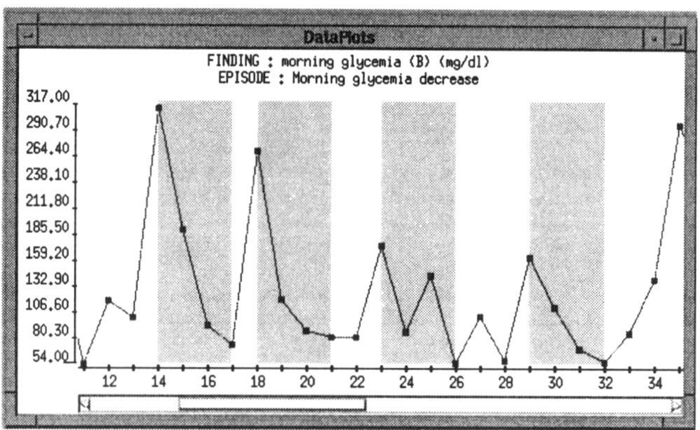

Figure 5.5 BGL decrease episodes in the breakfast time slice around day 23, corresponding to the decreasing pattern detected with the RAE technique.

intersection between the two curves, we easily detect five non-stationary patterns: three of type c), from day 1 to day 18, from day 23 to 36, and from day 51 to 70, and two of type b), from day 37 to 46 and after day 70.

These situations are not easily explainable on the basis of the insulin dosage analysis only. In particular, the two alternate patterns from day 35 to 77 correspond to situations in which the insulin dosage is approximately constant. In this example, the raw data and the detected trends should be communicated to the MU for a more accurate analysis.

The MU starts searching for the Before Breakfast episodes related with non-stationarity conditions. The first step of the MU analysis is to focus on the non-stationarity episodes found by the PU. Figure 5.5 shows the analysis of the data around day 23, corresponding to the decreasing pattern c) detected by the PU over the interval 23-36. The MU is able to find recurrent decreasing trends before day 23, that can be joined in a single BGL *Decrease* episode, lasting for a period slightly different than the one found with the RAE method. Moreover two episodes of *Induced Hypoglycemia*, the complex TA that associates an hypoglycemic episode with an high evening insulin dose, mark out the inappropriateness of the insulin regimen that the patient is following (see Figure 5.6).

The BG-MD over the period lasting from day 1 to day 36 can be derived from Table 5.2. In particular, the probability of hypoglycemia is about 11%, that is remarkably high from a clinical point of view. Moreover, this action is supported by the CA-MD, that shows a high NPH insulin dose for the 77.8% of the monitoring time. The reasoning module of the MU detects a problem at the

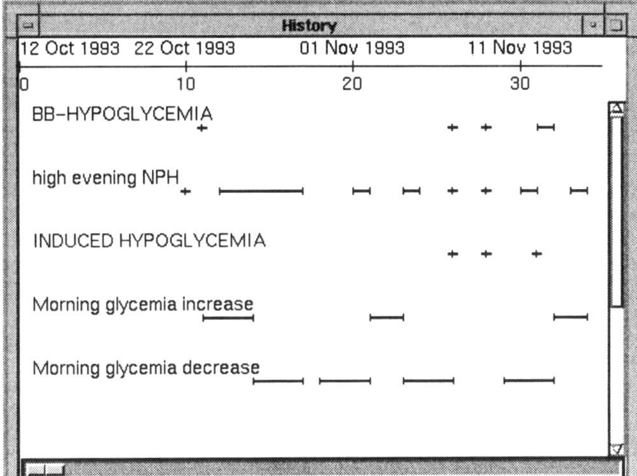

Figure 5.6 A set of relevant TAs in the breakfast time slice around day 23. It is possible to notice that during the last ten days there is an high concentration of "Induced Hypoglycemia" episodes.

Before Breakfast time-slice, and triggers the decision making module to suggest a protocol revision. The final result of the analysis is a list of protocols that may handle the problems detected, ordered on the basis of their relative distance from the current one. In this case, the most suitable choice is a protocol with three injections per day with a lower NPH insulin dose at dinner.

If the TA analysis is performed over the entire monitoring period, a very dangerous situation is detected, with a high probability of hypoglycemic episodes and presence of both Suspected Dawn and Somogy effects. Table 5.2 shows also the TAs performed on the Before Breakfast monitoring data. Seven hypoglycemic episodes were derived, with a total duration of 8 days, corresponding to 10% of the monitoring time. Five hypoglycemic episodes were associated to a *High Evening* NPH *Insulin* (*Induced Hypoglycemia* episodes). Six *Suspected Somogy effect* episodes and 5 *Suspected Dawn effect* episodes were also detected, and finally a succession of significant increasing and decreasing trends was found. The persistence of *High Evening* NPH *Insulin* episodes in the follow-up period revealed that the insulin dosages were increased with respect to the protocol, in spite of the high frequency of hypoglycemic episodes. Such increase was recognized to be the main cause of BGL instability.

Taking into account the entire monitoring period, the generated suggestion was again the selection of a therapeutic protocol with a lower NPH insulin dose

Table 5.2 A summary of the TAs episodes detected from day 1 to day 36 (upper table) and in the overall monitoring period (lower table) in the breakfast time slice. The BG-MD as well as the CA-MD can be easily derived from these tables. The high frequency of metabolic instability episodes and the relatively high number of induced hypoglycemia episodes reveal a potentially dangerous situation for the patient under study.

TAS (over days 1-36)	# Occurrences	Total Duration (days)	Percentage (%)
BASIC TAS			
Hypoglycemia	4	4	11.1
Hyperglycemia	5	5	16.7
High NPH Insulin	8	28	77.8
Low NPH Insulin	1	1	2.8
COMPLEX TAS			
Induced Hypoglycemia	2	2	5.6

TAS (over days 1-79)	# Occurrences	Total Duration (days)	Percentage (%)
BASIC TAS			
Hypoglycemia	7	8	10
Hyperglycemia	14	22	27.8
High NPH Insulin	11	68	86.0
Low NPH Insulin	2	2	2.5
BGL Increase	25	31	39.2
BGL Decrease	24	31	39.2
COMPLEX TAS			
Suspected Dawn Effect	5	15	18.9
Suspected Somogy Effect	6	7	8.9
Metabolic Instability	22	58	73.4
Induced Hypoglycemia	5	6	7.6

at dinner. The physician who performed the analysis with us, also prescribed a careful life-style check.

5.7 CONCLUSIONS

In this chapter we outlined the methodologies used to perform a distributed intelligent data analysis of pharmacodynamical time series coming from diabetic patients home-monitoring. The framework here presented exploits the cooperation between two hierarchically structured modules, in order to perform a useful and efficient interpretation of data even in the presence of incomplete information. The two modules should be able to assist patients and physicians in exploiting the whole clinical data-set collected over the follow-up, without losing meaningful information. Multiple are the implications of the above presented framework. First, the physician is assisted in recognizing in advance important clinical episodes, that can be associated to a patient's critical condition. This is a typical example of how a tele-monitoring system can successfully improve the quality of treatment in out-patients, through an immediate intervention that can avoid patient hospitalizations. Second, the patients can increase their autonomy and improve their ability to implement the protocol and manage the disease. From a methodological point of view, we believe that the mechanisms defined in our system to perform D-IDA represents an efficient and flexible framework that can be usefully exploited in a variety of long-term monitoring applications which require an active role of the patients.

The above described architecture represents a simple Distributed Artificial Intelligence scheme, where two application agencies [Smith et al., 1996] (the PU and MU modules) cooperate in order to control the patient blood glucose metabolism. At present, the overall system is being tested within a telecommunication system that relies on the HTTP protocol, while user interaction takes place using the HTML language.

References

Bellazzi, R., Cobelli, C., Gomez, E., and Stefanelli, M. (1995a). The T-IDDM project: Telematic management of Insulin Dependent Diabetes Mellitus. In Bracale, M. and Denoth, F., editors, *Health Telematics '95*, pages 271–276.

Bellazzi, R., Siviero, C., Stefanelli, M., and De Nicolao, G. (1995b). Adaptive controllers for intelligent monitoring. *Artificial Intell. in Med.*, 7:515–540.

The Diabetes Control and Complication Trial Research Group (1993). The effect of intensive treatment of diabetes on the development and progression of long-term complications in insulin-dependent diabetes mellitus. *The New England Journal of Medicine*, 14-329:977–986.

Deutsch, T., Lehmann, E.D., Carson, E.R., Roudsari, A.V., Hopkins, K.D., and Sönksen, P. (1995). Time series analysis and control of blood glucose levels in diabetic patients. *Comp. Meth. and Programs in Biomed.*, 41:167–182.

Frees, E.W. (1996). *Data Analysis using Regression Models.* Prentice Hall.

Gomez, E.J., Del Pozo, F., Arredondo, M.T., Sanz, M., and Hernando, E. (1992). A Telemedicine Distributed Decision-Support System for Diabetes Management. *IEEE–14th Ann. Int. Conf. of the IEEE Eng.in Med. and Biol. Soc., Paris*, CH3207-8, pages 1238–1239.

Hovorka, R., Svacina, S., Carson, E.R., Williams, C.D., and Sonksen, P.H. (1990). A consultation system for insulin therapy. *Comp. Meth. and Prog. in Biomed.*, 32:303-310.

Keravnou, E.T. (1995). Modelling medical concepts as time objects. In Barahona, P., Stefanelli, M., and Wyatt, J., editors, *Lecture Notes in Artificial Intelligence 934*, pages 67–90, Springer Verlag.

Larizza, C., Bernuzzi, G., and Stefanelli, M. (1995). A General Framework for Building Patient Monitoring Systems. In Barahona, P., Stefanelli, M., and Wyatt, J., editors, *Lecture Notes in Artificial Intelligence 934*, pages 91–102, Springer Verlag.

Riva, A. and Bellazzi, R. (1995). High level control strategies for diabetes therapy. In Barahona, P., Stefanelli, M., and Wyatt, J., editors, *Lecture Notes in Artificial Intelligence 934*, pages 185-196, Springer Verlag.

Riva, A. and Bellazzi, R. (1996). Learning Temporal Probabilistic Causal Models from Longitudinal Data. *Artificial Intell. in Med.*, 8:217–234.

Shahar, Y. and Musen, M.A. (1996). Knowledge-Based Temporal Abstraction in Clinical Domains. *Artificial Intell. in Med.*, 8:267–298.

Smith, R.G. and Davis, R. (1981). Frameworks for Cooperation in Distributed Problem Solving. *IEEE Trans. Systems Man and Cybernetics*, 11:1.

Smith, D.C., Cypher, A., and Sporher, J. (1994). Programming agents without a programming language. *Commun. of the ACM*, 37:55–67.

Zhong, N. and Ohsuga, S. (1995). Toward a Multi-Strategy and Cooperative Discovery System. *Proc. of the First International Conference on Knowledge Discovery & Data Mining*, pages 337–342, AAAI Press, Menlo Park.

6 PTAH: A SYSTEM FOR SUPPORTING NOSOCOMIAL INFECTION THERAPY

Marko Bohanec,
Miran Rems,
Smiljana Slavec,
and Božo Urh

Abstract: This chapter presents Ptah, a system for supporting medical doctors in making decisions related to the therapy of nosocomial (hospital-acquired) infections. The system is based on a chronologically organized database of infections and therapies. It facilitates four data analysis methods related to the effectiveness of antibiotics and resistance of bacteria to antibiotics. The methods construct time series of resistance vectors from the database, and present their results graphically.

6.1 INTRODUCTION

One of the most widely used medical information systems in the Republic of Slovenia is called InfoMed [Slavec, et al., 1992]. It supports activities such as patient management, billing, order entry and management, and reporting. Currently, InfoMed is operative in 12 out of 15 General Hospitals in the country.

Recently, InfoMed has evolved in the direction of decision support. A software module has been developed that enables its users—hospital staff—to design their own specific databases, and monitor and analyze collected data. In this way, a database of nosocomial infections and therapies was designed in the General Hospital Jesenice [Kramar and Rems, 1992, Rems, et al., 1995]. In 1994, they started to collect data on infections of surgical wounds, vein catheters and aspirate trachea. A preliminary analysis [Bohanec, et al., 1995] has shown that the collected data provides valuable information that can contribute to the improvement of therapeutic and decision-making activities.

Due to the importance of the problem and the availability of data, we decided to develop a decision support system called Ptah[1]. The system is designed as an on-line tool for a medical doctor. It performs four types of analyses of microbiological findings regarding bacterial resistance to antibiotics and effectiveness of antibiotics. Special attention is given to the following:

- *Visualization*: The results of all the analyses are presented graphically.
- *Comprehensibility*: The methods were carefully selected so that they involve only data and concepts that are familiar to and commonly used by physicians.
- *Simplicity and uniformity*: To facilitate easy learning and use of the system, the methods are controlled by a small and uniform set of parameters.

Ptah is implemented on personal computers running Microsoft Windows. Currently, it is being evaluated in the General Hospital Jesenice.

In the next section, nosocomial infections and issues related to their therapy are briefly introduced. This is followed by a presentation of Ptah. Section 6.3 describes the data that is used in various analyses supported by the system. Sections 6.4 and 6.5 demonstrate methods for the analysis of bacterial resistance and effectiveness of antibiotics, respectively. The chapter is concluded by an evaluation of the system, guidelines for further work, and summary.

6.2 NOSOCOMIAL INFECTION

Nosocomial, or *hospital-acquired*, infection is a disease that develops during the admission to the hospital and is a consequence of treatment, procedures of treatment or work of hospital staff [Gardner and Arnow, 1987]. About 5 to 10%

of patients admitted to the hospital develop a nosocomial infection, and 3% of them die of consequences [Santamaria, 1990].

Infections that occur at critically ill patients in intensive care units are particularly acute. The immune system of these patients is usually strongly deficient, therefore the therapy must be appropriate and timely. Studies of nosocomial infections mainly stress the need of permanent control of procedures and therapy at intubated patients and patients with central vein catheters [Cercenado, et al., 1990, Kamal, et al., 1991, Snowdon, 1994, Reed, et al., 1995].

A clinical manifestation of disease depends on at least three factors:

- patient's resistance,
- bacterial aggressiveness and resistance to antibiotics, and
- environment in which the patient is treated.

All the three factors behave biologically and vary extremely fast. For this reason, the therapy itself should be fast and predefined [Hemmer, 1993]. A proper treatment requires:

- permanent microbiological supervision,
- monitoring bacterial resistance, and
- permanent control of diagnostic and therapeutic procedures.

Particularly dangerous initiators of nosocomial infections are aggressive bacteria that are developed and transmitted within the hospital. Since they are permanently exposed to antibiotics, they adapt, develop a high level of resistance and become very difficult to cure. Such bacteria have to be detected as soon as possible, and their further development must be prevented by appropriate procedures.

Apart from saving lives, a proper procedure can also considerably affect the cost of therapy. In a recent study with over 160.000 patients [Pestotnik, et al., 1996], it was shown that the antibiotic costs could be reduced to about a half without affecting antimicrobial resistance patterns and even decreasing the mortality. Such a result was achieved only by applying a decision support system for antibiotic management, and not by constraining the physicians' access to antibiotics.

6.3 DATABASE OF NOSOCOMIAL INFECTIONS

The decision support system Ptah is based on a database of infections of surgical wounds, vein catheters and aspirate trachea, which has been collected in the General Hospital Jesenice since 1994. The data include:

- *infection*: type and date of infection, successive day of treatment, date of specimen;
- *activity* in which the infection arose: operation, intubation, catheter insertion;
- microbiological findings (*antibiogram*);
- *therapy*: prescribed antibiotics;
- *general data*, such as patient's temperature and local symptoms.

Among these, Ptah primarily focuses on antibiograms, which contain microbiological findings of specimen taken from patients. For each isolated bacterium, the antibiogram displays a *resistance vector*: each element of the vector corresponds to an antibiotic and represents the resistance of the bacterium to that antibiotic. There are four possible levels of resistance: *Resistant, Intermediary, Sensitive*, and *Unknown*. In Ptah, these levels are denoted '`R`', '`I`', '`S`', and '`.`', respectively.

All the analyses implemented in Ptah are based on *time series* of resistance vectors. These are constructed from the database using various criteria that can be defined by the user in order to focus only on data relevant for the problem at hand. First, a set of bacteria can be defined that determines the antibiograms that are taken (filtered) from the database. Similarly, the elements of resistance vectors can be freely positioned by defining an ordered set of antibiotics. The construction of time series can be additionally constrained by some other parameters, such as the age and sex of patients, type of activity, and/or organizational unit.

For the presentation that follows in the next two sections, we constructed a time series of all the resistance vectors of *Staphylococcus aureus* in the years 1994 and 1995. This series consists of 127 vectors in total. Each vector contains 13 elements that correspond to 13 most frequently prescribed antibiotics in the hospital; for instance, the first element corresponds to *ampicillin*, and the last one to *penicillin*. Thus, the vector '`S...R.R.R...R`' denotes that the corresponding bacterium is sensitive to ampicillin, but resistant to penicillin and three other antibiotics. The resistance to all the remaining antibiotics is unknown. Some other resistance vectors that occur in this time series are shown in Table 6.1.

6.4 ANALYSIS OF BACTERIAL RESISTANCE

When examining an antibiogram and selecting the most appropriate therapy, one of the key concepts used by the doctor is the *level of bacterial resistance* to

Table 6.1 Some resistance vectors of Staphylococcus aureus.

Date	Resistance vector
2-Nov-95	`..R.R...R...R`
9-Nov-95	`..S.S...SS..R`
13-Nov-95	`........S...R`
14-Nov-95	`..R.S...SS..R`
17-Nov-95	`..S.....S...R`

antibiotics. It is defined as a number (or proportion) of antibiotics to which the bacterium is resistant. The higher the number, the more dangerous and difficult the infection is to cure. The decision also depends on whether a highly resistant bacterium has been found in only one patient, or it occurred at more patients or more frequently in the near past. The latter may indicate a particularly dangerous infection that is caused by bacteria that develop within the hospital.

In Ptah, the *level* of bacterial resistance is acquired from time series by simply counting `R`'s in resistance vectors and graphically displaying them on a time axis. There is also an alternative graph of the *proportion* of `R`'s with respect to the elements of resistance vectors that are known (i.e., '`R`', '`S`' and '`I`', excluding '`.`').

A graph of the level of bacterial resistance that has been obtained from the time series defined above is shown in Figure 6.1. There are two types of bars in the graph that correspond to two types of activities: operations and intubations. The graph clearly shows occasional and partly periodic occurrence of highly resistant bacteria. Some occur only in one of the activities and they are successfully eliminated there. There are two such peaks in the graph: February and March 1995 for intubations, and the last quarter of 1995 for operations. Even more difficult cases occur when the therapy is unsuccessful and bacteria are transmitted from one activity to another. According to Figure 6.1, this happened in November 1994.

Another important set of questions related to bacterial resistance is: which types of resistance vectors occur in time series, how frequently, and whether it is possible to classify them in any way.

For this purpose, we use hierarchical clustering of resistance vectors. The difference of two vectors is defined as the number of different corresponding elements. The hierarchy is constructed by the McQuitty's method [McQuitty, 1966]. Initially, each vector is considered an elementary cluster. The method

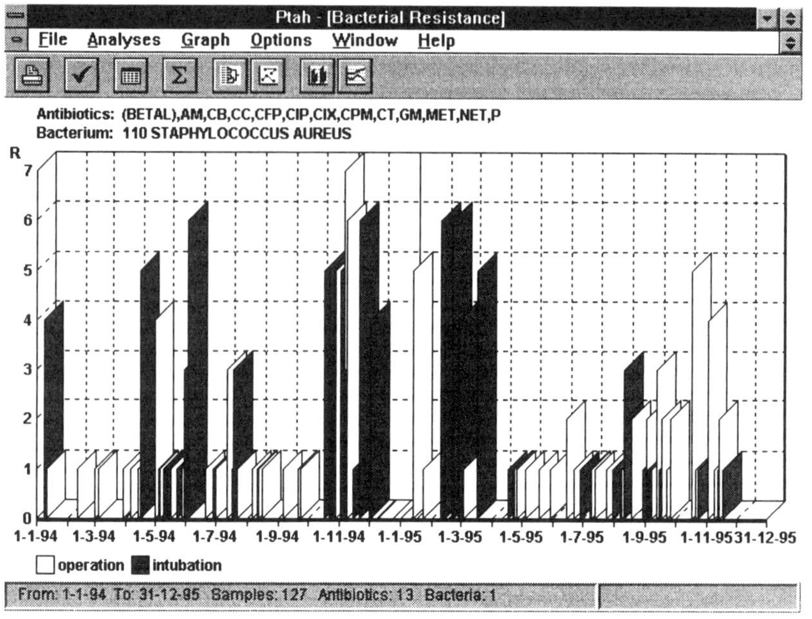

Figure 6.1 Resistance levels of Staphylococcus aureus.

then gradually joins vectors into clusters so that two vectors (or already constructed clusters) that differ the least are joined in each step. The difference between a newly created cluster $C_i \cup C_j$ and an existing cluster C_k is defined as:

$$d(C_i \cup C_j, C_k) = \frac{d(C_i, C_k) + d(C_j, C_k)}{2}$$

The result of clustering is represented by a dendrogram (Figure 6.2) that shows the hierarchy of vectors and the frequency of each vector in the time series. The thickness of lines in the graph approximately corresponds to this frequency. Note that only the 'R' elements occur in the resistance vectors. This is according to one of the options of Ptah that allows the user to define which vector elements (levels of resistance) are taken into account in clustering. Usually, dendrograms based on vectors containing only R's are considerably simpler, but as useful as the complete ones.

In Figure 6.2, the vectors are classified into two main groups. The first one occurs in the upper part of the figure and consists of bacteria whose resistance is relatively low. Among these, the most frequent case is that the bacteria are resistant only to penicillin. The second group is smaller in number, but

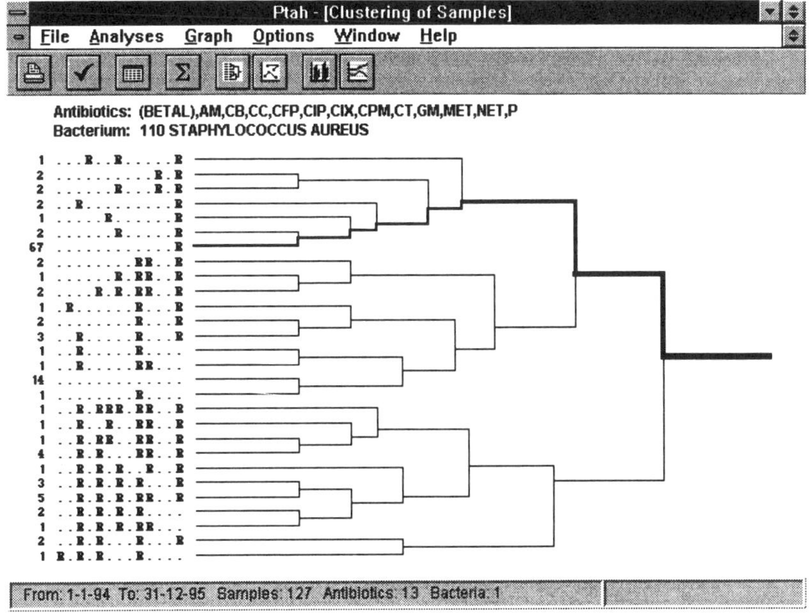

Figure 6.2 A dendrogram of resistance vectors.

contains various combinations of highly resistant bacteria. These are the ones that definitely need special attention in prescribing the therapy.

The third type of analysis is related to bacteria that are developed and transmitted within the hospital, which may in time reach a high level of resistance. The identification of such bacteria is based on the fact that these bacteria occur simultaneously at several patients and have similar characteristics. Therefore, their antibiograms and corresponding resistance vectors are similar.

We define that two vectors are similar when they differ in at most one element. Then, the approach is to present the vectors as points in a graph (Figure 6.3) and connect those that are similar and whose time difference is less than a chosen threshold (250 days in Figure 6.3). The vectors are arranged so that the most resistant ones are presented at the top.

Most of the vectors in Figure 6.3 are resistant to at most two antibiotics. However, there are bursts of related highly resistant bacteria, most notably in October and November 1994, and the first quarter of 1995. In October 1995, two bacteria with similar characteristics reappeared. At approximately the same time, there was a group of somewhat less resistant bacteria that also occurred in relation with operations. This clearly indicates that a new dangerous

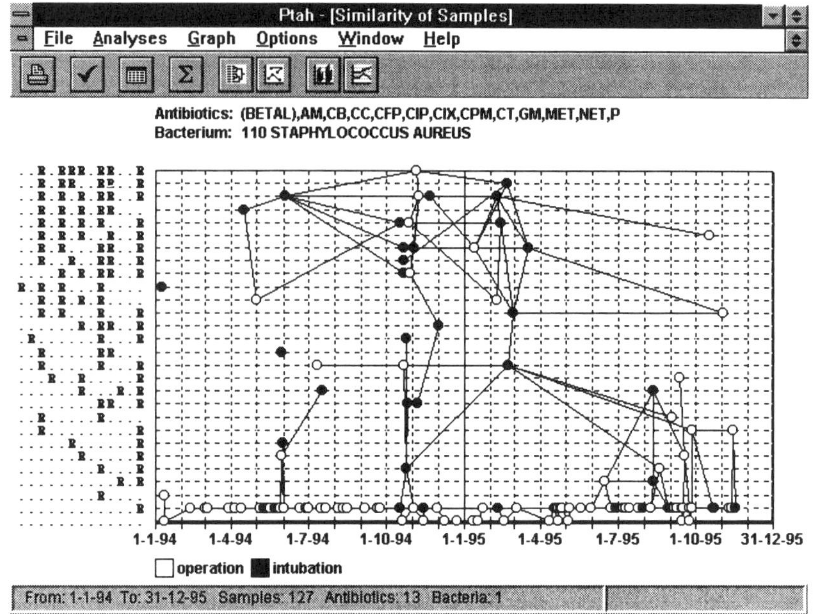

Figure 6.3 Similarity of resistance vectors.

organism was developing within the hospital at that time. On this basis, the hospital staff could have been warned and special measures undertaken for its prevention.

6.5 ANALYSIS OF ANTIBIOTICS' EFFECTIVENESS

The next important issue in the therapy of nosocomial infections concerns the expected results of therapy, which is in close connection with the *effectiveness* of antibiotics. This varies because bacteria adapt fast and become resistant to antibiotics, particularly to those that are regularly prescribed. When the effectiveness of an antibiotic becomes too low, its further use has to be discontinued for medical and financial reasons.

The *ineffectiveness* of antibiotics can be assessed statistically from time series as a cumulative or moving average percentage of resistance in a given period. For Staphylococcus aureus and four selected antibiotics, the cumulative average is shown in Figure 6.4. There, the ineffectiveness of cefotaxim is relatively low and stable. The remaining three antibiotics are less effective; they differ by about 5 to 10% and perform similarly in time. The peak of clyndamycin's ineffectiveness is close to 30%, which is considered an approximate limit for

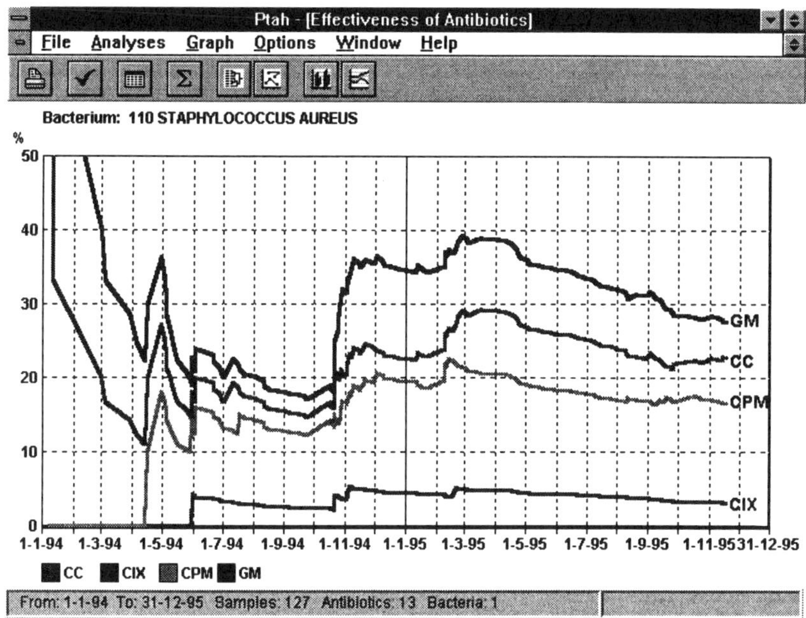

Figure 6.4 Cumulative ineffectiveness (in %) of gentamycin (GM), clyndamycin (CC), cefpiramide (CPM), and cefotaxim (CIX).

abandoning the antibiotic. The fourth antibiotic, gentamycin, was well above this limit in a considerable period of time.

6.6 EVALUATION OF THE SYSTEM

6.6.1 Design of Ptah

Ptah was designed as an on-line decision support system to be regularly used by physicians. Special attention was therefore given to the relevance and comprehensibility of the information it provides. The implemented methods are all well-known and fairly simple. However, they are combined together so as to allow the user to investigate the problem from various viewpoints. All the methods in one way or another deal with concepts that are familiar to and already used by the physician. Moreover, the methods were deliberately selected so that they can be controlled by a uniform set of parameters and that their results can be presented graphically.

In the design stage, we evaluated a number of data analysis methods other than those presented here. For example, we investigated the similarity of antibiotics by comparing the columns of time series. We tested methods such as Correlation Coefficients, Principal Component Analysis [Massart, et al., 1988] and Kohonen Neural Networks [Zupan and Gasteiger, 1993]. Although the results seemed quite interesting at first, the collaborating physicians considered these methods either too difficult to interpret, or irrelevant for the support of therapeutic activities. Consequently, such methods were excluded from the implementation in Ptah.

Another key factor that influenced the design was a strong preference of collaborating physicians towards simple, flexible and graphically-supported methods. In particular, they were not interested in methods that would make decisions on their behalf. Rather, they wanted the *support* of *their own* decisions. The key requirement was to provide an easy access to information they "knew it was there", but difficult to obtain.

6.6.2 Practical experience

Ptah is currently being evaluated in the Intensive Care and Surgery Units of General Hospital Jesenice. At this stage, it is somewhat early to make general conclusions about the system and its contributions to the therapy of nosocomial infections. Nevertheless, it has been well accepted by physicians who test it; some of them have already decided to use it on a regular basis. Also, some lessons have been learned that may be of interest for further development of this and similar systems.

As expected, physicians tend to consult Ptah only for sufficiently difficult decisions, i.e., when the patient is seriously ill, or the bacterium is either highly resistant, or has some unusual resistance pattern. In such cases, the physicians usually look at the bacterial resistance levels (Figure 6.1) and similarity of vectors (Figure 6.3). Among these two, the latter seems to be more informative, as it can serve a dual purpose: (1) early identification of dangerous organisms, and (2) identification of similar cases in the past. Also, by listing all the resistance vectors that occur in a given time series, this graph well supplements the dendrogram developed by clustering (Figure 6.2).

A general comment on the clustering of resistance vectors (Figure 6.2) is that although in most cases the generated structure well reflects the characteristics of a given bacterium, the graph is often too detailed and difficult to memorize. Therefore, it seems necessary to simplify the display, which we intend to achieve by pruning the dendrogram and representing the resulting clusters only by most typical resistance vectors.

The tests of Ptah have already confirmed the importance of visualization. Namely, some interesting regularities in data have been found only by inspecting various graphs. For example, some resistance level analyses (such as the one in Figure 6.1) indicate that highly resistant organisms occur periodically, at least in part. So, the question is whether is it possible to predict such behavior and take it into account in therapeutic procedures. The methods currently implemented in Ptah are not intended for this type of scientific discovery. However, they can—by means of visualization—provoke questions and provide a basis for the development of specialized methods.

6.7 FURTHER WORK

Further development of Ptah will first address the quality of underlying data. Currently, the data is entered manually, which not only is tedious, but results in errors and gaps in time series. In order to improve both data quality and quantity, we wish to automate data entry by means of electronic data interchange between the remote laboratory and the hospital.

Next, we intend to enhance the data analysis methods. Two possible improvements have already been mentioned above: (1) modification of the clustering algorithm in order to obtain more compact dendrograms, and (2) implementation of specialized methods for the analysis of periodical occurrence of highly resistant bacteria. Furthermore, because of the importance of an early detection of dangerous organisms, we intend to enhance the displays so as to highlight 'suspicious' newly developed organisms. We believe this can be achieved by appropriate pattern analysis methods. Also, we are investigating the need and possibility of developing an autonomous alerting mechanism.

Currently, Ptah focuses mainly on antibiograms and uses the remaining database items merely as filters for the construction of time series. However, the remaining items also contain valuable information that could be used in medical decision making. For example, the data could be used to establish a relation between a diagnosis, therapeutic procedure and its outcome. We intend to use machine learning methods for this purpose, and generate models for suggesting and verifying the most appropriate therapy.

6.8 SUMMARY

The described decision support system demonstrates the possibility of visually presenting information that can substantially help the doctor at deciding about nosocomial infection therapy. The system provides information about bacterial resistance and effectiveness of antibiotics that is required in decision making, but was difficult to obtain so far. The key factor that made this possible was the availability of data on infections, which serves for the construction of time series of resistance vectors.

There are four data analysis methods implemented in Ptah. The first three deal with bacterial resistance: (1) analysis of bacterial resistance level, (2) hierarchical clustering of resistance vectors, and (3) analysis of the similarity of resistance vectors. The fourth method is aimed at the analysis of the (in)effectiveness of antibiotics.

All the methods are relatively simple, but flexible. They were selected so as to facilitate the investigation of the decision-making problem from various viewpoints, provide information that is both relevant and comprehensible for the physician, and allow a graphical representation of the results.

A longer evaluation period is required to fully assess the impact of the system to the quality of decision making and therapeutic procedures. However, we expect that the system will improve the quality of therapy and possibly decrease the costs of antibiotic treatment. The most important facilities it provides for this purpose are: (1) an overview of bacterial resistance in the hospital, (2) comparison of an antibiogram with similar cases in the past, (3) early detection of highly resistant bacteria in different organizational units and/or therapeutic activities, and (4) early identification of ineffective antibiotics.

Further work on Ptah will proceed in three main directions: (1) improving the quality of the underlying database, (2) enhancing the data analysis methods, and (3) developing models that suggest and verify the most appropriate therapy.

Acknowledgments

The work reported here was financially supported by the Ministry of Science and Technology of the Republic of Slovenia.

Notes

1. Ptah is an acronym for the description of the system in Slovene: P*odpora* t*erapevtskih* a*ktivnosti pri* h*ospitalnih infekcijah* (*Support of Therapeutic Activities for Hospital-Acquired Infections*). It is also the name of an Ancient Egyptian god, the protector of craftsmen and artists.

References

Bohanec, M., Rems, M., and Urh, B. (1995). Design of an information system for supporting therapeutic activities of hospital infections (in Slovene). In Lavrač, N., editor, *Computer-Aided Data Analysis in Medicine*, pages 64–75. IJS Scientific Publishing IJS-SP-95-1.

Cercenado, E., et al. (1990). A conservative procedure for the diagnosis of catheter related infections. *Archive of Internal Medicine*, 150.

Gardner, P. and Arnow, P.M. (1987). Hospital-acquired infections. In Braumwald, E., editor, *Harrison's Principles and Practice of Internal Medicine*, pages 470–474.

McGraw-Hill.

Hemmer, M. (1993). Nosocomial pneumonia in mechanically ventilated patients. *Critical Care Medicine*, 8:591–597.

Kamal, G.D., Pfaller, M.A., Rempe, L.E., and Jebson, P.J. (1991). Reduced intravascular catheter infection by antibiotic bonding: A prospective randomized controlled trial. *Journal of American Medical Association*, 265:2364–2368.

Kramar, Z. and Rems, M. (1992). Computer evidence of hospital infections in General Hospital Jesenice (in Slovene). In *Proc. Medicinska informatika MI-92*, Bled, pages 161–165.

Massart, D.L., Vandeginste, B.G.M., Deming, S.N., Michotte, Y., and Kaufman, L. (1988). *Chemometrics: A Textbook. Data Handling In Science and Technology*, Vol. 2, Elsevier.

McQuitty, L.L. (1966). Similarity analysis of reciprocal pairs for discrete and continuous data. *Educ. Psychol. Measur.*, 26:55–67.

Pestotnik, S.L., Classen, D.C., Evans, R.S., and Burke, J.P. (1996). Implementing antibiotic guidelines through computer-assisted decision support: Clinical and financial outcomes. *Ann. Internal Medicine*, 124:884–890.

Reed, C.R., Sessler, C.N., Glauser, F.L., and Phelan, B.A. (1995). Central venous catheter infections concepts and controversies. *Intensive Care Medicine*, 21:177–183.

Rems, M., Kramar, Z., and Zupančič, M. (1995). Computer-assisted surveillance of nosocomial infections in intensive care unit. In *Proc. Eighth Anaesthesia A-A Symposium*, Portorož, pages 165–167.

Santamaria, J. (1990). Nosocomial infections. In Oh, T.E., editor, *Intensive Care Manual*, pages 409–416. Butterworths, Sydney.

Slavec, S., Zupan, I., and Saksida, I. (1992). InfoMed: Information systems in medicine (in Slovene). In *Proc. Medicinska informatika MI-92*, Bled, pages 307–311.

Snowdon, S.L. (1994). Hygiene standards for breathing systems. *British Journal on Anaesthesiology*, 72.

Zupan, J. and Gasteiger, J. (1993). *Neural Networks for Chemists*. Verlang Chemie, Weinheim.

II Data Mining

7 PROGNOSING THE SURVIVAL TIME OF PATIENTS WITH ANAPLASTIC THYROID CARCINOMA USING MACHINE LEARNING

Matjaž Kukar,
Nikola Bešič,
Igor Kononenko,
Marija Auersperg,
and Marko Robnik-Šikonja

Abstract: Anaplastic thyroid carcinoma is a rare but very aggressive tumor. Many factors that might influence the survival of patients have been suggested. The aim of this study was to determine which of the factors, known at the time of admission to the hospital, might predict survival of the patients with anaplastic thyroid carcinoma. Our aim was also to assess the relative importance of the factors and to identify potentially useful decision and regression trees generated by machine learning algorithms. Our study included 126 patients with anaplastic thyroid carcinoma treated at the Institute of Oncology Ljubljana from 1972 to 1992. In this chapter, we compare the machine learning approach with previous statistical evaluations of the problem (univariate and multivariate analysis) and show that it can provide a more thorough analysis and improve the understanding of the data.

7.1 INTRODUCTION

Anaplastic thyroid carcinoma is a very aggressive tumor with poor prognosis [Aldinger et al., 1987, Jereb et al., 1975]. Mean survival time is from 2.5 [Jereb et al., 1975] to 7 months [Venkatesh et al., 1990]; only occasionally, patients survive beyond five years [Aldinger et al., 1987, Auersperg et al., 1990, Tallroth et al., 1987]. Many factors that might influence the survival of patients have been suggested. They are the following: presence of metastases [Bešič et al., 1996, Venkatesh et al., 1990], growth rate of the tumor [Bešič et al., 1996], age [Venkatesh et al., 1990], focal anaplastic carcinoma [Aldinger et al., 1987, Bešič et al., 1996], tumor size [Bešič et al., 1996], and treatment [Bešič et al., 1996]. In the clinical setting, several factors together influence the survival. In order to determine them, multivariate statistical analysis [Cox, 1972], which allows the analysis of many factors simultaneously, is required [Stare, 1989]. As anaplastic thyroid carcinoma is a rare disease [Jereb et al., 1975], till now, only a few series of patients with anaplastic thyroid carcinoma large enough to enable multivariate statistical analysis of prognostic factors and survival have been published [Aldinger et al., 1987, Auersperg et al., 1990, Bešič et al., 1996, Junor et al., 1992, Nel et al., 1985, Venkatesh et al., 1990]. Of them, only [Nel et al., 1985] and [Bešič et al., 1996] used Cox's proportional hazard survival model [Cox and Oakes, 1984, Cox, 1972]. However, both of them included in their studies also the factors that were not known at the admission to the hospital [Bešič et al., 1996, Nel et al., 1985], so their results could not be pertinent to making decisions before treatment. Our goals were to determine which of the factors, that are known at the time of the admission to the hospital, predict the survival of patients with anaplastic thyroid carcinoma, to find out the relative importance of the factors, and to identify potentially useful decision and regression trees generated by selected machine learning algorithms [Breiman et al., 1984, Karalič, 1992, Kononenko, 1994, Robnik-Šikonja and Kononenko, 1996, Albus, 1975a].

7.2 PATIENTS AND DATASET

According to the hospital's cancer registry, a total of 137 patients with anaplastic thyroid carcinoma were admitted to the Institute of Oncology in Ljubljana, Slovenia, from 1972 to 1992. Complete documentation and follow-up data as well as cytomorphologic and/or histomorphologic slides were available for 126 of these patients. These 126 patients were included in the present retrospective study. There were 90 females and 36 males; mean age was 66.7 years, range 35-84 years. Altogether 93 concomitant diseases were found in 88 of the 126 patients. In all the cases, the diagnosis of anaplastic thyroid carcinoma was confirmed by the histopathology and/or cytopathology. All cytologic and histologic specimens were reexamined and the diagnosis was verified. For 75 patients the diagnosis was confirmed by both cytomorphology and histomorphology, for 37 only by cytomorphology, and for 14 patients only by histomorphology.

The patients were described with 11 attributes (see Table 7.1). The *rapid* value of the growth rate (attribute 3) comprised the patients with a history of tumor growth shorter than three months and the *slow growth rate* the patients with a history of tumor growth longer than three months. On admission, the patients were examined in order to determine the presence of distant metastases (attribute 9). Their presence was confirmed by X-ray investigations of the chest and bone, scintigrafic, ultrasound investigations and/or computed tomography. Tumors were described as focal or massive (attribute 10). Patients with an inoperable thyroid tumor, in whom fine needle aspiration biopsies from several places of the tumor showed anaplastic thyroid carcinoma, were described massive. As the diagnosis was confirmed in 89% by cytomorphology, cytomorphological classification of tumor type was used (attribute 11). The meaning of the remaining attributes is quite obvious and needs no further explanation.

Table 7.1 Description of the dataset.

	Attribute	*Values*
1	Sex	male, female
2	Age (interval in years)	<60, 60-70, 70-80, ≥80
3	Growth rate of tumor	rapid, slow
4	Previously enlarged thyroid gland	yes, no
5	Prior radioactive iodine therapy	yes, no
6	Tumor size (interval in cm)	<5, 5-10, 10-15, ≥15
7	Primary tumor confined to thyroid gland	yes, no
8	Enlarged neck lymph nodes	yes, no
9	Distant metastases	yes, no
10	Focal anaplastic carcinoma	yes (focal), no (massive)
11	Cytomorphological type of the anaplastic thyroid carcinoma	round cell, spindle cell, pleomorphous cell

The survival data were calculated from the time of the first admission to the Institute of Oncology for the treatment of anaplastic thyroid carcinoma. Median duration of survival of the patients (treated and non treated) was three months (Figure 7.1).

The original dataset consisted of patients with *continuous* classes (survival time in months). We experimented with classification and regression trees. In

Table 7.2 Grouping of the survival time and the entropy of the dataset.

Survival time	*No. of patients*
Less than 1 month	31
1 to 2 months	27
3 to 4 months	26
5 to 10 months	27
More than 10 months	15
Total patients	126
Entropy of the dataset (after grouping)	2.29 bit

the first case we grouped the patients into 5 groups, each containing approximately the same number of patients (Table 7.2). In the second case we used the original continuous classes (the distribution can be seen in Figure 7.1).

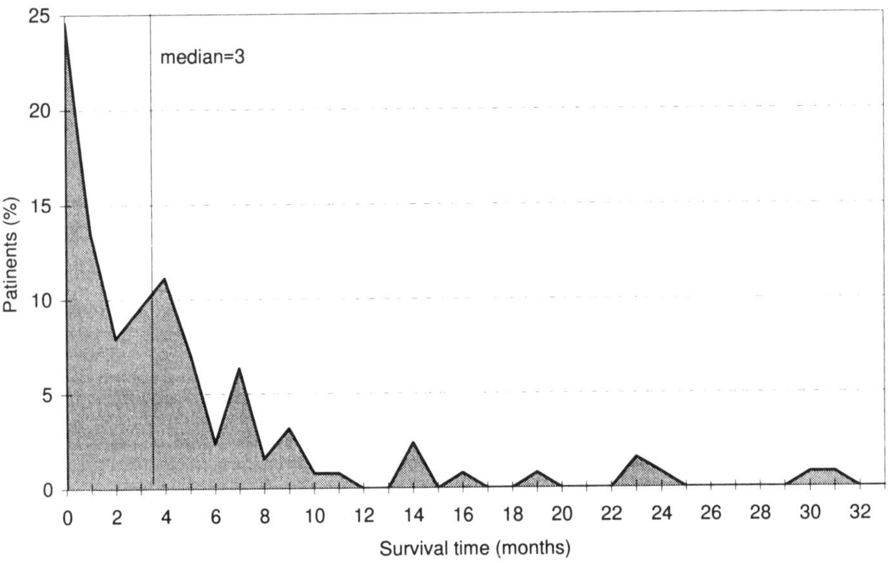

Figure 7.1 Distribution of the survival time (months).

7.3 THE ALGORITHMS USED

7.3.1 Classification trees

Assistant-R and Assistant-I. Assistant-R [Kononenko et al., 1997] is a reimplementation of the Assistant learning system for top-down induction of decision trees [Cestnik et al., 1987]. The basic algorithm goes back to CLS (Concept Learning System) developed by Hunt et al. [Hunt et al., 1966] and reimplemented by several authors (see [Quinlan, 1986] for an overview). The main features of the original Assistant algorithm are the binarization of attributes, decision tree pruning [Niblett and Bratko, 1986], handling of incomplete data and the use of naive Bayesian classifier when there are some attribute values for which no training instances are available.

The main difference between Assistant and its reimplementation Assistant-R is the use of the ReliefF heuristic for attribute selection instead of the information gain heuristics. ReliefF [Kononenko, 1994] is an extension of Relief [Kira and Rendell, 1992a, Kira and Rendell, 1992b]. The key idea of Relief is to estimate attributes according to how well their values distinguish between the instances that are near to each other. For that purpose, for the given attribute Relief evaluates the difference between the two probabilities:

- the probability that two similar instances from different classes have different values of that attribute,
- the probability that two similar instances from the same class have different values of that attribute.

Although the original Relief can deal with discrete and continuous attributes, it cannot deal with incomplete data and is limited to the two-class problems only. Kononenko [Kononenko, 1994] developed an extension of Relief, called ReliefF, that improves the original algorithm by estimating probabilities more reliably and extends it to deal with incomplete and multi-class datasets.

Assistant-R also uses the the m-estimate [Cestnik, 1990, Cestnik and Bratko, 1991] for reliable estimation of the probabilities during building and pruning of a decision tree. In our experiments, the parameter m was set to 2. This setting is usually used as default and, empirically, gives satisfactory results [Cestnik, 1990, Cestnik and Bratko, 1991] although, with tuning, better results can be expected. The m-estimate is also used in the naive Bayesian formula and for postpruning instead of the Laplace's law of succession (as proposed in [Cestnik and Bratko, 1991]).

Assistant-I is a variant of Assistant-R that, instead of ReliefF, uses the information gain as the selection criterion, as does the original Assistant. However, the other differences remain (m-estimate of probabilities).

7.3.2 Regression trees

Regression analysis is a technique for modeling relations between independent variables (attributes) and a dependent continuous variable (class). In the context of machine learning it is also referred to as learning of a continuous class. The majority of the current propositional inductive learning systems predict discrete classes. Although they can also solve continuous class problems by discretizing the values of the class variable in advance, this approach is often inappropriate. On the other hand, regression learning systems, e.g., CART [Breiman et al., 1984], Retis [Karalič, 1992] and CORE [Robnik-Šikonja and Kononenko, 1996] predict continuous classes directly with a function that assignes a value to the class variable.

In our experiments, we used the CART, Retis and CORE systems. Both CART and Retis use the mean squared error for attribute estimation.

The experimental system CORE (COntinuous RElief) uses an extended version of ReliefF – RReliefF [Robnik-Šikonja and Kononenko, 1996] – which is capable of correctly estimating the quality of attributes in continuous class problems with strong dependencies between attributes. RReliefF is a cousin of ReliefF working on continuous class problems and is capable of detecting conditional dependencies between the attributes. Similarly to ReliefF, for each attribute it estimates the probability of separating different from similar near instances. ReliefF and RReliefF provide an unified view to the attribute estimation in learning of discrete and continuous classes.

Retis and CORE perform postpruning of the induced regression tree by using the m-estimate of probability, while CART utilizes the cost-complexity postpruning.

In all our experiments the quality of regression trees was measured by the rooted *mean squared error* (MSE) – mean squared difference between the predicted and actual values.

$$\sqrt{MSE} = \sqrt{\frac{1}{N}\sum_{i=1}^{N}(\text{actual}_i - \text{predicted}_i)^2} \tag{7.1}$$

7.3.3 CMAC neural networks

The Cerebellar Model Articulation Controller – CMAC [Albus, 1975a, Albus, 1975b] is an associative neural network in which only a small subset of the network influences any instantaneous output, and this subset is determined by the input to the network. It accepts real-valued inputs and produces real-valued outputs. The associative mapping built into CMAC assures local generalization: similar inputs produce similar outputs, while distant inputs produce nearly independent outputs. As the result of the built-in associative properties, the number of training passes required for network convergence is orders of magnitude smaller with CMAC than with some other types of neural networks (e.g., backpropagation) on real-world problems.

The associative mapping is defined for the N-dimensional input, each dimension discretized into predefined number of intervals [Ellison, 1991]. For any given input it activates the subset of weights which are used to calculate the output of the CMAC. The cardinality of the active subset is fixed and given in advance as a learning parameter. The active weights are then modified according to the LMS (least mean squares) rule [Widrow and Stearns, 1985].

7.4 EXPERIMENTS

The algorithms were tested by using the 10-fold cross-validation method. The dataset was partitioned in 10 equally sized subsets. Testing was repeated 10 times: in each step nine subsets were used for training and the remaining one for testing.

The results of both classification and regression algorithms are provided in Table 7.3. For regression algorithms, we measured the *mean squared error* (MSE). For classification algorithms, we measured the classification accuracy (percentage of correctly classified patients) and the average information score [Kononenko and Bratko, 1991]. This measure eliminates the influence of prior probabilities and deals appropriately with the probabilistic answers of the classifier. The average information score is defined as:

$$\mathrm{Inf} = \frac{\sum_{i=1}^{\#testing\ instances} \mathrm{Inf_i}}{\#testing\ instances} \tag{7.2}$$

where the information score of the classification of the i-th testing instance is defined by:

$$\mathrm{Inf_i} = \begin{cases} -\log_2 P(Cl_i) + \log_2 P'(Cl_i), & P'(Cl_i) \geq P(Cl_i) \\ -(-\log_2(1 - P(Cl_i)) + \log_2(1 - P'(Cl_i))), & P'(Cl_i) < P(Cl_i) \end{cases} \tag{7.3}$$

where Cl_i is the correct class of the i-th testing instance, $P(Cl)$ is the prior probability of class Cl and $P'(Cl)$ the probability provided by the classifier.

7.4.1 *Results of Assistant-I and Assistant-R*

Results of 10-fold cross-validation of Assistant-I and Assistant-R are quite similar (Table 7.3). Although the classification accuracy does not seem very high,

Table 7.3 Classification accuracy, information score and the square root of the MSE.

Algorithm	*Class. accuracy*	*Inf. score*	$\sqrt{MSE}$
Assistant-I	41.7%	0.56 bit	–
Assistant-R	38.3%	0.56 bit	–
Retis	–	–	11.2
CART	–	–	11.3
CORE	–	–	9.0
CMAC	–	–	10.7

we have to keep in mind that the majority class is only 24.6%. Also the information score (0.56 bit) suggests that the decision tree provides useful information.

In order to evaluate how meaningful the induced decision trees are for experts (physicians), trees were induced from all the available data. Both decision trees (but especially that of Assistant-R in Figure 7.3) in upper levels correspond very well to the physicians' knowledge.

The upper two levels of the Assistant-R tree (Figure 7.3) suggest the conditional dependence (with respect to the survival time) between the distant metastases and the growth rate of the tumor. This dependence was only partially detected by Assistant-I an was not detected by other algorithms.

The top four attributes and their estimations, as ranked by ReliefF at the root of the tree, are presented in Table 7.4.

Table 7.4 Attributes' estimation by ReliefF.

Attribute	*Quality*
Distant metastases	0.078
Age (interval)	0.020
Prior radioactive iodine therapy	0.008
Growth rate of tumor	0.004

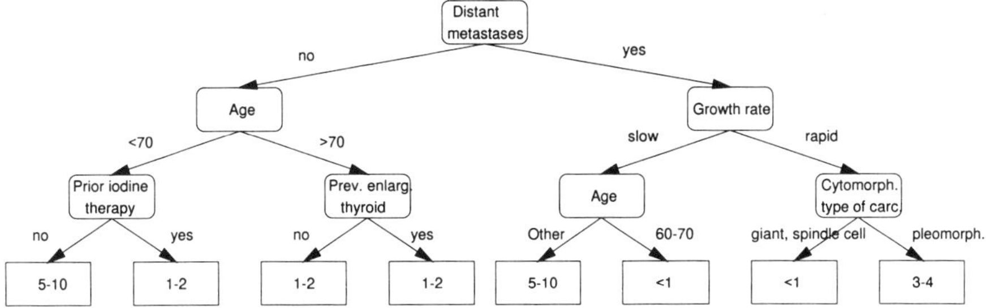

Figure 7.2 Decision tree generated by Assistant-I.

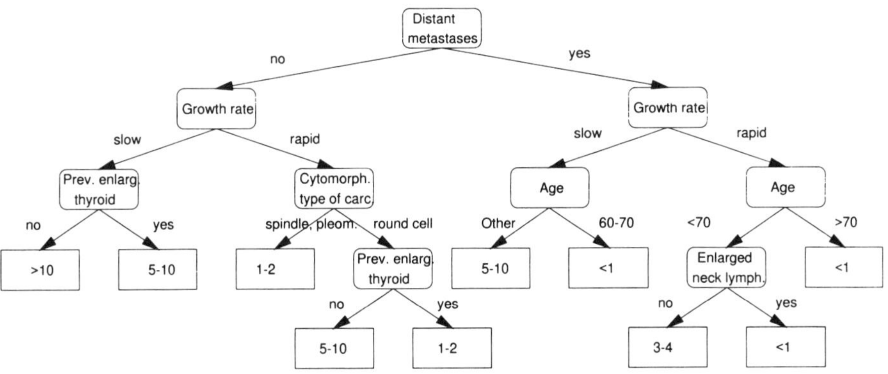

Figure 7.3 Decision tree generated by Assistant-R.

7.4.2 Results of CART, CORE and Retis

Regression trees generated by CART and CORE are shown in Figures 7.4 and 7.5. From Table 7.3 it can be seen that for the regression algorithms the $\sqrt{MSE}$ is quite high (about 10 months).

The problem with the MSE (Eq. 7.1) is that it squares the differences between actual and predicted values. So only a few badly missed results can dramatically affect the total result. On the other hand, one can also observe some other estimations of the central value, such as the median value of the absolute error. In the case of CORE it was 2.2 months, and for the 68.3% of the patients the absolute error (non-squared) was less than three months. The $\sqrt{MSE}$ was so high (9 months) because of a few outliers, whose survival times were actually mispredicted for more than 20 months.

It is interesting to note the similarity between CART and CORE, as they use quite different criteria for attribute selection (the mean squared error and

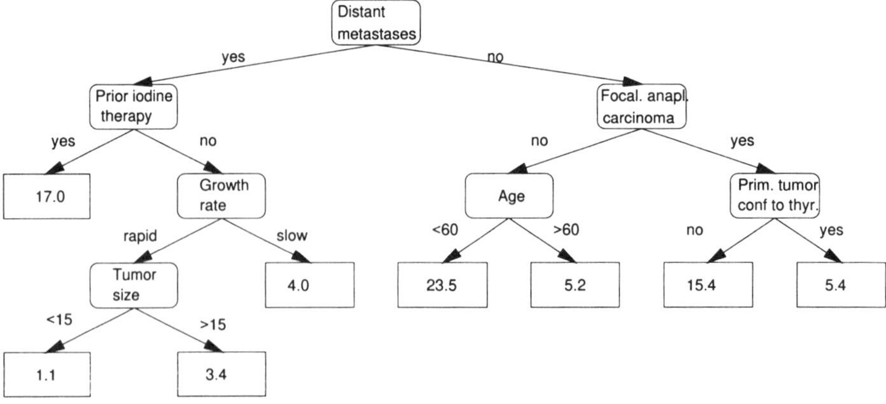

Figure 7.4 Regression tree generated by CART.

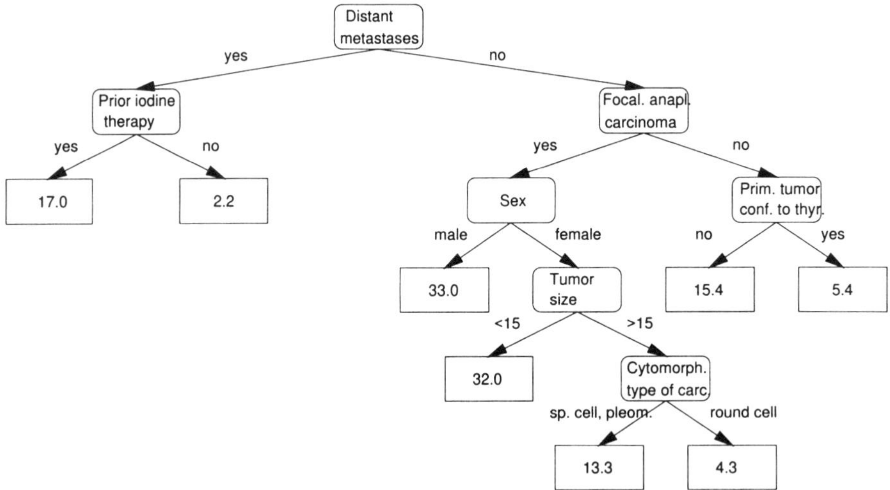

Figure 7.5 Regression tree generated by CORE.

RReliefF, respectively). This could be due to the fact that no strong conditional dependencies can be found in the regressional variant of the problem.

One would also expect similar trees of Assistant-R and CORE because they use similar selection criteria (ReliefF and RReliefF, respectively). However, the structural difference between the classification tree of Assistant-R and the regression tree of CORE suggest that the metrics of the discretized class and the continuous class differ significantly (as can be seen from Table 7.2, the discretized classes use roughly a logarithmic scale). This problem could possibly be overcome by changing the CORE to use the logarithmic (instead of the linear) scale for the continuous class.

7.4.3 Statistical methods and results from univariate and multivariate analysis

Each of the 11 potential prognostic factors (Table 7.1) was evaluated by univariate statistical analysis (confidence level = 0.95). Survival curves of the attributes were compared by means of the *log-rank* test [Bešič et al., 1996]. The relative importance of factors influencing the survival time of patients was multivariately analyzed by means of the Cox proportional hazards model [Cox, 1972]. All statistically significant factors from the univariate analysis were analyzed multivariately in the Cox model. The calculations were made by statistical packages SOLO and BMDP2L (BMDP Statistical Software Inc, 1992) on a personal computer. Univariate analysis identified the potential prognostic factors. Of the eleven factors analyzed by the univariate analysis, six were the potentially prognostic factors (Table 7.5). Of the six factors obtained by the univariate analysis, multivariate analysis found out three prognostic factors: distant metastases, growth rate of tumor and age of patients (Table 7.6; the better prognostic factor are those with the greater difference to 1.0). Similar results can also be found in [Bešič et al., 1996].

Table 7.5 Attributes' estimation by the univariate analysis.

Attribute	*P*
Distant metastases	<0.001
Focal anaplastic carcinoma	<0.001
Primary tumor confined to thyroid gland	0.002
Growth rate of tumor	0.005
Age (interval)	0.045
Tumor size	0.050

7.5 DISCUSSION

The obtained results are largely in accordance with the physicians' prior knowledge about the problem. The highly ranked attributes are those as expected.

Table 7.6 Attributes' estimation by the multivariate analysis.

Attribute	*exp(coef)*
Distant metastases	0.3803
Growth rate of tumor	0.5879
Age (interval)	1.0193

However, the experts' speculation that the prior radioactive therapy causes cancer a few years later, was not confirmed.

The attribute estimation of multivariate analysis [Bešič et al., 1996] is also very similar to our results (compare Tables 7.4 and 7.6).

The most successful of the applied algorithms seems to be Assistant-R. This is not surprising, since it was shown before [Kukar et al., 1996] that it performs very well in medical problems. Although the achieved classification accuracy was slightly lower than that of Assistant-I (see Table 7.3), it has some other advantages:

- the physicians preferred its decision tree to that of Assistant-I,
- it detected an interesting dependency between distant metastases and growth rate of the tumor (see also Section 7.4.1). The mutual presence of distant metastases and rapid growth of the tumor suggest very short survival time. On the other hand, the absence of distant metastases and slow growth rate of the tumor suggest much longer survival. This is not entirely new to physicians; they have already speculated that this might be the case [Bešič et al., 1996], and
- it efficiently pointed out the *unfair* attributes, as explained below.

The original dataset consisted of 13 attributes. However, two attributes were evaluated during (or after) the treatment period and were therefore not present at the admission (treatment and its adequacy). Assistant-I and Assistant-R have positioned these attributes at the root of the trees, achieving a 75-80% classification accuracy.

It is controversial if treatment is a prognostic factor at all because it is not present at the admission [Bešič et al., 1996]. The aim of our study was to determine which factors, known at the admission to hospital, can predict the survival of patients with anaplastic thyroid carcinoma, so we decided not to include treatment in our analysis.

After the elimination of unfair attributes, the classification accuracy of the classification trees decreased from 75% to only about 40%. This suggests the following:

- present attributes are not sufficient to reliably predict the survival time,
- it would be possible to extract some other useful attributes from the retrospective database of the patients, such as:
  - general health condition of the patient on admission, and
  - performance status and concomitant diseases of the patient.

We believe that the classification accuracy could be improved by including the attributes that describe general condition of patients. These factors have impact on the treatment: if the patient is in bad condition, he can not tolerate specific therapy and the prognosis is dismal. If the new attributes cause the classification accuracy raise to at least 70%, the classification trees could find good use in the everyday practice. However, it is unclear how the new attributes could affect the regression trees, since the impact of the *unfair* attributes on them was not as high as on the classification trees.

In further work we hope to include different types of metrics in the regression systems. We will improve the description of the patients with new attributes and replace a few pre-discretized continuous attributes from the original dataset (age and tumor size) with their continuous versions. This may help the classification and especially the regression systems to decrease errors in their predictions. Providing a general method for estimating the reliability of algorithms' answers and including a cost-benefit analysis (misclassification costs) may also turn out to be very useful.

Acknowledgments

We thank Prof. Dr. Marija Us-Krašovec and Prof. Dr. Rastko Golouh for reviewing cytologic and histologic specimens. Assistant-I and Assistant-R were implemented by Edvard Šimec. This work was supported by the Ministry of Science and Technology of Slovenia.

References

Albus, J. S. (1975a). A new approach to manipulator control: The cerebellar model articulation controller (CMAC). *Journal of Dynamic Systems, Measurement and Control*, 97(3):220–227.

Albus, J. S. (1975b). Data storage in the cerebellar model articulation controller (CMAC). *Journal of Dynamic Systems, Measurement and Control*, 97(3):228–233.

Aldinger, K., Samaan, N., Ibanez, M., and Hill, S. J. (1987). Anaplastic carcinoma of the thyroid. A review of 84 cases of spindle and giant cell carcinoma of the thyroid. *Cancer*, 41:2267–2275.

Auersperg, M., Us-Krašovec, M., Petrič, G., Pogačnik, A., and Bešič, N. (1990). Results of combined modality treatment in poorly differentiated and anaplastic thyroid carcinoma. *Klin. Wochenschr.*, 9:267–270.

Bešič, N., Auersperg, M., Vrecl, R., Us-Krašovec, M., Stare, J., and Golouh, R. (1996). Prognosenfaktoren fuer das anaplastische schilddruesenkarzinom - eine multivariate analyse von 126 patienten. In Reinwein, D. and Weihheimer, B., editors, *Schilddruese 1996*. Walter de Gruyter-Verlag.

Breiman, L., Friedman, J. H., Olshen, R. A., and Stone, C. J. (1984). *Classification and Regression Trees*. Wadsworth International Group, Belmont CA.

Cestnik, B. (1990). Estimating probabilities: A crucial task in machine learning. In *Proc. European Conference on Artificial Intelligence 1990*, pages 147–149, Stockholm, Sweden.

Cestnik, B. and Bratko, I. (1991). On estimating probabilities in tree pruning. In Kodratoff, Y., editor, *Proc. European Working Session on Learning*, pages 138–150, Porto, Portugal. Springer Verlag.

Cestnik, B., Kononenko, I., and Bratko, I. (1987). ASSISTANT 86: A knowledge elicitation tool for sophisticated users. In Bratko, I. and Lavrač, N., editors, *Progress in Machine Learning*. Sigma Press, Wilmslow, England.

Cox, D. (1972). Regression models and life tables. *Journal of Royal Stat. Soc. (B)*, 34:187–220.

Cox, D. R. and Oakes, D. (1984). *Analysis of Survival Data*. Chapman and Hall, London.

Ellison, D. (1991). On the convergence of the multidimensional Albus perceptron. *The International Journal of Robotocs Research*, 10(4):338–357.

Hunt, E., Martin, J., and Stone, P. (1966). *Experiments in Induction*. Academic Press, New York.

Jereb, B., Stjernsward, J., and Lowhagen, T. (1975). Anaplastic giant-cell carcinoma of the thyroid. *Cancer*, 35:1293–1295.

Junor, E., Paul, J., and Reed, N. (1992). Anaplastic thyroid carcinoma: 91 patients treated by surgery and radiotherapy. *European Journal of Surgical Oncology*, 18:83–88.

Karalič, A. (1992). Employing linear regression in regression tree leaves. In Neumann, B., editor, *Proceedings of ECAI'92*, pages 440–441. John Wiley & Sons.

Kira, K. and Rendell, L. (1992a). The feature selection problem: traditional methods and new algorithm. In *Proc. AAAI'92*, San Jose, CA.

Kira, K. and Rendell, L. (1992b). A practical approach to feature selection. In Sleeman, D. and Edwards, P., editors, *Proc. Intern. Conf. on Machine Learning*, pages 249–256, Aberdeen, UK. Morgan Kaufmann.

Kononenko, I. and Bratko, I. (1991). Information based evaluation criterion for classifier's performance. *Machine Learning*, 6:67–80.

Kononenko, I., Šimec, E., and Robnik-Šikonja, M. (1997). Overcoming the myopia of inductive learning algorithms with ReliefF. *Applied Intelligence*, 7:39–55.

Kononenko, I. (1994). Estimating attributes: Analysis and extensions of RELIEF. In De Raedt, L. and Bergadano, F., editors, *Proc. European Conf. on Machine Learning*, pages 171–182, Catania, Italy. Springer Verlag.

Kukar, M., Kononenko, I., and Silvester, T. (1996). Machine learning in prognosis of the femoral neck fracture recovery. *Artificial Intelligence in Medicine*, 8:431–451.

Nel, C., Heerden, J. V., and Goellner, J. (1985). Anaplastic carcinoma of the thyroid: A clinicopathologic study of 82 patients. In *Mayo Clin. Proc.*, volume 1-2, pages 51–58.

Niblett, T. and Bratko, I. (1986). Learning decision rules in noisy domains. In *Proc. Expert Systems 86*, Brighton, UK.

Quinlan, J. (1986). Induction of decision trees. *Machine Learning*, 1:81–106.

Robnik-Šikonja, M. and Kononenko, I. (1996). Non-myopic attribute estimation in regression. Technical report, University of Ljubljana, Slovenia, Faculty of computer and information science.

Stare, J. (1989). *Statistical analysis of survival and its aplication in patients after acute myocardial infarction.* Master's Thesis. University of Ljubljana, Slovenia.

Tallroth, E., Wallin, G., Lundell, G., Lowhagen, T., and Einhorn, J. (1987). Multimodality treatment in anaplastic giant cell thyroid carcinoma. *Cancer*, 60:1428–1431.

Venkatesh, Y., Ordonez, G. N., and Schultz, P. (1990). Anaplastic carcinoma of the thyroid. A clinicopathologic study of 121 cases. *Cancer*, 66:321–330.

Widrow, B. and Stearns, S. D. (1985). *Adaptive Signal Processing.* Prentice-Hall, Englewood Cliffs, NJ.

8 DATA ANALYSIS OF PATIENTS WITH SEVERE HEAD INJURY

Iztok A. Pilih,
Dunja Mladenić,
Nada Lavrač,
and Tine S. Prevec

Abstract: This chapter presents an application of decision tree induction to the problem of the prediction of outcome after a severe head injury. This study shows that induced decision trees are useful for the analysis of the importance of clinical parameters and of their combinations for the evaluation of the severity of brain injury and for outcome prediction. Due to a small number of patient data available for this study the induced decision trees cannot yet be considered as a reliable prognostic tool. Nevertheless, meaningful regularities have been discovered that help in the analysis of this difficult prognostic task.

8.1 INTRODUCTION

The prediction of the outcome of severe head injury is a difficult and complex problem since it depends on a large number of factors: those defining the condition of a patient before an injury, the ones acting during the injury, as well as the numerous factors acting in the period after the injury. Limitations of the early clinical evaluation of the brain injury (at the site of the accident or on admission to the hospital) and the long period of recovery make the problem even more demanding [Vollmer, 1993]. In spite of these limitations, the outcome prediction is needed and is useful for several reasons. It provides the insight into the pathophysiological events after head injury that makes therapeutic decisions easier, it is needed to inform the relatives, it helps in the evaluation of the effectiveness of the medical care and enables the timely selection of the most suitable rehabilitation program [Vollmer, 1993, Braakman, 1992].

Traditional approaches to the problem consist of a systematic collection of a large number of relevant factors, the statistical analysis of their prognostic values, and the search for the most valuable combinations of factors that influence the actual outcome after a severe head injury. Such approaches are based on large homogeneous populations of data of patients with severe head injury and on the application of statistical methods [Braakman, 1992]. Several prognostic models have been created by such approaches. They can provide more reliable prognosis than the lifelong personal experience [Braakman, 1992]. Prognostic models are usually presented as mathematical models, graphs or tables. Choi and co-workers [Choi et al., 1991] presented a prognostic model in the form of a decision tree.

This work presents an application of machine learning [Quinlan, 1986, Michie et al., 1994] to the problem of outcome prognosis after a severe head injury [Pilih et al., 1995, Pilih et al., 1996]. The chapter is organized as follows. Section 8.2 presents the prognostic problem: the available dataset, the prognostic classes and the clinical parameters are described. The machine learning methodology of decision tree induction is briefly described in Section 8.3. The experiments and results of decision tree induction are presented in the next three sections. Sections 8.4 and 8.5 deal with the problem of outcome prediction, whereas Section 8.6 deals with the analysis of the brainstem syndrome which is one of the most important parameters for outcome prediction. The chapter concludes with a summary and directions for further work.

8.2 PATIENT DATA

This study is based on the data of patients who were referred to the Celje General Hospital, Slovenia, after a severe head injury in the period from October 1992 till April 1993, first treated in the Intensive Care Unit and later at the

Department of Trauma Surgery. In this period, 38 patients were admitted to the hospital.

All the patients were submitted to a diagnostic protocol used as the doctrinary procedure for the patients with severe head injury at the Department of Trauma Surgery. In addition to the general clinical examination and standard laboratory tests, the diagnostic protocol includes computer axial tomography (CT), and the evaluation of coma according to the Glasgow coma scale (GCS) [Teasdal and Jennett, 1974]. The neurological evaluation of brainstem functions separating brainstem affection into seven brainstem syndromes (BSS) according to Gerstenbrand and co-workers [Gerstenbrand and Lücking, 1970, Gerstenbrand and Rumpl, 1983, Gerstenbrand et al., 1990] was also applied.

8.2.1 Prediction classes: Glasgow outcome scale

The outcome was evaluated six months after the injury according to the Glasgow outcome scale (GOS). Patients were classified into five groups: GOS1 - fatal outcome, GOS2 - persistent vegetative state (patients with complete expression of apallic syndrome according to [Gerstenbrand and Rumpl, 1992] were included in this group), GOS3 - severely disabled patients needing much support for their personal care and daily activities due to their mental and physical handicaps, GOS4 - moderately disabled patients, able of taking care of themselves in their daily life, GOS5 - patients with a good outcome (able to continue their education, professional and social engagements similar as before the head injury) [Jennett and Bond, 1975].

Eighteen out of the 38 patients (47%) died in the first six months after the injury, their survival time being from 5 hours to 97 days. More than half of these patients (25% of all the patients) died during the first week. Six months after the injury, among the 20 patients that survived (53% of all the patients), one patient was in the persistent vegetative state (GOS2), three in the severe disability group (GOS3), five were moderately disabled (GOS4), and eleven had a good outcome (GOS5).

8.2.2 Description of clinical parameters

Age. The mean value of the patients' age was 46 (standard deviation 19), within the range 16–81 years. In the group of the youngest patients ($\leq$ 20 years) most had a good outcome (66.7%), the death rate of patients aged under 40 was 18.7%, whereas above 40 it was much higher: 68.2%.

Computer axial tomography (CT). CT was performed by a Siemens Somatom HiQ. Only the CTs recorded upon admission were considered in this study. Six types of abnormalities were evaluated: epidural haematoma, subdural haematoma, intracerebral haematoma or contusion, subarachnoidal haemorrhage, intraventricular haemorrhage, and midline displacement larger than 5 mm. `CT score` was computed as a simple sum (the range is from 0 to 6) of these CT abnormalities. Five patients who had no CT abnormalities all survived with a good outcome, whereas the death rate of patients with more than one CT abnormality was over 50%.

Glasgow coma scale (GCS). The score based on `GCS` is an estimate of the affection of consciousness. Verbal responsiveness (range 1–5), eye opening (range 1–4) and motor responses (range 1–6) are evaluated. `GCS` score is computed as a sum of the above estimates, expressed in the range from 3 (the most severe affection) to 15 (no affection) [Teasdal and Jennett, 1974]. This study includes only patients with `GCS` $\leq$ 8 which we used as a definition of a severe head injury. The death rate of patients with `GCS` below 5 was 83.3%, whereas above 5 the death rate was much lower: 17.6%.

Brainstem syndromes (BSS). `BSS` [Gerstenbrand and Lücking, 1970, Gerstenbrand and Rumpl, 1983, Gerstenbrand et al., 1990] separate brainstem dysfunction into seven stages, from 1 to 7, where stage 7 corresponds to the slightest affection of the brainstem `MS1` (Mesencephalic Syndrome 1), stage 6 is `MS2a`, stage 5 is `MS2b`, stage 4 is `MS3`, stage 3 is `MS4`, whereas stages 2 and 1 are Bulbar Syndromes 1 and 2 (`BS1` and `BS2`), respectively. `BS2` is the most severe brainstem affection; patients do not recover if this state lasts for more than 20 minutes [Gerstenbrand et al., 1990]. The patients with `MS1` were not included in this study because they do not fulfill the criterion of a severe head injury (`GCS` $\leq$ 8). Brainstem syndromes are estimated from the basic clinical signs (see below) [Gerstenbrand and Lücking, 1970, Gerstenbrand and Rumpl, 1983, Gerstenbrand et al., 1990], in accordance with Table 8.A.1 given in the appendix.

Basic clinical signs. The basic clinical attributes used in the descriptions of patient records include [Gerstenbrand and Lücking, 1970, Gerstenbrand and Rumpl, 1983, Gerstenbrand et al., 1990]: `Vigilance`; reaction parameters: `Reaction to acoustic stimuli`, `Reaction to pain stimuli` (also called reaction to nociceptive stimuli); optomotoricity parameters: `Position of bulbi`, `Motility of bulbi`, `Pupillary diameter`, `Pupillary reaction to light`; parameters of body motility: `Body posture`, `Muscle tone`, `Pyramidal signs`; vegetative parameters: `Respiration rate`, `Heart rate`, `Systolic blood pressure`, `Diastolic blood pressure`, `Body temperature`.

For illustration, we list the values of some clinical attributes: `Vigilance` (0 - coma, 1 - sopor, 2 - somnolence); `Reactions to pain stimuli` (0 - no motor reaction, 1 - rest of extension of upper and lower extremities, 2 - extension of upper and lower extremities, 3 - flexion of upper and extension of lower extremities, 4 - rest of non-finalized defense reaction, 5 - delayed nonpurposeful defense reaction, 6 - prompt finalized defense reaction); `Body posture` (0 - flaccid posture, 1 - rest of extension of upper and lower limbs, 2 - extension of upper and lower limbs, 3 - flexion of upper and extension of lower limbs, 4 - mass movements of upper limbs and extended position of lower limbs, 4 - mass movements of upper limbs and extension trend in lower limbs, 5 - mass movements and rotations). Note that since two values of `Body posture` are very hard to be distinguished, they were merged into a single value (value 4). Such merging of values occurred also in some other attributes (see Appendix, Table 8.A.1).

8.3 INDUCTION OF DECISION TREES

In supervised machine learning, a set of examples with known classifications is given. An example is described by an outcome (class) and the values of a fixed collection of parameters (attributes). Each attribute can either have a finite set of values (discrete attribute) or take real numbers as values (continuous attribute). For instance, in our prediction problem the examples are patient records that comprise both continues (e.g., `Age`) and discrete attributes (e.g., `GCS`).

Machine learning tools [Quinlan, 1986, Michie et al., 1994] have been applied in a variety of medical domains to help to solve diagnostic and prognostic problems [Kononenko and Kukar, 1995]. These tools enable the induction of diagnostic and prognostic knowledge in the form of rules or decision trees.

In this study, the program Magnus Assistant [Mladenić, 1990] was used to construct decision trees. Magnus Assistant is a descendant of the program Assistant [Cestnik et al., 1987] and belongs to the ID3 family of systems for top-down induction of decision trees [Quinlan, 1986]. The system recursively builds a binary decision tree. The nodes of the tree correspond to attributes, arcs correspond to values or sets/intervals of values of attributes, and leaves (terminal nodes) correspond to prognostic classes. In each recursive step of the decision tree construction, an attribute is selected and a subtree is built. Algorithm 8.1 is an outline of the Magnus Assistant algorithm.

At each recursion step, the selection of the best attribute is based on the informativity of the attribute [Quinlan, 1986] aimed at minimizing the expected number of tests needed for the classification of new cases. Tree construction is thus heuristically guided by choosing the most informative attribute at the current node of a partially built tree. *Informativity* (usually referred to as *information gain*) measures the information gained by partitioning a set of

```
if all examples belong to the same class then
    this node becomes a leaf labeled with the class of examples
else
    if any of the pre-pruning criteria is satisfied then
        this node becomes a leaf labeled with the majority class of examples
    else
        for the next node select the best attribute (which minimizes the
            expected entropy of the training set)
        split the set of examples in the node into disjoint subsets according
            to binarized values of the attribute
        recursively repeat the whole algorithm for each subset
    end if
end if
```

Algorithm 8.1 The Magnus Assistant algorithm.

examples according to the values of the attribute A:

$$info(A,E) = entropy(E) - \sum_{v} p_v(E) \times entropy(E_v)$$

In the above formula, E denotes the set of examples on the current node of the decision tree, $p_v(E)$ denotes the probability of attribute value v in example set E, and E_v denotes the subset of examples for which attribute A has value v. The summation is over all the values of attribute A.

The definition of *entropy* is taken from the information theory and in our case it can be described as the average amount of information needed to identify the class of an example taken from the set of *Examples*:

$$entropy(E) = \sum_{c} p_c(E) \times \log_2 p_c(E)$$

In the above formula, $p_c(E)$ stands for the probability of class c in a set of examples E and is usually calculated as the proportion of examples belonging to class c. The summation is over all the classes.

Magnus Assistant incorporates also mechanisms for dealing with noisy data (i.e., data comprising errors). The main idea underlying this mechanism is to prune a decision tree [Cestnik et al., 1987] in order to avoid overfitting the dataset of examples which may be erroneous. Magnus Assistant uses two kinds of tree pruning techniques to deal with noisy data: post-pruning and pre-pruning. Post-pruning is used after the tree induction to substitute some of the subtrees with terminal nodes (leaves). In post-pruning, the expected quality (predicted classification accuracy) of each internal node is compared with the expected quality of its subtrees to decide whether to prune the subtrees. On the other hand, pre-pruning is used during tree induction and enables noise handling by means of stopping the generation of a subtree and making a leaf node labeled with the majority class of the current examples. There are three pre-pruning criteria used by the above algorithm: (1) stop if the number of examples in the current node is smaller than the threshold value; (2) stop if the majority class in the current example set has a higher probability than the threshold probability (the so-called minimal weight threshold); (3) stop if the informativity of the best attribute is below the threshold value. Threshold values for all the three pre-pruning parameters are set by the user and should reflect the expected level of noise in the data.

To classify a new case, a path from the root of the tree is selected on the basis of the values of attributes of the new patient to be classified. In this way, for a given patient record, the path leads to a leaf which assigns a class that labels the leaf. The selected path may be viewed as a generalization of the specific patient record for which the prediction is being determined. If a leaf is labeled with more than one class, each with the probability of class prediction, then the class with the highest probability is selected for the classification of a new case.

The entire decision tree reflects the detected regularities in the data, describing the properties that are characteristic for subsets of examples belonging to subtrees. The ordering of attributes (from the root towards the leaves of the tree) reflects also the importance of attributes for the outcome class in the leaf. The measure of attribute informativity is the selected measure of importance.

8.4 OUTCOME PREDICTION FOR TWO OUTCOME CLASSES

The main goal of these experiments was to predict the outcome six months after a severe head injury based on clinical findings on admission, and to study the prognostic values of the attributes. For this purpose, the Magnus Assistant program was used. Experiments were done by employing different tree pruning parameters. The two decision trees reported in this section were generated by Magnus Assistant using pre-pruning (minimal weight threshold = 40%).

Due to the small number of training examples available (38), we first decided to reduce the number of attributes to three only (either `GCS` or `BSS`, `CT score`, and `Age`) and the number of outcome categories to two: `GOS1`, `GOS2` and `GOS3` were grouped into the `Bad outcome` category, and `GOS4` and `GOS5` into the `Good outcome` category.

8.4.1 Experiments using GCS, CT score and Age

In this experiment, GCS, CT score and Age were the only attributes used. The decision tree induced by Magnus Assistant is shown in Figure 8.1.

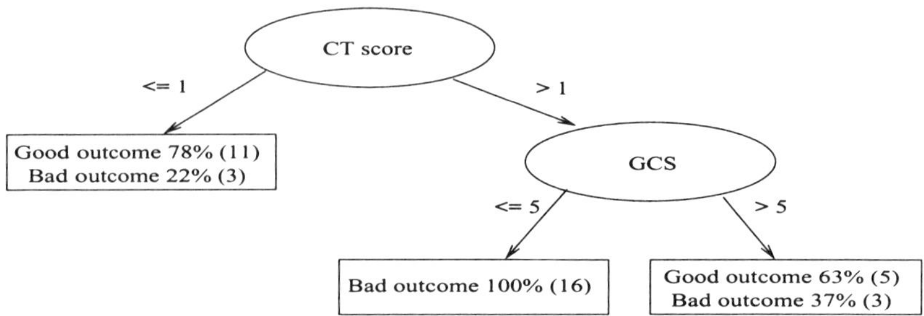

Figure 8.1 Decision tree generated with three attributes (GCS, CT score, Age) and two outcome classes (Bad, Good). The percentages indicate the probabilities of class assignment, and the numbers in parentheses the number of patients in each outcome class.

CT score was selected by Magnus Assistant as the most informative attribute among the three attributes used. It was therefore used in the root of the tree, and the patients were split into two subsets, according to CT score values. Eleven out of 14 patients with CT score 0 or 1 had a good outcome. Patients with CT score > 1 were separated according to GCS. All the 16 patients with GCS ≤ 5 had a bad outcome. Patients with a higher GCS had better, but still uncertain outcomes.

In this decision tree only 16 patients out of 38 are located in the leaf with only one outcome category and 22 patients belong to the leaves with both outcome categories. The impurity of the leaves is unfavorable. When a tree is used for classification, such leaves provide the classification as if the leaves were labeled with the most probable class, according to the probability of this class in the leaf.

In order to test the prognostic accuracy of the induced decision tree, we used the so-called *leave-one-out method*: the outcomes predicted by decision trees generated from the data of 37 patients were compared with the actual outcome of the patient that was eliminated from the training set of examples. Thirty-eight such tests were made. The proportion of correct classifications represents the measure of prognostic accuracy. Decision trees using the selected three parameters and two outcome classes had a relatively high prognostic accuracy (82%).

8.4.2 *Experiments using BSS, CT score and Age*

In these experiments, BSS was used instead of GCS. The decision tree generated with three attributes (BSS, CT score and Age) and two outcome classes (Bad and Good) is shown in Figure 8.2.

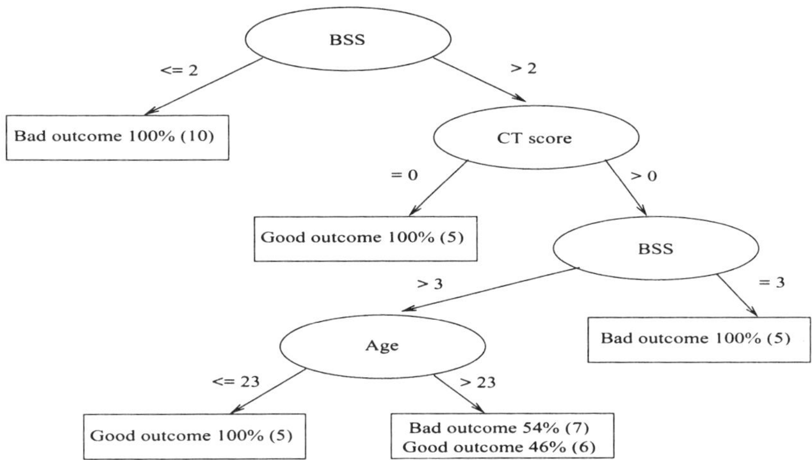

Figure 8.2 Decision tree generated with three attributes (BSS, CT score, Age) and two outcome classes (Bad, Good).

The splitting of the decision tree root is based on BSS which is the most informative attribute among the three attributes used. All the 10 patients with the most severe brainstem dysfunctions (values $\leq$ 2: 1 - BS2 and 2 - BS1) died. The other 28 patients were further separated according to CT score. Five patients with CT score 0 had good outcomes, whereas patients with CT abnormalities had worse outcomes, and were further separated according to BSS. All five patients with the most severe midbrain syndrome (value 3 - MS4) died. Patients with a less severe brainstem dysfunction (values > 3: MS3, MS2b, MS2a) were further separated according to Age: five patients with Age $\leq$ 23 had good outcomes. The outcome of older patients was worse and more uncertain.

In this decision tree, 25 patients (out of 38) are located in the leaves with only one outcome category and 13 patients belong to the leaf with both outcome categories.

The decision trees induced in this experiment again have a relatively high prognostic accuracy (79%) when tested by the leave-one-out method.

8.4.3 Analysis of results

These experiments show that induced decision trees are useful for the analysis of the importance of clinical parameters and their combinations for the prediction of the outcome. BSS has the highest informativity. It is followed by the sum of CT abnormalities. Next is the GCS score, and the last is the age of patients. Similar observations were discussed in other studies [Benzer et al., 1987, Marosi et al., 1991, Rumpl et al., 1991]. Moreover, nonparametric correlation tests applied on the same dataset of 38 patients [Pilih et al., 1995] also show that BSS has the highest correlation value, followed by GCS, CT score and the age of patients.

In the decision trees, where outcome prediction is based on BSS, 25 out of 38 patients (66%) are in the leaves with only one outcome class (good or bad). On the other hand, in the decision trees where outcome prediction is based on GCS there are only 16 out of 38 patients (42%) in the leaves with a single class outcome. We believe that an important factor influencing the impurity of leaves of GCS-based decision trees is a consequence of the poor discrimination of GCS. Other authors [Benzer et al., 1987, Marosi et al., 1991, Rumpl et al., 1991] share this opinion. Marosi and co-authors [Marosi et al., 1991] suggested to supplement the GCS data with the information about the pupillary diameter and reaction to light, as well as the position and motility of bulbi. These (and some other) data are already included in the classification of BSS, which (in our opinion) leads to the advantage of BSS over GCS.

The prognostic accuracy of decision trees based on BSS and GCS is similar: 79% and 82%, respectively. This result is similar to the result of Choi et al. [Choi et al., 1991] who analyzed 555 patients with severe head injury with similar methods and have reported about 77.7% of correct prognoses. However, the similar amount of correct predictions based on BSS and GCS is somewhat unexpected since there is a larger amount of pure predictions in the leaves of decision trees based on BSS. This is probably mostly due to the limited number of outcome classes (two classes only) used for this analysis. In part, this may also be due to the small number of patients in our study, where a single patient may significantly influence the structure of the decision tree.

8.5 OUTCOME PREDICTION FOR FIVE OUTCOME CLASSES

These experiments were mainly designed to test whether it is possible to replace the complex BSS parameter with the basic clinical parameters that are used for BSS estimation.

8.5.1 Experiments using basic clinical signs

In the first experiment only the basic clinical attributes were used (`BSS` was not used). The decision tree, generated by Magnus Assistant using pre-pruning (minimal weight threshold = 20%), is shown in Figure 8.3.

The attribute `Reaction to pain stimuli` is used in the root of the decision tree since it has the highest informativity. According to this attribute, patients are divided into two subgroups: the patients with poor or no motor reaction (values 1 and 0) and the others with a better reaction (values 2 or more). Patients in the first left branch were further separated according to `Heart rate`. Those with a lower heart rate (60 beats/minute or less) had a good outcome (one patient), whereas patients with `Heart rate` > 60 mostly died: out of 16 patients 15 died (`GOS1`) and one survived (`GOS5`). The patients with better motor reactions to pain (values 2 or more) in the first right branch of the tree (21 patients) were further separated on the basis of the attribute `Systolic blood pressure`. The attribute `Respiration rate` was used in the next node of the tree. Patients with the respiration rate up to normal (16 respirations/minute or less) all survived (most with a good outcome and one severely disabled). The patients with higher respiration rates were separated in the next node according to the position of the body. The patients who showed mass movements and rotations had better outcomes than the others.

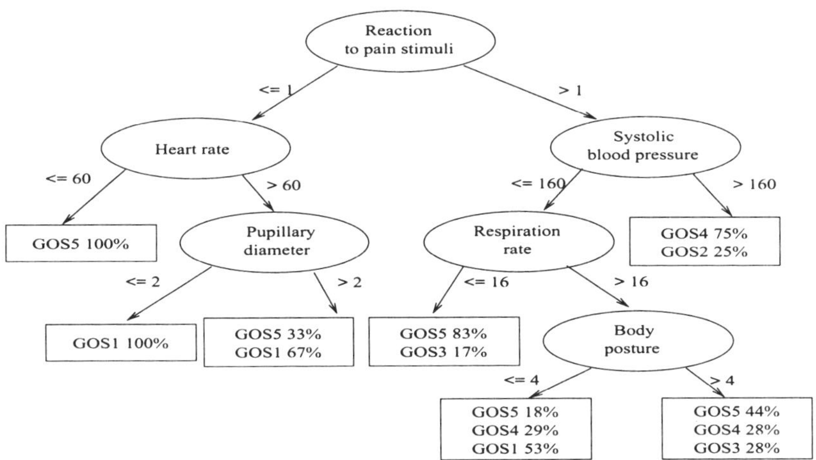

Figure 8.3 Decision tree generated with basic clinical attributes and five outcome categories.

8.5.2 Experiments using basic clinical signs and BSS

In the second experiment, `BSS` was used in addition to the basic clinical attributes. Unexpectedly, the generated decision tree was identical to the one generated without using `BSS`. Therefore, Figure 8.3 represents also the decision tree generated in this experiment.

When testing the informativity of the basic clinical attributes and `BSS`, `BSS` and `Reaction to pain stimuli` turned out to have an equal information score. This is the reason why the structure of the decision tree does not change if the root node `Reaction to pain stimuli` is replaced by `BSS`. However in this case, the left and right arcs leading from the root `BSS` are labeled by values ≤ 2 and > 2, respectively.

8.6 BRAINSTEM SYNDROME DETERMINATION

As shown in Sections 8.4 and 8.5, brainstem syndromes (`BSS`), as well as `Reaction to pain stimuli` are the most important for outcome prediction. However, it is sometimes difficult to determine `BSS` because of the numerous clinical signs that define them. In our study it also occurred that different clinical signs had values that belong to different brainstem syndromes. In such a situation it is not straightforward how to determine the actual `BSS`. Moreover, the searching for all the clinical signs which are needed for a formally complete determination of `BSS` (see Table 8.A.1 in the appendix) is also time consuming and is problematic in urgent situations at the admission of heavily injured patients when time, measured in minutes, is one of the most decisive factors for the outcome. Consequently, the experiments described in this section were intended to modify `BSS` determination by possibly reducing the present complex set of signs listed in Table 8.A.1 to the most essential (informative) ones for `BSS` determination, when the available time is limited.

To achieve this goal, two experiments for determining `BSS` were designed: the first one using the actual patient data for decision tree construction, and the second by generating training examples from the data about the main neurological signs of Table 8.A.1. The two decision trees for determining `BSS` were induced by Magnus Assistant using pre-pruning (minimal weight threshold = 20%).

8.6.1 BSS determination from patient data

This experiment was based on the available data of 38 patients and the `BSS` determination of the trauma surgeon, specially trained in head trauma. The induced decision tree for `BSS` determination is shown in Figure 8.4. Note that, for the reason of compactness, the tree has been rewritten by merging some of the branches.

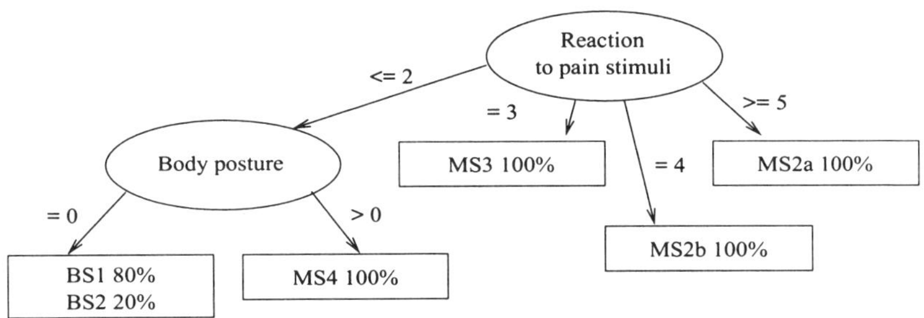

Figure 8.4 Decision tree for BSS determination using the actual patient data.

The analysis suggests that `Reaction to pain stimuli` and `Body posture` have the highest informative values for `BSS` determination. So both of them are used in the induced decision tree. The attribute `Reaction to pain stimuli` represents the root of the tree. It separates patients into midbrain syndromes `MS2a`, `MS2b` and `MS3`. The other patients are separated according to `Body posture` into `MS4` and into a common category comprising both bulbar syndromes `BS1` and `BS2`.

8.6.2 BSS determination from main neurological signs

In this experiment, Table 8.A.1 served as a source of training examples for `BSS` determination from the data about the main neurological signs determining `BSS` [Gerstenbrand et al., 1990]. Seven training examples were generated from Table 8.A.1, one for each brainstem syndrome (an example is a table column). The induced decision tree is shown in Figure 8.5. Again, the tree has been rewritten by merging some of the branches in order to get a simpler tree representation.

The attribute `Reaction to pain stimuli` again turns out to be the most important parameter for determining the brainstem syndromes. The induced decision tree determines both bulbar syndromes (`BS1` and `BS2`) and the midbrain syndrome 4 (`MS4`) solely on the basis of `Reaction to pain stimuli`. Less severely affected patients are further separated on the basis of `Vigilance`. Patients that show somnolence on admission are classified as `MS1`, and those with sopor as `MS2a`. For the patients with coma, `Reaction to pain stimuli` was considered again in order to distinguish between `MS2b` and `MS3`.

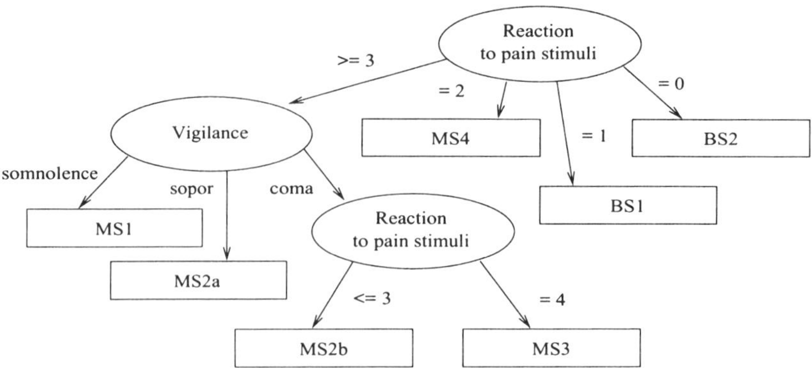

Figure 8.5 Decision tree for BSS determination from main neurological signs.

8.6.3 *Analysis of results*

The comparison of BSS determination using the two trees in Figures 8.4 and 8.5 shows some differences. The same syndrome was determined in 33 out of 38 patients (87%) using the actual patient data for tree construction, and in 23 out of 38 patients (61%) when the main neurological signs were used for tree construction. This speaks in favor of the decision tree in Figure 8.4 despite the fact that this decision tree (constructed from the actual patient data) joins BS1 and BS2 into a joint bulbar syndrome category (BS1 and BS2).

Most differences in decisions made by the two decision trees occur in the determination of the bulbar syndromes. In eight cases where the trauma surgeon determined BS1, the decision tree in Figure 8.5 proposes a more severe affection BS2. For three patients with MS2a evaluated by the trauma surgeon, the decision tree in Figure 8.5 proposes MS2b. For two other patients both trees determine BS2 instead of MS4. The analysis shows that in all the instances where the differences in classifications occur, the brainstem syndromes determined by decision trees are more severe than the ones determined conventionally using Table 8.A.1, despite the fact that also the conventional BSS assignment is based on the same knowledge source.

8.7 SUMMARY

This chapter presents an application of decision tree induction to the problem of the outcome prediction six months after a severe head injury. The study shows that induced decision trees are useful for the analysis of the importance of clinical parameters and of their combinations for the prediction of the outcome. Among the parameters studied, the brainstem syndromes (BSS) turn out to be the most informative. However, the experiment in which BSS was replaced by the basic clinical attributes from which BSS is estimated has shown that BSS can successfully be replaced by Reaction to pain stimuli in the specific conditions of this experiment.

The use of decision tree induction methods turns out to be useful for improving the insight into the complex problem of severe head injury. The nature of the traumatic brain disease [Grčević, 1988], where different factors influence the course of recovery, makes the problem very difficult. By using the attributes available upon admission of patients included in this study, the precision level of about 80% can be achieved, when considering two outcome classes. Results of previous studies, based on often much larger groups of patients than ours, have also almost all reached a similar prediction accuracy. It seems that this is the approximate prediction accuracy of the data available on admission of patients with severe head injury. The rest of the outcome variability depends on the influence of factors guiding the course of the traumatic brain disease [Grčević, 1988]. Only the consideration of these factors by following the course of recovery of patients after severe head injury can complete the information needed to increase the reliability of the outcome prediction.

In further work, new cases will be added to the patient record database. The experiments in outcome prediction using the enlarged dataset will be repeated and the results compared. We are also planning to provide new training examples for the BSS estimation experiments in order to derive simple rules for fast BSS determination, that can, despite their simplicity, provide for more reliable diagnosis in time limiting conditions on admission to a hospital.

Acknowledgments

This work was funded by the Ministry of Science and Technology of Slovenia.

References

Benzer, A., Mitterschiffthaler, G., Prugger, M., and Rumpl, E. (1987). Innsbruck Coma Scale versus Glasgow Coma Scale. *Notfallmedizin*, 13:41–50.

Braakman, R. (1992). Early prediction of outcome in severe head injury. *Acta Neurochir.*, 116:161–163

Cestnik, B., Kononenko, I., and Bratko, I. (1997). ASSISTANT 86: A knowledge elicitation tool for sophisticated users. In Bratko, I., Lavrač, N., editors, *Progress in Machine Learning*, pages 31–45. Sigma Press, Wilmslow.

Choi, S.C., Muizelaar, J.P., Barnes, T.Y., et al. (1991). Prediction tree for severely head-injuried patients. *J. Neurosurg.*, 75:251–255.

Gerstenbrand, F. and Lücking, C. (1970). Die akuten traumatischen Hirnstammschaden. *Arch. Psychiat. Nervenkrankh.*, 213:264–281.

Gerstenbrand, F. and Rumpl, E. (1983). Das prolongierte Mittelhirnsyndrom traumatischer Genese. In Neumärker, K.J., editor, *Hirnstammläsionen. Neurologische, psychopatologische, morphologische, neurophysiologische and computertomographische Aspekte*, pages 236–248. Hirzel, Leipzig.

Gerstenbrand, F., Saltuari, L., Kofler, M., and Formisano, R. (1990) Clinical evaluation of severe head injury. *Neurologija*, 39: Suppl. 1:71–88.

Gerstenbrand, F. and Rumpl, E. (1992). Apallisches Syndrom. In Hornbostel, H., Kaufmann, W. and Siegenthaler, editors, (1992). *Innere Medizin in Praxis und Klinik*, pages 763–8. Georg Thieme Verlag, Stuttgart, New York.

Grčević, N. (1988). Head injury. The concept of inner cerebral trauma. *Scand. J. Rehab. Med.*, Suppl. 17:25–31.

Jennett, B. and Bond, M. (1975). Assessment of outcome after severe brain damage. *Lancet*, 1:480–487.

Kononenko, I. and Kukar, M. (1995) Machine learning for medical diagnosis. In Lavrač, N., editor, *Computer Aided Data Analysis in Medicine*, pages 9–30. IJS Scientific Publishing, Ljubljana.

Marosi, M.J., Gerstenbrand, F., Luef, G.J., Zimmermann, S., and Schmutzhard, E. (1991). Innsbruck coma rating scale. *Lancet*, 337:1043.

Michie, D., Spiegelhalter, D.J., and Taylor, C.C., editors, (1994). *Machine Learning, Neural and Statistical Classification.* Ellis Horwood, Chichester.

Mladenić, D. (1990). *The learning system Magnus Assistant.* BSc Thesis. Faculty of Computer and Information Sciences, University of Ljubljana (in Slovenian).

Pilih, I.A., Mladenić, D., Lavrač, N., and Prevec, T.S. Using decision trees to predict the outcome after a severe head injury. In Lavrač, N., editor, *Computer Aided Data Analysis in Medicine*, pages 221–233, IJS Scientific Publishing, Ljubljana (in Slovene).

Pilih, I.A., Mladenić, D., Lavrač, N., and Prevec, T.S. (1996) Data analysis of patients with severe head injury: Outcome prediction with decision trees. In Lavrač, N., Keravnou, E., and Zupan, B., editors, ECAI-96 Workshop Proceedings *Intelligent Data Analysis in Medicine and Pharmacology*, pages 69–72.

Quinlan, J.R. (1986) Induction of decision trees. *Machine Learning*, 1:81–106.

Rumpl, E., Gulle, H.D., Stadler, C., Millonig, H., and Prugger, M. (1991). Die Innsbrucker Koma-Skala beim schweren Schädel-Hirn-Trauma. *Intenziv- und Notfallbehandlung*, 16:7–13.

Teasdale, G. and Jennett, B. (1974). Assessment of coma and impaired consciousness: A practical scale. *Lancet*, 2:81–84.

Vollmer, D.G. (1993) Prognosis and outcome of severe head injury. In Cooper, P.R., editor, *Head injury*, 3rd edition, pages 553–581, Williams & Wilkins, Baltimore.

Appendix: Clinical characteristics of brainstem syndromes

Table 8.A.1 presents seven brainstem syndromes described in terms of basic clinical signs. This table, taken from [Gerstenbrand et al., 1990], is slightly modified and rewritten for the needs of our study: for instance, attribute values that are hard to be distinguished are merged into a single value, which increases the robustness and simplicity of induced trees.

Table 8.A.1 Clinical characteristics of brainstem syndromes.

	7 - MS1	6 - MS2a	5 - MS2b	4 - MS3	3 - MS4	2 - BS1	1 - BS2
Vigilance	2 somno.	1 sopor	0 coma	0 coma	0 coma	0 coma	0 coma
Reaction to acoust. stimuli	1 slightly delayed	0	0	0	0	0	0
Reaction to pain stimuli	6 prompt finaliz. defence reaction	5 delayed non purpose. defence reaction	4 rest of a non finaliz. defence reaction	3 flexion of upper extens. of lower limbs	2 ext. of upper and lower limbs	1 rest of extens. of upper and lower limbs	0 no
Position of bulbi	2 normal	1 slight. diverg.	0 diverg.	0 fixed diverg.	0 fixed diverg.	0 fixed diverg.	0 fixed diverg.
Motility of bulbi	3 swaying	2 oscil.	1 disconj.	0 no	0 no	0 no	0 no
Pupillary diameter	3 normal	3 normal	3 normal	2 small	2 small	1 very large	0 large
Pup. reac. to light	2 normal	2 normal	2 normal	1 weak	1 weak	1 weak	0 no
Body posture	5 mass movem. and rotat.	4 mass movem. of upper, extens. trend in lower limbs	4 mass movem. of upper, extended position of lower limbs	3 flexion of upper, extens. of lower limbs	2 extens. of upper and lower limbs	1 rest of extens. of upper and lower limbs	0 flaccid posture
Muscle tone	4 normal	3 slight. incr. in lower limbs	3 incr. in lower limbs	1 incr.	2 mark. incr.	1 slight. incr.	0 flaccid
Respir. rate	4 normal	4 normal	3 Cheyne Stokes	2 rapid regular hyper-ventil.	2 regular hyper-ventil.	1 ataxic	0 no
Heart rate	1 slight. incr	3 normal	1 incr.	1 incr.	2 mark. incr.	1 incr.	0 decr.
Blood pressure	1 normal	1 normal	1 normal	2 slight. incr.	2 incr.	1 normal	0 decr.
Body temp.	3 normal	3 normal	1 slight. incr.	1 incr.	2 mark. incr.	1 incr.	0 decr.

9 DEMENTIA SCREENING WITH MACHINE LEARNING METHODS

William R. Shankle,
Subramani Mani,
Michael J. Pazzani,
and Padhraic Smyth

Abstract: Machine learning algorithms were applied to an electronic patient database generated by the UC Irvine Alzheimer's clinic to learn the simplest and most accurate patient parameters that would discriminate 244 very mildly demented from 198 normally aging subjects. Attributes included age, sex and education plus responses to the Functional Activities Questionnaire, the Mini-Mental Status and Blessed Orientation, Memory and Concentration tests. The machine learning algorithms included decision tree learners (C4.5, CART), rule inducers (C4.5Rules, FOCL) and naive Bayes. Stepwise logistic regression was used to compare results. The sample was randomly split into training and testing sets, and the results were validated over 30 runs. Although the Functional Activities Questionnaire has been used since 1980, the machine learning algorithms were the first to identify that a single attribute, measuring forgetfulness, equaled or exceeded the accuracy of any other scoring method of this test. Post hoc inspection of the odds ratios obtained by stepwise logistic regression confirmed this finding. The application of machine learning has identified an extremely simple, yet accurate screen for very mild dementia.

9.1 INTRODUCTION

With the advent of Electronic Medical Records (EMR) the size of patient databases has greatly increased. Traditional methods are not sufficient to analyze and interpret the enormous amounts of data being generated. Machine learning (**ML**) techniques can be valuable in this context for extracting useful information from large medical data sets. In this chapter, we apply ML methods to the detection of the earliest stages of dementia due to Alzheimer's disease and other causes.

Machine learning can generate classification rules where the data include the known classification of each case. The application of ML methods in the domain of medicine has been relatively infrequent, partly because of past difficulties in accessing medical data electronically. Artificial intelligence approaches to medicine started with knowledge-based systems, constructed from knowledge provided by human experts, not data. Beginning with the expert systems of the seventies (MYCIN [Shortliffe, 1976], PUFF [Aikins et al., 1982]), followed by Bayesian systems of the late eighties and early nineties (ACORN [Wyatt, 1989], PATHFINDER [Heckerman et al., 1992]), these knowledge-based systems generated much enthusiasm. But there are very few such actual systems in routine clinical use. Another approach starting in the mid eighties sought to make use of real data and a domain model for knowledge acquisition and rule learning [Cestnik et al., 1987, Michalski et al., 1986, Lavrač and Mozetič, 1992]. KARDIO [Bratko et al., 1989] is an expert system for evaluation of electrocardiograms based on this approach. With increasing availability of electronic medical records, machine learning has the potential to become a valuable adjunct to clinical decision-making. There has been some recent effort in this direction [Ohmann et al., 1995].

Dementia is defined as multiple cognitive impairments with loss of related functional skills without altered consciousness. A simple, unobtrusive method for detecting dementia early in the disease's course would help get patients to seek early evaluation and treatment, resulting most probably in preserving the existing quality of life and reducing the financial burden to family and health care providers. The Agency for Health Care Policy Research (**AHCPR**) clinical practice guidelines for the assessment and recognition of Alzheimer's disease and related disorders [Williams and Costa, 1995] recommends two simple tests, the Functional Activities Questionnaire (**FAQ** [Pfeffer et al., 1982]), and the six-item Blessed Orientation, Memory and Concentration test (**BOMC** [Fillenbaum et al., 1987]), to screen for dementia after excluding delirium and depression. We recently reported that the use of ML methods in conjunction with the FAQ and the BOMC markedly improved sensitivity in detecting dementia in a sample of 609 normal, cognitively impaired, and demented subjects when compared with published scoring criteria [Shankle et al., 1996].

In this chapter, we focus on discriminating the effects of normal aging on cognition from the very early stages of dementia because early detection is potentially very important for improving quality of life, and reducing total health care costs to family and society. To do this, we used the AHCPR-recommended screening instrument, the FAQ, plus the Folstein Mini-Mental Status Exam [Folstein et al., 1975] and two items from the BOMC not included in the MMSE (we henceforth use **MMSEBOMC** to denote this particular combination of tests) in conjunction with several ML methods and stepwise logistic regression, and compared these results to those using published scoring criteria for the same set of data from the same set of subjects. Other items of the BOMC did not need to be considered in addition to the MMSE since the rest of the BOMC is a subset of the MMSE. See Section 9.2 for a description of these tests.

9.2 DESCRIPTION OF THE DATA SET

9.2.1 Sample description

The total sample consisted of the initial visits of 198 cognitively normal and 244 cognitively impaired or very mildly demented (Clinical Dementia Rating Stage ≤ 0.5) subjects seen at the University of California, Irvine Alzheimer's Disease Research Center (ADRC). Patients received a complete diagnostic evaluation consisting of patient and caregiver interviews, general physical and neurological exam, two hours of cognitive testing including the CERAD [Welsh et al., 1994] neuropsychological battery and other selected tests, routine laboratory testing for memory loss, and magnetic resonance neuroimaging with or without single photon emission with computed tomography. Control subjects were either community volunteers or unaffected spouses of patients, and received an abbreviated, 45 minute version of the patient cognitive battery, which consisted of the CERAD plus measures of activities of daily living. They did not receive a medical exam, laboratory testing or neuroimaging unless cognitive or functional testing suggested an impairment. The number of subjects available for the various analyses varied somewhat because of missing data. The sample sizes for each screening test appears in Table 9.1.

9.2.2 Classification of dementia status

The diagnosis of dementia status, using DSM-IV criteria [DSM-IV, 1994], was based on a review of all the data by the neurologist and neuropsychologist during their diagnostic review session. Each subject was categorized as ei-

Table 9.1 Characteristics of the UCI ADRC Sample of this study.

Attribute	Normal			Impaired			Total		
	N	M	SD	N	M	SD	N**	M	SD
Age*	196	67.2	11.8	278	68.2	10.9	474	67.6	11.3
% Female*	198	71	–	274	43	–	472	59	–
Yrs Education	140	15.0	2.7	274	15.3	3.2	414	15.2	3.0
FAQ	137	0.2	0.8	211	7.6	6.2	348	5.1	6.1
MMSE	198	29.2	0.9	227	24.8	5.5	425	26.6	4.8

* T-test for normal vs. impaired groups (unpaired samples with unequal variances) was significant at $P < 0.001$

** Sample size varies due to missing data

ther unimpaired, cognitively impaired but not meeting criteria for dementia, or demented. A classification of *dementia* required the presence of multiple cognitive impairments plus functional impairments resulting from the cognitive impairments in the absence of delirium or other non-organic etiologies such as major depression. They were also classified by dementia severity using standard criteria for the Clinical Dementia Rating Scale (**CDRS** [Morris, 1993]), in which 0 = normal, 0.5 = questionably or very mildly demented, and 1–5 indicate increasing severity of dementia. Control subjects showing cognitive impairment or very mild dementia (CDRS ≤ 0.5) were included in the cognitively impaired/very mildly demented sample, which we will refer to as the *impaired* group. Patients who tested normally were included in the cognitively normal sample; subjects with delirium were excluded from the analysis. Table 9.1 shows the sample characteristics.

9.2.3 FAQ and MMSEBOMC tests

The FAQ consists of ten questions about basic and more complex activities of daily life. The total score ranges from 0 (normal) to 30 (severely disabled). The answers to these questions were extracted from the UCI ADRC relational database of over 1,200 variables per subject-visit to compute the FAQ total and item scores. The AHCPR recommends using total FAQ scores of 9 or higher for detecting impairment. [Pfeffer et al., 1982] found a total FAQ score of 5 or higher to be most sensitive as a second stage screen in discriminating normal vs. questionably demented subjects. We examined the sensitivity and specificity of total FAQ scores from 1 to 30 without ML methods. With ML methods, we used age, sex, education, and all FAQ attributes with and without the FAQ total score. The description for how these runs were performed is in the machine learning methods section.

The MMSEBOMC consists of 11 questions from the MMSE regarding orientation for time and place, registration, attention, short-term recall, language, and drawing, plus two questions from the BOMC test (recall of an address and number of trials to correctly repeat the address twice), which we were added because of their potential sensitivity in detecting early dementia. To avoid overfitting the data, we held the proportion of attributes relative to group sample size to about 10% by aggregating the individual MMSE attributes reflecting short-term recall, orientation to time, and orientation to place into three aggregate attributes respectively. The MMSEBOMC attributes therefore consisted of the three MMSE aggregate attributes, individual MMSE attributes reflecting registration, attention and drawing, and the two BOMC attributes. These attributes plus age, sex and education were used with ML methods to classify normal and impaired subject samples. The MMSE ranges from 0 (severely impaired) to 30 (no impairment). The occurrence of dementia increases with advancing age and decreases with increasing educational level. Depending upon a subject's age and education, a total MMSE score of 24 or higher is used to classify a subject as normal [Oconnor et al., 1989, Crum et al., 1993]. We examined the sensitivity and specificity of total MMSE scores from 1 to 30 without ML methods.

9.3 METHODS

9.3.1 Specific algorithms

We concentrated on decision tree learners, rule learners and the naive Bayesian classifier. Decision trees and rules generate clear descriptions of how the ML method arrives at a particular classification. The naive Bayesian classifier was included for comparison purposes. MLC++ (Machine Learning in C++) is a software package developed at Stanford University [Kohavi et al., 1994] which implements commonly used machine learning algorithms. It also provides standardized methods of running experiments using these algorithms. C4.5 is a decision tree generator and C4.5Rules produces if-then rules from the decision tree [Quinlan, 1993]. Naive Bayes is a classifier based on Bayes Rule. Even though it makes the assumption that the attributes are conditionally independent of each other given the class, it is a robust classifier and serves as a good comparison in terms of accuracy for evaluating other algorithms [Duda and Hart, 1973]. FOCL [Pazzani and Kibler, 1992] is a concept learner which can incorporate a user provided knowledge of two types. First, when provided with a guideline or protocol directly, FOCL has the capacity for revision if the guidelines produce better classification rules than that produced from exploration of the data. Second, FOCL can accept information on each nominal variable indicating which values of the variable increase the probability of belonging to a class (such as impaired) and information on each continuous variable on whether higher or lower values of the variable increases the probability of belonging to a class. We call this, "constrained FOCL", in the experimental results. FOCL can also learn from the data only, without an initial input of constraints or guidelines. We call this, "unconstrained FOCL", in the experimental results. CART [Breiman et al., 1984] is a classifier which uses a tree-growing algorithm that minimizes the standard error of the classification accuracy based on a particular tree-growing method applied to a series of training subsamples. We used Caruana and Buntine's implementation of CART [Buntine and Caruana, 1992] (the "IND" package), and ran CART 10 times on randomly selected 2/3 training sets and 1/3 testing sets. For each training set, CART built a classification tree where the size of the tree was chosen based on cross-validation accuracy on this training set. The test accuracy of the chosen tree was then evaluated on the unseen test set.

9.3.2 Treatment of missing data

We used each ML algorithm's particular approach for handling missing data. In C4.5 missing attributes are assigned to both branches of the decision node, and the average of the classification accuracy is used for these cases. In the naive Bayesian classifier, missing values are ignored in the estimation of probabilities. In FOCL, any test on a missing value is treated as false. Therefore, it attempts to learn a set of rules that tolerates missing values in some variables. CART uses surrogate tests for missing values.

9.3.3 Generation of training and testing samples

The samples for the FAQ, and MMSEBOMC ML and stepwise logistic regression analyses mostly overlapped but the sizes differed due to different patterns of missing data. For the FAQ there were 348 instances—137 cognitively normal and 211 impaired; for the MMSEBOMC there were 425 instances—198 normal and 227 impaired. We cross-validated the analytical results in the following manner. The complete sample of each screening test was used to randomly assign subjects to either the training or testing set in a 2/3 to 1/3 ratio. This was done 30 times with the complete sample of subjects to generate 30 pairs of training and testing sets.

9.3.4 *ML analyses*

We ran experiments in which data from the FAQ and MMSEBOMC tests were used separately by each learning algorithm. The ML algorithms were trained on the training set and the resulting decision tree then classified the unseen testing set. The classification accuracy of each ML algorithm is hence the mean of the accuracies obtained for the 30 runs of the testing set. An example of one decision tree rule-set appears in Figure 9.1.

Rule 1: age $>$ 56 *and* job $>$ 2 $\Rightarrow$ class **impaired**

Rule 2: money $>$ 0 *and* forget $>$ 0 $\Rightarrow$ class **impaired**

Rule 3: gender $=$ 0 *and* age $>$ 56 *and* forget $>$ 0 $\Rightarrow$ class **impaired**

Rule 4: age $>$ 56 *and* age $\leq$ 64 *and* forget $>$ 0 $\Rightarrow$ class **impaired**

Rule 5: age $>$ 73 *and* forget $>$ 0 $\Rightarrow$ class **impaired**

Rule 6: forget $\leq$ 0 $\Rightarrow$ class **normal**

Rule 7: Default $\Rightarrow$ class **impaired**

Figure 9.1 A C4.5Rule set.

9.3.5 *Stepwise logistic regression analyses*

Data from the FAQ and the MMSEBOMC were separately regressed against dementia status in the following manner (demographic attributes were included in both regressions). We applied Stata's [Stata, 1993] stepwise logistic regression package (swlogis) to each randomly generated training set to obtain models consisting of the attributes' coefficients (odds ratios). We then tested each model's classification accuracy (swlogis was run with options *lstat, all*) with the testing set corresponding to the given training set. For the FAQ testing set, we assigned *lstat's* cutoff parameter value to be 39% for the proportion of normal cases; for the MMSEBOMC, the *lstat* cutoff parameter lstat was set to 47%. These cutoff values properly reflected the sample's prior probabilities. The means and standard deviations of the classification accuracy, sensitivity and specificity were computed for the 30 samples.

Using the same training and testing set pairs previously described, we also performed logistic regression using the FAQ's forgetting question as the only independent variable; this allowed a more direct comparison to the ML results obtained by CART. The means and standard deviations of the classification accuracy, sensitivity and specificity were computed for the 30 samples.

9.3.6 Nonsense rules

It is possible for ML methods to generate a rule which makes no domain sense, i.e., a "nonsense rule". The rule sets generated by the various ML methods were inspected for their clinical sense by an ADRC staff neurologist. After identifying the nonsense rules, we used FOCL to incorporate domain-specific knowledge that would prevent (constrain) such rules from occurring. We then compared classification performance of the constrained vs. unconstrained runs using FOCL to see how performance was affected. An example of a decision tree with a nonsense component follows:

```
forget > 0 (having trouble):
|   age <= 52 :
|   |   edulevel > 16 : normal (4.0)
|   |   edulevel <= 16 :
|   |   |   SHOP <= 0 (no trouble shopping): impaired (5.6)
|   |   |   SHOP > 0 (having trouble shopping): normal (2.0)
```

In this example, eight persons (5.6+2.0) were forgetful, 52 years old or younger, and had 16 or fewer years of education. Among them, those who could shop were classified as impaired while those who required assistance to shop were classified as normal: this is a *nonsense rule*, which arises because of insufficient examples covering the circumstances specified by the nonsense rule. As becomes apparent later, the appearance of such nonsense rules should encourage one to look for logical errors in the data, gather more data, constrain the ML method with domain-specific knowledge, or to search for a reduced rule-set using pruning techniques.

9.4 RESULTS

9.4.1 Machine learning results

We examined the sensitivity (probability of correctly classifying an impaired subject) and specificity (probability of correctly classifying a cognitively normal subject) for each ML run of the testing samples. For each run, the same statistics were also generated for the cutoff values of the total scores of the FAQ and MMSE without the use of ML methods, and for the stepwise logistic regression. Figures 9.2 and 9.3 respectively show the receiver operating characteristic (ROC) curves for the FAQ and MMSE total scores without ML methods, as well as the performance of the best results using various ML algorithms. In the ROC plot, the X-axis is the false alarm rate (1 minus specificity) and the Y-axis is the detection rate (sensitivity). Table 9.2 shows the classification results of each ML method and of published criteria for total MMSE and FAQ scores. A number of strategies were used to select an optimal decision tree for

Table 9.2 Sensitivity and Specificity of each Screening test by algorithm and published scoring criteria.

FAQ (Normal = 137, Impaired = 211)							
%	CART	C45	C45R	FOCL	NB	FAQ>8	FAQ>4
Ss	93	92	89	94	67	20	49
Sp	80	78	79	80	97	99	96
Ac	88	88	85	89	83	51	68

MMSEBOMC (Normal = 198, Impaired = 227)						
%	C45	C45R	FOCL	NB	MMSE>24	MMSE>27
Ss	77	70	79	66	30	62
Sp	80	86	70	87	100	81
Ac	79	77	75	75	63	71

Ss – Sensitivity, Sp – Specificity, Ac – Accuracy, C45R – C45Rules, and NB – naive Bayes

clinical use. We ordered pruned decision tree rule-sets by their frequency of occurrence across the different ML methods and runs. We examined the cross-validation procedure of CART, which selects the best single decision tree for a specified number of runs; we repeated this procedure 10 times. Each time, CART selected the same best decision tree.

With regard to possible biases between the normal and impaired samples, only age and sex showed statistically significant differences. However, the age difference between normal and impaired subjects was less than one year, which is not a clinically significant difference. Therefore, only sex showed a clinically and statistically significant difference, with a preponderance of females in the normal group. This possible bias can be evaluated by examining whether gender had a significant role in the ML or stepwise logistic regression results. Our analyses show that gender only affected the classification accuracy of the MMSEBOMC test. For the FAQ test, Figure 9.2 shows that the FAQ with ML methods outperformed the best of the published cutoff criteria for the total FAQ score. It is interesting to note that the cutoff score of 9 or higher, recommended by the AHCPR, has a considerably poorer sensitivity for discriminating

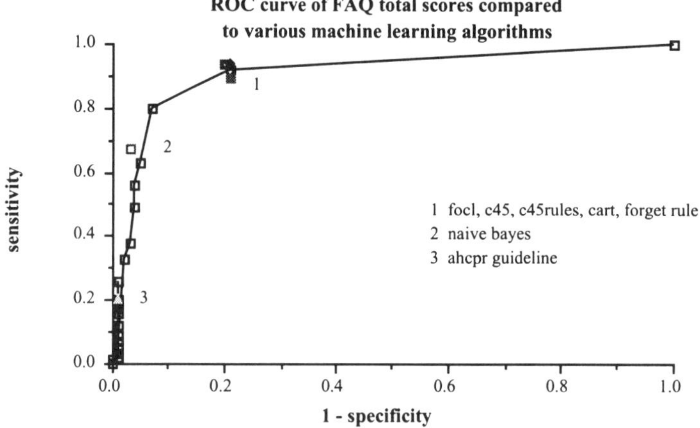

Figure 9.2 FAQ ROC.

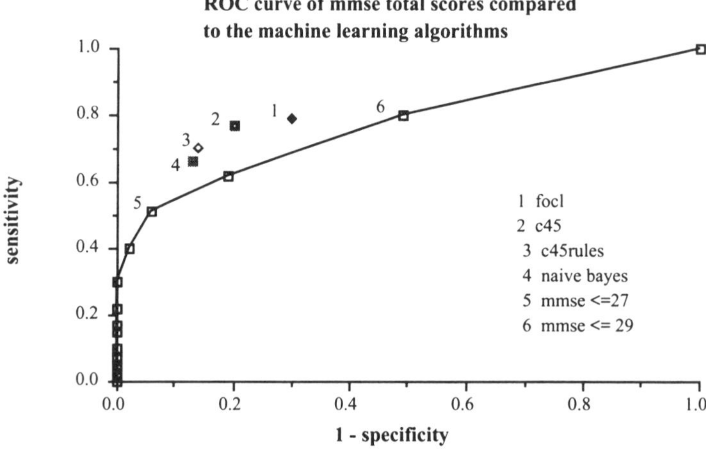

Figure 9.3 MMSE ROC.

very mildly demented from normal subjects (20%) than that obtained for the ML methods, FOCL, C4.5, C4.5Rules, and CART (93%).

One should also note that the number of questions needed to achieve accurate classification with ML methods is markedly reduced. In the case of CART, only one question is required (*"Do you require assistance remember-*

ing appointments, holidays, family occasions, or taking medications?"). For the MMSEBOMC test, Figure 9.3 shows that, when used with ML methods, classification accuracy is always higher than that obtained using any published cutoff values of the total MMSE score. Using constrained vs. unconstrained analysis of the data with FOCL, there did not appear to be a significant improvement in classification accuracy, but no nonsense rules were generated when constraining FOCL with domain-specific knowledge. Given the various search strategies for finding the best decision tree or rule-set for clinical use, all approaches converged on one main conclusion: the response to a single question from the FAQ test gave classification accuracy as good as any other rule set and better than any published criteria. This question, *"Do you require assistance remembering appointments, family occasions, holidays or taking medications?"*, we call the **forgetting rule**. All runs for all ML algorithms studied included this rule in the decision tree/rule-set; no other attribute was included in every decision tree/rule-set. Using CART's cross-validation procedure, this single rule decision tree was selected as the best tree on 10 out of 10 runs.

9.4.2 Logistic regression results

Stepwise logistic regression using the FAQ attributes gave a mean classification accuracy of $86.5 \pm 4.4\%$, which was similar to that obtained using ML methods (88%). The sensitivity ($84.1 \pm 6.8\%$) was lower than ML methods (93%), and the specificity ($88.8 \pm 5.3\%$) was higher than that obtained from ML methods (80%). The forgetting attribute had the largest odds ratio on 23 of 30 runs (11.9 ± 7.6), and was the only attribute included in all 30 models.

Logistic regression using the FAQ's forgetting attribute alone for the 30 randomly sampled training and testing sets gave a sensitivity of $92.7 \pm 2.0\%$ and specificity of $80.8 \pm 5.5\%$, which is significantly higher in sensitivity ($p < 0.00001$, two-sample t-test) and significantly lower in specificity ($p < 0.00001$, two-sample t-test) than that obtained by the stepwise logistic regression model.

For the MMSEBOMC, mean classification accuracy, $75.1 \pm 4.2\%$, sensitivity ($74.2 \pm 6.2\%$) and specificity ($76.5 \pm 6.8\%$) were not statistically different from those obtained by ML methods. In the logistic regression models, the attributes, *sex* and *repeating the months of the year in reverse order*, appeared in all 30 models; the attributes, *# of trials to obtain 2 correct repetitions of a previously unlearned address*, and *orientation to place*, appeared in 29 of 30 models; and the attribute, *delayed recall of a previously unlearned address*, appeared in 25 of 30 models. All other attributes appeared in less than 19 models. Among these five attributes, no one attribute had a distinctly larger odds ratio (range=1.4 to 6.4).

Comparison of sensitivity and specificity for the forgetting attribute logistic regression vs. the MMSEBOMC stepwise logistic regression using a two-sample t-test with unequal variances shows that the forgetting attribute alone gives statistically higher sensitivity ($p < 0.00001$) and specificity ($p < 0.0094$).

9.5 DISCUSSION

There are four main findings of the present analysis. *First*, the ML methods can be interfaced with an electronic medical record system to learn directly from the data. The feasibility of this is also demonstrated by the work described in, for example, [Ohmann et al., 1995] and [Gierl and Stengel-Rutkowski, 1994]. This feature contrasts with that of knowledge-based systems, in which human experts design the decision rules and then test the data. Whereas humans usually select a few rules by which they make decisions, a machine can consider a larger number of rules if needed. When supplemented by a review of the ML-generated rules or by incorporation of domain-specific knowledge into the ML algorithm, specific rules that violate domain knowledge can be minimized, thus enhancing the power and comprehensibility of rules obtained from ML methods. This approach also identifies subtle logical errors in the electronic medical record that could be overlooked. For example, after reviewing a nonsense rule using job performance as a criterion, we discovered that some normal subjects had misinterpreted the question about their ability to perform a job, answering that they could no longer perform their job because they had retired. In fact, they were fully able to perform their job given the need to do so. The inconsistency in the attribute values was discovered, and corrected. Re-running the ML algorithm verified that the nonsense rule had been eliminated by this correction of the data.

The *second* important finding of this chapter is that ML methods used in conjunction with the MMSEBOMC test attributes outperform any published criteria for using total MMSE score to classify normal and cognitively impaired or very mildly demented subjects. They also do much better than any cutoff possible using the ROC curve. This supports the idea that some attributes of the MMSEBOMC are more important than others, and that the less important attributes may actually confuse classification. The findings of the logistic regression analyses also supported these conclusions.

The *third* important finding of this chapter is clinical: when used with ML methods, a single question from the FAQ (the forgetting question) classifies cognitively normal aging subjects and subjects with very mild dementia as well as or better than any other combination of attributes from the FAQ and the MMSEBOMC with and without total score, and out-performs any of the recommended scoring criteria for the FAQ or the MMSE total scores. The logistic regression results confirm the ML finding that the FAQ forgetting attribute alone compared to the other best models from stepwise logistic regression of either the FAQ or the MMSEBOMC test gives the highest sensitivity (93%) for discriminating normal aging from the earliest stages of dementia. As expected, when both ML and logistic regression methods use only the information from the FAQ forgetting attribute to classify subjects, they give essentially identical sensitivity and specificity.

The similarity of the ML and logistic regression results also occurred in analyzing MMSEBOMC attributes. A recent study comparing Concept Formation ML methods with logistic regression also found highly similar classification results in predicting survival of injured patients entering the emergency department [Hadžikadić et al., 1996]. This suggests that other features of these methods besides classification accuracy are important in deciding which to use. In this study, ML methods more directly indicated the minimal set of attributes which accurately predicted normal aging vs. early stages of dementia. Inspection of the odds ratio of the FAQ forgetting attribute confirmed the ML finding. The presence of missing data also limited the number of cases available for analysis by logistic regression but not by ML methods. Unless one can easily perform calculations in a clinical setting, it is also easier to use the classification rules derived from ML methods than it is to work with regression coefficients in classifying subjects. The FAQ forgetting attribute alone gave a higher specificity than the MMSEBOMC stepwise logistic regression results, but resulted in a lower specificity than that obtained from the stepwise logistic regression using the entire set of FAQ attributes. Therefore, compared to the best results obtained from all other permutations of the FAQ and MMSEBOMC test attributes, the forgetting attribute used alone for screening would incorrectly classify about 8% more normal aging individuals as cognitively impaired, and it would correctly classify about 6.6% more cognitively impaired persons as cognitively impaired. Given the ease and applicability of the FAQ forgetting attribute for screening, we think that the tradeoff for higher sensitivity is preferable, since one can apply a second screen in a clinical setting to eliminate normal aging individuals misclassified as impaired.

It is interesting to note that the AHCPR-recommended criteria for impairment using a total FAQ score of 9 or higher, is much higher than the score of a person answering positively only to the forgetting question (their FAQ total = 1–3 in that case). The higher total FAQ score recommended by the AHCPR is based on studies which included all levels of dementia severity. Using this criterion for the very mildly demented subjects in the present study resulted in only a 20% sensitivity, which implies that responses to other questions of the FAQ actually reduce the sensitivity for detecting very mild stages of dementia (compared to the forgetting rule alone). This is why inclusion of the total FAQ score as an attribute in the ML runs reduced the specificity and sensitivity when compared with the results obtained from analyses of the FAQ item attributes alone. The FAQ attributes therefore contribute unequally to dementia classification, with the forgetting question being the most contributory. This is our *fourth* significant finding.

The only demographic variable which differed to a clinically significant extent between normal and cognitively impaired subjects was sex. Since the decision rule sets obtained from the FAQ test plus demographic attributes rarely included gender in any of the ML runs, we conclude that FAQ decision rules are not biased by sample differences in gender. However, gender was a significant attribute in classifying subjects using the MMSEBOMC test. The findings here are restricted to the population represented, which consists of individuals, mostly over 65 years and with more than a high school education. Previous studies showing the insensitivity of the FAQ to educational level suggests that the results of this study also apply to persons 65 or over, regardless of education.

9.6 CONCLUSIONS

The dementia screening tests recommended by the Agency for Health Care Policy Research were analyzed with machine learning and stepwise logistic regression methods. Compared to the most accurate cut-off criteria published for the total scores of these tests, machine learning methods increased the accuracy significantly, for the FAQ, by a wide margin of more than 30%. Furthermore, they reduced the number of test questions needed to obtain this accuracy to just one question. Stepwise logistic regression not only confirmed the machine learning results, but also assisted in the logical pruning of the decision trees through the inspection of the odds ratios of each attribute which participated in a rule-set. Despite the use of these tests in dementia evaluation for over 20 years, these findings have not been previously discovered, suggesting a useful role for machine learning in the evaluation of commonly used medical tests.

Also, machine learning methods discovered subtle errors in the electronic medical record which were due to misinterpretation of what was being asked of the subject. The rule set derived from the full data can be used on paper or as software in various clinical settings to enhance the detection of very early stages of a dementing illness. This should result in less disability per patient and better quality of life for both caregiver and patient through early intervention. The utility of ML-derived protocols with some human supervision has general applicability to many important medical areas, including cancer, heart disease, and stroke.

Acknowledgments

We thank professor Carl Cotman for helping establish a working relation with the AHCPR. This work was supported by the Alzheimer's Association Pilot Research Grant, PRG-95-161, *The Alzheimer's Intelligent Interface: Diagnosis, Education and Training.*

References

Aikins, J., Kunz, J., Shortliffe, E., and Fallat, R. (1982). PUFF: An expert system for interpretation of pulmonary function data. Technical report, Stanford University.

Bratko, I., Mozetič, I., and Lavrač, N. (1989). *KARDIO: A Study in Deep and Qualitative Knowledge for Expert Systems.* MIT Press, Cambridge, MA.

Breiman, L., Friedman, J., Olshen, R., and Stone, C. (1984). *Classification and Regression Trees.* Wadsworth, Belmont.

Buntine, W. and Caruana, R. (1992). *Introduction to IND Version 2.1 and Recursive Partitioning.* NASA.

Cestnik, G., Konenenko, I., and Bratko, I. (1987). Assistant-86: A knowledge-elicitation tool for sophisticated users. In Bratko, I. and Lavrač, N., editors, *Progress in Machine Learning*, pages 31–45. Sigma Press.

Crum, R., Anthony, J., Bassett, S., and Folstein, M. (1993). Population-based norms for the mini-mental state examination by age and educational level. *JAMA*, 269(18):2386–2390.

DSM-IV (1994). *Diagnostic and Statistical Manual of Mental Disorders.* American Psychiatric Association, Washington, D. C., 4th edition.

Duda, R. and Hart, P. (1973). *Pattern Classification and Scene Analysis.* John Wiley, New York.

Fillenbaum, G., Heyman, A., Wilkinson, W., and Haynes, C. (1987). Comparison of two screening tests in Alzheimer's disease—The correlation and reliability of the mini-mental state examination and the modified blessed test. *Archives of Neurology*, 44(9):924–7.

Folstein, M., Folstein, S., and McHugh, P. (1975). Mini-mental state: A practical method for grading the cognitive state of patients for the clinician. *Journal of Psychiatric Research*, 12(3):189–98.

Gierl, L. and Stengel-Rutkowski, S. (1994). Integrating consultation and semi-automatic knowledge acquisition in a prototype based architecture: Experiences with dysmorphic syndromes. *Artificial Intelligence in Medicine*, 6:29–49.

Hadžikadić, M., Hakenewerth, B., Bohren, B., Norton, J., Mehta, B., and Andrews, C. (1996). Concept formation vs. logistic regression: Predicting death in trauma patients. *Artificial Intelligence in Medicine*, 8:493–504.

Heckerman, D., Horvitz, E., and Nathwani, B. (1992). Towards normative expert systems: Part I The Pathfinder Project. *Methods of Information in Medicine*, (31):90–105.

Kohavi, R., John, G., Long, R., Manley, D., and Pfleger, K. (1994). MLC++: A machine learning library in C++. In *Tools with Artificial Intelligence*, pages 740–743. IEEE Computer Society Press. Available by anonymous ftp from: `starry.stanford.edu:pub/ronnyk/mlc/toolsmlc.ps`.

Lavrač, N. and Mozetič, I. (1992). Second generation knowledge acquisition methods and their application to medicine. In Keravnou, E., editor, *Deep Models for Medical Knowledge Engineering*, pages 177–198. Elsevier.

Michalski, R., Mozetič, I., Hong, J., and Lavrač, N. (1986). The multi-purpose incremental learning system AQ15 and its testing application to three medical domains. In *Proceedings of the Fifth National Conference on Artificial Intelligence*, pages 1041–1045, Philadelphia, PA. Morgan Kaufmann.

Morris, J. (1993). The clinical dementia rating (CDR): Current version and scoring rules. *Neurology*, 43(11):2412–4.

Oconnor, D., Pollitt, P., Treasure, F., Brook, C., and Reiss, B. (1989). The influence of education, social class and sex on mini-mental state scores. *Psychological Medicine*, 19:771–776.

Ohmann, C., Yang, Q., Moustakis, V., Lang, K., and Elk, v. P. (1995). Machine learning techniques applied to the diagnosis of acute abdominal pain. In Barahona, P. and Stefanelli, M., editors, *Lecture Notes in Artificial Intelligence: Artificial Intelligence in Medicine AIME95*, volume 934, pages 276–281. Springer Verlag.

Pazzani, M. and Kibler, D. (1992). The utility of knowledge in inductive learning. *Machine Learning*, (9):57–94.

Pfeffer, R., Kurosaki, T., Harrah, C., Chance, J., and Filos, S. (1982). Measurement of functional activities in older adults in the community. *Journal of Gerontology*, 37:323–9.

Quinlan, J. (1993). *C4.5: Programs for Machine Learning.* Morgan Kaufmann, Los Altos, California.

Shankle, W., Datta, P., Dillencourt, M., and Pazzani, M. (1996). Improving dementia screening tests with machine learning methods. *Alzheimer's Research*, 2(3).

Shortliffe, E. (1976). *Computer-Based Medical Consultations: MYCIN.* Elsevier/North-Holland.

Stata (1993). *STATA Release 3.1.* Stata Corporation, 6th edition.

Welsh, K., Butters, N., Mohs, R., Beekly, D., Edland, S., and Fillenbaum, G. (1994). The Consortium to Establish a Registry for Alzheimer's Disease (cerad) part V—A normative study of the neuropsychological battery. *Neurology*, 44(4):609–14.

Williams, T. and Costa, P. (1995). Recognition and initial assessment of alzheimer's disease and related dementias: Clinical practice guidelines. Technical report, Department of Health and Human Services.

Wyatt, J. (1989). Lessons learned from the field trials of ACORN, a chest pain advisor. In Barber, B., Cao, D., Qin, D., and Wagner, F., editors, *Proceedings MedInfo*, pages 111–115. Elsevier.

10 EXPERIMENTS WITH MACHINE LEARNING IN THE PREDICTION OF CORONARY ARTERY DISEASE PROGRESSION

Branko Šter,
Matjaž Kukar,
Andrej Dobnikar,
Igor Kranjec,
and Igor Kononenko

Abstract: Fourteen classifiers were applied to the problem of coronary artery disease progression. The classifiers were taken from different paradigms of machine learning (symbolic, statistical and neural) in order to encapsulate the different approaches. The unsolved problem of coronary artery disease progression consists of predicting the stenosis (narrowing of the coronary artery) change on the basis of clinical, laboratory and epidemiological attributes. A total of 263 patients belonging to two classes (stenosis changed vs. non-changed) were described with 25 attributes. The overall results are not promising and suggest that the attributes used are not sufficiently relevant to enable the prediction of coronary artery disease progression. It should also be pointed out that the simplest classifiers (the naive Bayesian classifier and linear discriminant method) generally yield the best results. This phenomenon seems to be typical for medical data and is consistent with our previous experience.

10.1 INTRODUCTION

In recent years a series of machine learning algorithms have been developed which can be used as efficient tools for the analysis of databases and for extracting the classification knowledge that can be used to solve new problems from the given problem domain [Michie et al., 1994, Dietterich and Shavlik, 1990]. The technology of inductive learning is already appropriate for routine use. Several commercial systems are available with advanced user interfaces that enable the development of applications in various fields. Furthermore, the artificial neural networks have recently been developed which follow the relevant learning principles: perform the network design task, robustness, efficiency and generalization in learning. Several algorithms satisfy these brain-like properties [Rumelhart and McClelland, 1986, Hecht-Nielsen, 1990].

It seems that these technologies are well suited for medical diagnosis in small specialized diagnostic problems. Data about correct diagnoses are often available in medical archives in specialized hospitals or their departments. All that has to be done is to input the data into the computer in the appropriate form and run the system for inductive learning. The derived set of decision rules can be used to reveal the basic relations and laws in the problem domain in an explicit and transparent form and, of course, can be used for diagnosing new patients. In several medical domains the inductive learning systems [Kononenko et al., 1984, Horn et al., 1985, Quinlan et al., 1987, Roškar et al., 1986, Pirnat et al., 1989, Kukar et al., 1996] and neural network based algorithms [Alpsan et al., 1995, Baxt, 1991, Brouwer, 1994, Roy et al., 1995, Šter et al., 1995, Šter and Dobnikar, 1995] were applied.

As medical prognosis is a difficult task for physicians due to large time delays (several years) in recognizing the correct prognosis, machine learning may be more acceptable for solving prognostic rather than diagnostic problems. Our aim in this study was to use machine learning to try to solve the unsolved problem of predicting the progression of coronary artery disease based on a certain set of non-invasive measurements. The final goal is to reduce the number of invasive measurements which are expensive, painful and dangerous for the patient. The database was obtained from Dr. Igor Kranjec, M.D., of the Department of Cardiology, University Medical Center in Ljubljana, Slovenia.

We used several machine learning algorithms in order to try to develop a reliable predictor from the given database. We used four algorithms for top-down induction of decision trees, two versions of the Bayesian classifier, four versions of neural networks, three versions of discriminant functions and two variants of nearest neighbor algorithms. In total we tried fourteen different algorithms. The results indicate that the given set of measurements does not provide enough useful information for the given task.

In the next section the prognostic problem is described and in Section 10.3 the fourteen algorithms are briefly outlined. Section 10.4 presents the results of the experiments and the next two sections describe further experiments which clarify the poor information content of the given set of measurements. Section 10.7 concludes this study.

10.2 CORONARY ARTERY DISEASE (CAD)

The database includes patients suffering from Coronary Artery Disease (CAD). Coronary Heart Disease (CHD) and Coronary Artery Disease are synonyms. The progression of coronary atherosclerosis induces the narrowing of the coronary artery by a thickening of the vessel wall. This thickening is described as a "plaque" which can eventually grow to such a size that it impinges on the artery lumen and so decreases the blood flow. This results in ischemia (deficiency of blood) of the tissues supplied by that artery, i.e., a certain part of the heart muscle (myocardium) does not receive enough blood. At total occlusion blood flow is interrupted and necrosis (infarction) occurs.

The coronary arteriography is an invasive intervention by which the diameter of an artery can be measured (note: the angiography is a broader term than the arteriography, but may be used in this context with the same meaning). By two successive arteriographies (with a certain time interval) the progress of CAD (narrowing of the artery) can be stated. However, coronary arteriography cannot be repeated several times because it is dangerous, expensive and not widely available (only two laboratories in Slovenia). So the problem is to predict the change in the artery diameter on the basis of clinical, laboratory and epidemiological factors. Table 10.2 provides a brief description of the attributes used in the database and Table 10.3 shows the basic statistics of the data.

The change in the artery diameter between two angiographies (ddme=dme2-dmel) defines the class to which the patients are assigned. Critical values of ddme define class borders. In principle, because ddme for each patient is known, the categories can be defined in different ways. The progress of CAD is defined as the decrease of dme (i.e., negative ddme). Two reasonable groupings, defined by means of numerical variable ddme, are the following (see Tables 1.1a and 1.1b).

MCAD. A significant border of ddme lies around -0.3mm (short-term variability).

ECAD. Two approximately equally large categories; decrease and increase of dme. This task has no profound medical meaning, it is rather an attempt to redefine the problem (as we shall see, the results on MCAD are hopeless). The meaning is rather intuitive: widening and narrowing of the artery.

Table 10.1a The MCAD grouping.

Class	*Class borders*	*Number of cases*	*Proportion*
0	ddme < -0.27	41	15.6%
1	ddme >= -0.27	222	84.4%

Table 10.1b The ECAD grouping.

Class	*Class borders*	*Number of cases*	*Proportion*
0	ddme < 0.0	133	50.6%
1	ddme >= 0.0	130	49.4%

10.3 MACHINE LEARNING METHODS

Lookahead Feature Construction (LFC) [Ragavan and Rendell, 1993] is an algorithm for the induction of binary decision trees. At each node LFC uses a feature which is constructed from several attributes using logical operators (conjunction, disjunction and negation). The feature should capture significant dependencies between attributes. In this way it is easier to describe the class boundaries in problems with mutually dependent attributes. From the constructed binary features the best feature is selected and the process is recursively repeated on two subsets of training instances, corresponding to the two values of the selected feature. This approach is convenient for decision trees because fewer nodes are required to describe the class, therefore smaller trees with better statistical support are obtained. Searching for features is a computationally demanding problem. LFC possesses the valuable property of efficiently limiting the problem space. The space of possible useful constructs is restricted, due to the geometrical representation of the conditional entropy which is the estimator of an attribute's quality. To further reduce the search space, the algorithm also limits the width and the depth of the search. The lookahead depth limits the length of the logical expressions. Information gain is used as the splitting criterion.

Assistant-I [Cestnik et al., 1987] is an algorithm for top-down induction of binary decision trees using information gain for estimating the quality of attributes. Other features of Assistant-I binarization of attributes, pruning of

Table 10.2 Description of the attributes (N-numerical, C-categorical, L-logical).

Attribute description	*Type and values*
age, years	N (28 .. 81)
sex	C (M, F)
hypertension	L(yes,no)
high blood sugar	L(yes,no)
smoking	L(yes,no)
total cholesterol, mmol/l	N (2.1..9.2)
high-density lipoproteins, mmol/l	N (0.2..5.1)
low-density lipoproteins, mmol/l	N (0.7..8.1)
triglyceride, mmol/l	N (0.4..9.0)
recent Angina Pectoris (AP) (<= 1 month ago)	L (yes, no)
spontaneous AP before 1st angiography	L (yes, no)
myocardial infarction before 1st angiography	L (yes, no)
recent myocardial infarction (<= 1 month ago)	L (yes, no)
interval between both angiographies, days	N (1..999)
spontaneous AP between both angiographies	L (yes, no)
myocard. infarction between both angiographies	L (yes, no)
patient was prescr. nitrates between both angio.	L (yes, no)
patient was prescribed beta-blocker	L (yes, no)
patient was prescribed calcium-blocker	L (yes, no)
patient was prescribed aspirin	L (yes, no)
diseased coronary artery	C (LCX, RCA, LAD)
artery segment	N (1, 2, ..., 13)
obstructive (medial) diameter of the artery at 1st ang., mm	N (0.14..1.84)
% diameter stenosis at 1st angio.	N (54%..95%)

decision trees, dealing with incomplete data and classification in combination with the naive Bayesian classifier.

Assistant-R uses the ReliefF measure [Kononenko and Šimec, 1995] for attribute selection, which is derived from Relief [Kira and Rendell, 1992]. The idea of ReliefF is to estimate the difference of two probabilities: the probability that two similar instances from different classes have different values of the given attribute and the probability that two similar instances from the same class have different attribute values. ReliefF is able to correctly estimate the quality of attributes even if the attributes are strongly conditionally dependent, which is not the case with other measures, such as information gain. Instead of the relative frequency Assistant-R uses the m-estimate of probability, which was shown to often significantly increase the performance of machine learning algorithms [Cestnik, 1990]. The parameter m trades off between the contribu-

Table 10.3 The basic statistics of the dataset.

Attribute	*Total(n=263)*	*Progres.(134)*	*Regres.(129)*
age	56 ± 9	57 ± 9	55 ± 10
sex	male 216 (82%)	male 103 (77%)	male 113 (88%)
hypertension	71(27%)	34(25%)	37(29%)
diab.	166(63%)	88(66%)	78(60%)
smoking	127(48%)	67(50%)	60(47%)
cholesterol	5.9 ± 1.1	6.0 ± 1.1	5.8 ± 1.6
hdl	0.9 ± 0.4	0.9 ± 0.4	0.9 ± 0.5
ldl	4.1 ± 1.0	4.2 ± 1.0	4.0 ± 1.1
trigl.	2.0 ± 1.1	2.1 ± 1.0	1.9 ± 1.1
recent AP	66 (25%)	34 (25%)	32 (25%)
spontaneous AP1	127 (48%)	73 (54%)	54 (42%)
MI1	115 (44%)	63 (47%)	52 (40%)
recent mi	34 (13%)	17 (13%)	17 (13%)
interval	40	49	31
spontaneous AP2	68 (26%)	38 (28%)	30 (23%)
MI2	4 (2%)	2 (1%)	2 (2%)
nitrates	166 (63%)	82 (61%)	84 (65%)
beta-blocker	165 (63%)	89 (66%)	76 (59%)
calcium-blocker	176 (67%)	90 (67%)	86 (67%)
aspirin	208 (79%)	106 (79%)	102 (79%)
diseased artery	46, 72, 14	29, 36, 69	17, 36, 76
artery segment	6 ± 3	7 ± 3	6 ± 3
medial diameter 1	0.8 ± 0.3 mm	0.8 ± 0.4	0.7 ± 0.3
diameter stenosis 1	75.9 ± 9.5%	74.8 ± 9.7%	77.0 ± 9.2%

tions of the relative frequency and the prior probability $P_a(X)$. The default setting of m is usually 2.

The naive Bayesian classifier estimates the probability of each class given the values of all attributes by assuming the conditional independence of attributes. Although the assumption seems unrealistic, the naive Bayesian classifier often outperforms other classifiers in real-world problems. In particular, in medical diagnostic problems it usually performs the best [Kononenko and Šimec, 1995].

The semi-naive Bayesian classifier [Kononenko, 1991] is an extension of the naive Bayesian classifier. Instead of assuming the complete independence of attributes, the semi-naive version searches for dependencies. The detected significant dependencies are taken into account during classification of new cases.

CART (Classification And Regression Trees) is an algorithm for building decision trees (the regression part was not used in this study) [Breiman et al., 1984]. Binary trees are grown by induction from the learning sample cases. At each node the best split is searched for, taking into consideration all the attributes. Two different split measures are considered: Twoing criterion (not impurity-based) and Gini index (impurity based). The tree is built until no more splitting is sensible. The tree is pruned using the method called Minimal Cost-Complexity pruning.

Fisher's linear discriminant described in [Schalkoff, 1992], attempts to find an optimal discrimination hyperplane between two classes. It is assumed that each class forms one cluster. A direction (vector w) is searched for such that, when samples are projected onto it, the maximum separability (Fisher's measure) is obtained. The next thing is to determine a hyperplane (perpendicular to w) which yields the lowest classification error. This method in its original form is suited only for two-class domains.

The linear discriminant method (maximum likelihood approach) [Duda and Hart, 1973, Michie et al., 1994] provides M linear discriminant functions, where M stands for the number of classes. Each sample is classified as $argmaxd_i(x), i = 1, ..., M$, where $d_i(x)$ is the i-th discriminant function $d_i(x) = ln[P(x|C_i)P(C_i)]$, where $P(C_i)$ denotes the apriori probability of class i and $P(x|C_i)$ is the probability density function of class i. If normal distribution is assumed for $P(x|C_i)$, we obtain quadratic functions in terms of x. In case of equal covariance matrices, the functions become linear in terms of x. Linear discriminant method assumes the common covariance matrix Σ, so instead of class covariance matrices Σ_i, the "pooled" covariance matrix is used. When the actual parameters of the population $(\Sigma_i, m_i, P(C_i))$ are unknown, they are, of course, estimated from the sample set.

The quadratic discriminant method (maximum likelihood) [Duda and Hart, 1973, Michie et al., 1994] can be derived similarly as linear discriminant analysis, except that original covariance matrices and therewith quadratic functions are kept.

The k-nearest neighbors (k-NN) is a well known non-parametric statistical method [Duda and Hart, 1973, Schalkoff, 1992] which is quite efficient and simple to implement. The method is used as a direct classifier. Each new sample is classified according to the majority class of the k nearest learning samples.

In our experiments two types of distance (to define the nearest neighbors) have been used: the Euclidean and Manhattan distance.

The learning vector quantization (LVQ) [Kohonen, 1984] is an iterative process, which sets codebook vectors that approximate the input vector by quantized values. In general, several codebook vectors are assigned to each class. An input vector is assigned to a class of the nearest codebook vector. The codebook vectors, set asymptotically by LVQ, approximately minimize the misclassification error in the nearest-neighbor sense.

The backpropagation algorithm (BP) (with momentum) is a well known method [Rumelhart and McClelland, 1986] for training a multi-layer feed-forward neural network. BP minimizes the mean squared error using the gradient descent. Backpropagation is an extension of the delta learning rule to multiple-layer architecture. The key feature of the algorithm is the use of the error term, already calculated at the higher level of neurons, for the gradient calculation at the lower level. Calculating the gradient in multi-layer networks would be otherwise much more time-consuming. Here we use a version with an additional internal test-sample. During the period of training, the classification accuracy on internal test-sample is measured and the best net considering this criterion is chosen. This is implemented to prevent overfitting.

The backpropagation with weight-elimination is a variant of the backpropagation algorithm with the complexity-regularization procedure [Weigend et al., 1991]. The complexity penalty is added to the error. Besides reducing the error, the tendency during the learning is also to reduce the complexity. Lower complexity requires smaller weights. Very small weights are practically eliminated from the network. On the other hand, small weights signify the more linear domain of the neuron's operation and the whole network may tend more to linearity. A simpler network has better generalization capabilities than a complex one, provided that it is able to solve the problem (i.e., the network is not too simple). The complexity parameter is incrementally adjusted during learning by a certain heuristic [Weigend et al., 1991].

The RBFL method [Roy et al., 1995] is based on the radial-basis function neural network (RBF). Linear programming (LP) models are used to train the RBF net. LP models are solved by the Simplex technique, developed by Dantzig in the 1940's. Gaussian functions are used for kernel functions in the RBF net. During training, several Gaussians of different centers and widths are created. The minimal width of a Gaussian is 0.001 in all dimensions of the normalized input space. The response of such a net for each output class is the weighted sum of its kernel function values in a point of the input space. An output

Table 10.4 Classification accuracy and information score of symbolic classifiers on the MCAD problem with default and "best" settings of parameters (s ... threshold for joining the values of attributes).

Method	*Parameters*	*Accuracy [%]*	*Inf [bit]*
LFC	beam=8, depth=2	82.1	0.0
LFC*	m=10, ts-pruning	84.4	-0.0
Assistant-I	m=2	78.3	-0.0
Assistant-I*	m=5, elimin. thr. =0.08	84.4	-0.1
Assistant-I′	m=0	74.5	0.2
Assistant-R	m=2	79.1	-0.1
Assistant-R*	m=5	84.4	-0.0
n-Bayes	m=2	84.8	0.0
n-Bayes*	m=10	84.8	0.1
sn-Bayes	m=2	81.8	0.1
sn-Bayes*	s=0.8, m=2	84.4	-
CART	-	82.9	-

* tuned on accuracy, ′ tuned on Inf, otherwise default parameters

class is obtained by taking the maximal class response. LP models are used to calculate the weights of Gaussians in order to minimize the classification error.

10.4 RESULTS

We used 10-fold cross-validation to estimate the classification accuracy of different classifiers [Michie et al., 1994, Haykin, 1994]. We present the results for the MCAD and ECAD problems separately. The classifiers were divided into two groups: the first group consists mainly of symbolic methods and the second of numerical, i.e., statistical and neural methods. For the first group we also measured the average information score [Kononenko and Bratko, 1991]. This measure takes also into account the prior probabilities of classes, which turns to be very important on the MCAD problem. For the second group of methods only classification accuracies are provided here, but further details on this subject can be found in [Šter et al., 1995] and [Šter and Dobnikar, 1995].

10.4.1 MCAD domain

For LFC, Assistant-I, Assistant-R, the naive and the semi-naive Bayesian classifier the data were discretized (for certain attributes the borders were set by physicians). The average number of values per attribute is four. The a priori probability of the majority class is 84.4%.

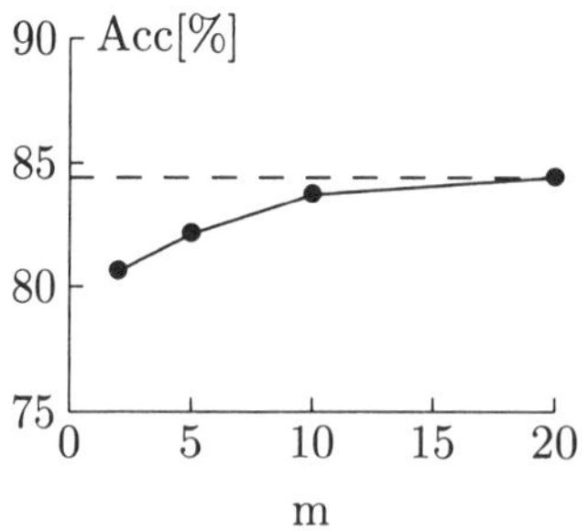

Figure 10.1 Effect of parameter m on the accuracy of LFC (dashed line ... majority class proportion) on the MCAD problem.

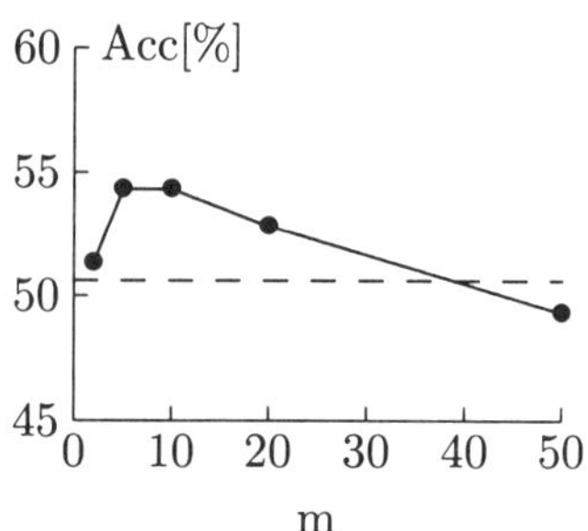

Figure 10.2 Effect of parameter m on the accuracy of LFC (dashed line ... majority class proportion) on the ECAD problem.

Table 10.4 shows the results of symbolic methods. For each of the classifiers (except CART) we show the results achieved with a default setting of parameters and the best results according to the classification accuracy and according to the information score achieved with parameter tuning. It is obvious that none of these classifiers is able to extract any useful information from the attributes. The average information score stays at around zero bits/answer in all cases, which indicates that on the average all classifiers provide zero information for the MCAD prediction problem. The best classification accuracy achieved does not exceed the probability of the majority class. Therefore, the default classifier (that classifies each testing instance into the majority class) would achieve the same result.

Figure 1.1 shows the influence of parameter m that controls the probability estimation during the tree-construction in LFC. With larger m (larger influence of the prior probabilities - the root node information) the classification accuracy increases but does not exceed the default accuracy. In fact, either the one-leaf-tree is obtained or all the leaves are assigned the same class, which is in both cases equivalent to the default classifier.

Figure 10.3a shows the effect of parameter m that controls the probability estimation used for calculating the attribute importance in ReliefF. Larger values of m support the prior information rather than the node information. Figure 10.3b shows the effect of tuning the elimination threshold in Assistant-R, that controls the number of attributes used for building the decision tree. A greater threshold eliminates more attributes. The best results are obtained with (almost) no attributes, therefore with the default classifier.

Table 10.5 Classification accuracy and information score of symbolic classifiers on the ECAD problem with default and "best" settings of parameters (s ... threshold for joining the values of attributes).

Method	*Parameters*	*Accuracy [%]*	*Inf [bit]*
LFC	beam=10, dep.=3, ts-prun.	51.3	0.0
LFC*	m=5, conj. 4,1, ts-prun.	56.6	0.1
Assistant-I	m=2	49.4	0.0
Assistant-I*	m=0, el. thr.=0.00	53.5	0.4
Assistant-I′	m=0	49.8	0.4
Assistant-R	m=2	44.8	-0.1
Assistant-R*	elim. el. thr.=0.00	54.3	0.1
Assistant-R′	m=0, el. thr.=0.0, k=20	53.3	0.4
n-Bayes	m=2	58.1	0.1
n-Bayes*	m=10	58.8	0.1
n-Bayes*	m=20	60.4♣	0.1
sn-Bayes	m=2	58.1	0.1
sn-Bayes*	m=20	59.3	0.1
sn-Bayes*	s=0.7, m=2	59.7	-
CART	-	49.4	-

* tuned on accuracy, ′ tuned on Inf, otherwise default parameters
♣ for m=20 leave-one-out estimate is 56.7 (Inf=0.1)

The naive Bayesian classifier yields the highest results, but even these are only in the default range. The more sophisticated methods all perform less successfully. This probably implies that the data are problematic (probably highly overlapping) and also that no important mutual dependency of the attributes seems to exist.

Results of statistical and neural methods are summarized in Table 10.6 and Figure 1.5. It is clear that none of the methods had any success in this domain. Very similar results were obtained with a version of this database, where the continuous attributes were discretized more densely (7 values per attribute on average). The only essential difference is that Assistant-I performs better (about 5 percent higher accuracy).

10.4.2 ECAD domain

The a priori probability of the majority class in this domain is 50.6%. The results are shown in Table 10.5. In Figure 10.2, the classification accuracy of the LFC again approaches the default value with larger parameter m, however smaller m yields a better result which indicates that there is some useful information provided by the attributes. Figure 10.4a shows that the estimation of attributes by ReliefF is much more reliable in the root of the tree than in the lower level nodes. Figure 10.4b shows that this time (ECAD) using less attributes causes a subsequent decrease in the degree of accuracy.

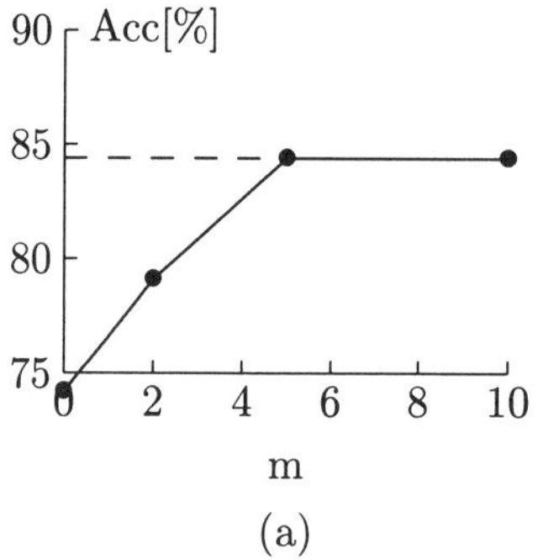

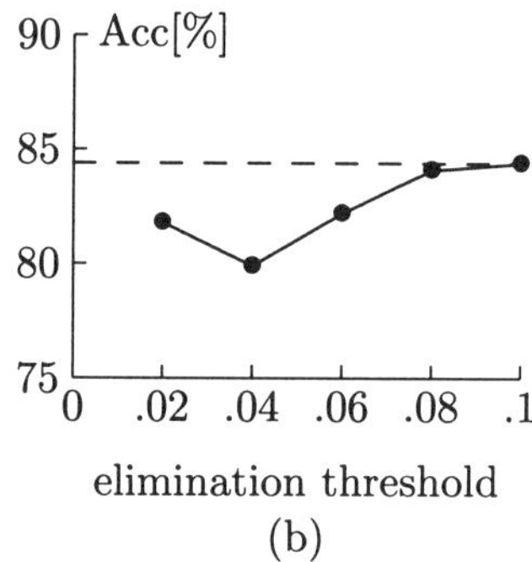

Figure 10.3 Influences of parameters m (a) and the elimination threshold (b) on the classification accuracy of Assistant-R on the MCAD problem.

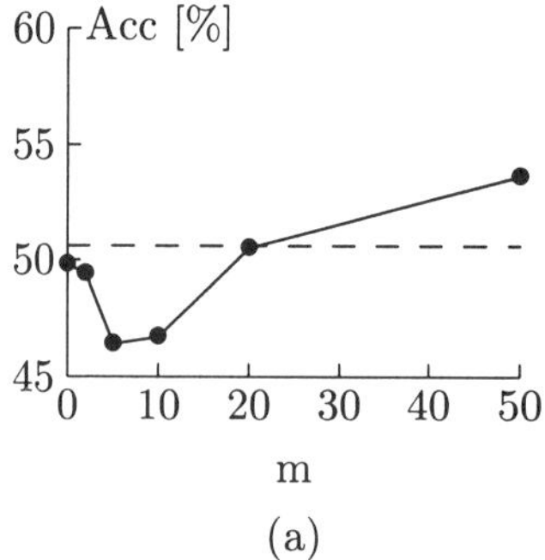

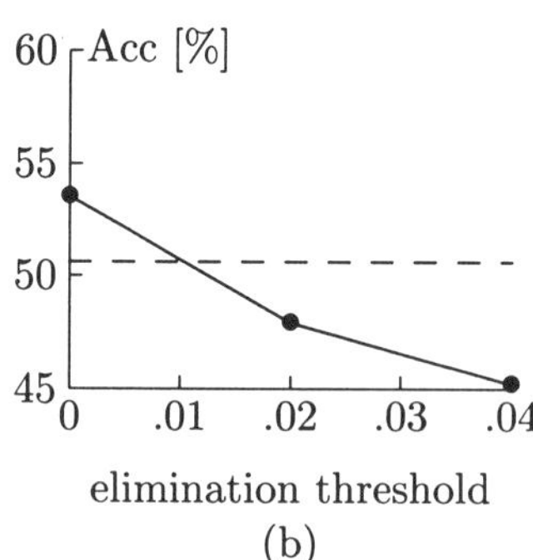

Figure 10.4 Influences of parameters m (a) and the elimination threshold (b) on the classification accuracy of Assistant-R on the ECAD problem.

It is obvious, that this domain yields better results than MCAD. That is to say that the highest accuracy is almost ten percent above the default, and the highest information score (Inf) reaches 0.4. Nevertheless, this prediction is still too weak to be useful in practice.

Results of the statistical and neural methods are summarized in Table 10.6 and Figure 10.6. The most successful method on the ECAD problem is the naive Bayesian classifier.

Table 10.6 Classification accuracy of statistical and neural classifiers on MCAD and ECAD.

Method	*Accuracy [%] on MCAD*	*Accuracy [%] on ECAD*
Fisher	83.2	54.5
Lin. discr.	84.4	56.0
Quad. discr.	83.6	49.8
k-NN	84.0	44.5
BP (10 hidden)	83.3	52.5
BP-weight el.	81.7	50.2
LVQ	82.1	49.0
RBFL	84.4	47.8
Default	84.4	50.6

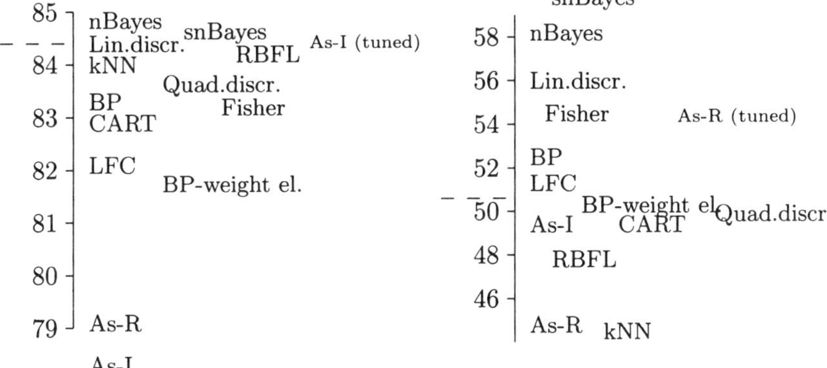

Figure 10.5 Classification accuracy of all classifiers on the MCAD problem (dashed line represents the default accuracy).

Figure 10.6 Classification accuracy of all classifiers on the ECAD problem (dashed line represents the default accuracy).

10.5 INCREASING THE LEARNING SET SIZE

We also experimented with learning sets of different sizes. We traced the tendency of the classification accuracy with the enlargement of the learning set.

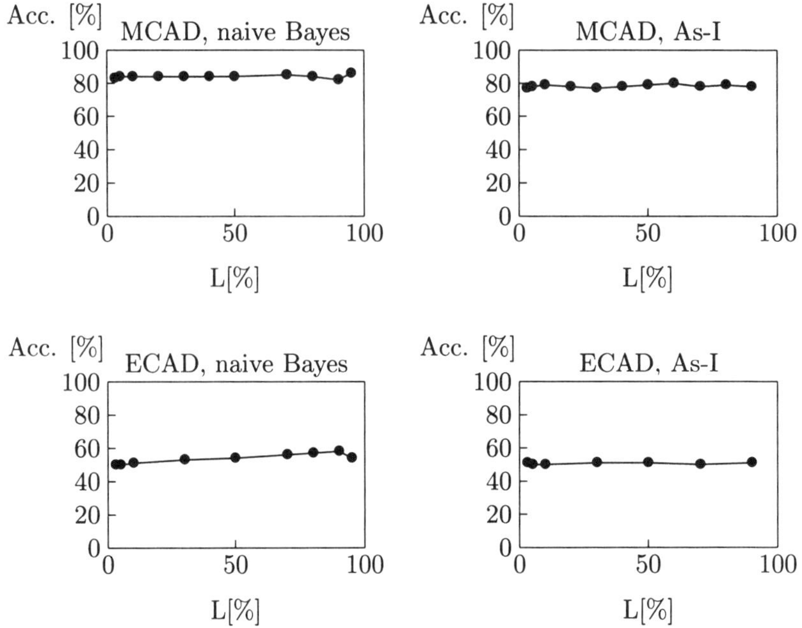

Figure 10.7 The effect of increasing the learning set size on the classification accuracy of two classifiers in the two problems.

The goal of this experiment was to determine whether the current number of cases (263) is too small to allow us to achieve a successful classification in the CAD problem. If accuracy increased continually we could conclude that the new cases continually contribute new relevant information and that additional cases are required.

Two classifiers on databases MCAD and ECAD were used: the naive Bayesian classifier and Assistant-I. Each database was partitioned several times in different proportions into a learning and a testing set. The percentage of learning cases is denoted by L (others are testing cases). For each partition (a point in the graph) the result is obtained as the average result of ten random splits in the specified proportion. The results are presented in Figure 10.7.

The results show that the classification accuracy is almost independent of the number of learning cases. Only on ECAD with the naive Bayesian classifier a slight increase can be observed. It can be concluded that additional cases would not essentially improve the results.

10.6 COMBINING DECISIONS OF DIFFERENT CLASSIFIERS

In recent years the concepts of multistrategy learning and multiple knowledge have emerged. With this approach, the answers given by several existing algorithms are combined, in the hope that the resulting combination will result in a better performance. A combined system could also offer better explanations and higher accuracy than any single classifier, no matter how finely tuned. There are many different methods for combining decisions. In other experiments it was shown [Kononenko, 1992, Kukar et al., 1996] that in most cases the naive Bayesian combination outperforms other methods. In essence, it is the same as that of the naive Bayesian classifier, except that instead of attributes we have the classifiers. In this case, the probability of an instance belonging to the j-th class (Cj) is calculated with:

$$P(C_j|Cl_1, ..., Cl_k) = P(C_j) \prod_{i=1}^{k} P(C_j|Cl_i)/P(C_j) \qquad (10.1)$$

where k is the number of classifiers and Cl_i is the i-th classifier. In our experiments we have chosen some typical algorithms from different fields (statistical, neural and machine learning). We combined Assistant-R, backpropagation neural network, CART, linear discriminant method, LFC, the naive Bayesian classifier and backpropagation with weight elimination.

For the sake of combinations, all the algorithms were run with their default settings, because we wanted to see whether the combined classifier can be compared with the best fine-tuned single classifier. The results are in Table 10.7.

Table 10.7 Classification accuracy of the combined classifier compared to single classifiers.

	MCAD		ECAD	
	Accuracy [%]	*Inf [bit]*	*Accuracy [%]*	*Inf [bit]*
Average single	82.5	-0.05	52.5	0.04
Best single	84.2	0.07	58.3	0.10
Naive Bayesian comb.	82.9	0.14	53.2	0.15

It is interesting to note that while the average classification accuracy increases only from 82.5% to 82.9% (MCAD) and from 52.5% to 53.2% (ECAD), the improvement of the information score is slightly better (from -0.05 bit up to the 0.14 bit for MCAD and from 0.04 bit up to the 0.15 bit for ECAD). This is consistent with our previous results [Kukar et al., 1996]. However, the overall results still remain disappointing.

10.7 CONCLUSIONS

In spite of applying a large number of classifier systems, in the presented problem of coronary artery disease progression we cannot obtain any useful results. This also corresponds to some of the statistical methods and previous conclusions of others. The database in this form is evidently not appropriate for useful prediction. The reasons for this are probably as follows:

- The lack of relevant attributes, which are either unknown, not measured nor collected (e.g., history of the disease in the family).
- If there exist very complex dependencies in data, the number of cases may be too small to reveal the dependencies. On the other hand, the results of the experiment with learning sets of different sizes do not support this assumption, but rather lead to the conclusion that the attributes are not sufficiently relevant.
- Measurement noise of angiography, which influences the measured diameters of the coronary artery.

Another important point of view concerns the fact that this intrinsically prognostic problem is converted here into a diagnostic one and is treated with classification methods. However, the problem was defined by the physicians in this way and the data available enable only such an approach. It could be advantageous to have temporal values of the attributes, but it is impossible to say whether this would make the problem easier or even more difficult to handle. Unfortunately, the time interval between the two angiographies varies and was set by physicians' decisions when to perform an angiography.

Although the result of this article is negative, we hope it may be valuable for the medical science. It shows the insufficiency of the present attributes for the prediction of CAD progression and indicates that there may be other important factors (perhaps still unknown) causing coronary artery disease progression.

Acknowledgments

The RBFL neural network was implemented by Ivan Gabrijel; the LFC method by Marko Robnik; Assistant-I, Assistant-R and the naive Bayesian classifier by Edvard Šimec, all from the Faculty of Computer and Information Science. We also thank Dr. Matjaž Klemenc, M.D., who contributed to the formulation of the presented problem.

References

Alpsan, D., Towsey, M., Ozdamar, O., Tsoi, A. C., and Ghista, D. N. (1995). Efficacy of modified backpropagation and optimisation methods on a real-world medical problem. *Neural Networks*, 8(6):945–962.

Baxt, W. G. (1991). Use of an artificial neural network for the diagnosis of myocardial infarction. *Annals of Internal Medicine*, 115:843–848.

Breiman, L., Friedman, J., Olshen, R., and Stone, C. (1984). *Classification and Regression Trees*. Wadsworth.

Brouwer, R. K. (1994). A method for training recurrent neural networks for classification by building basins of attraction. *Neural Networks*, 8(4):597-603.

Cestnik, B. (1990). Estimating probabilities: A crucial task in machine learning. In *Proc. European Conference on Artificial Intelligence 1990*, Stockholm.

Cestnik, B., Kononenko, I., and Bratko, I. (1987). Assistant 86: A knowledge-elicitation tool for sophisticated users. In Bratko, I. and Lavrač, N., editors, *Progress in Machine Learning, Proc. EWSL 87*. Sigma Press.

Dietterich, T. G. and Shavlik, J. W., editors, (1990). *Readings in Machine Learning*. Morgan Kaufmann.

Duda, R. O. and Hart, P. E. (1973). *Pattern Classification and Scene Analysis*. John Wiley & Sons.

Haykin, S. (1994). *Neural Networks*. Macmillan College Publishing Company.

Hecht-Nielsen, R. (1990). *Neurocomputing*. Addison-Wesley.

Horn, K. A., Compton, P., Lazarus, L., and Quinlan, J. R. (1985). An expert system for the interpretation of thyroid assays in a clinical laboratory. *The Australian Computer Journal*, 17(1):7-11.

Kira, K. and Rendell, L. (1992). A practical approach to feature selection. In Sleeman, D. and Edwards, P., editors, *Proc. Intern. Conf. on Machine Learning*, pages 249-256. Morgan Kaufmann.

Kohonen, T. (1984). *Self-Organization and Associative Memory*. Springer Verlag.

Kononenko, I. (1992). Combining decisions of multiple rules. In du Boulayand, B. and Sgorev, V., editors, *Artificial Intelligence V: Methodology, Systems, Applications*. Elsevier.

Kononenko, I. (1991). Semi naive Bayesian classifier. In Kodratoff, Y., editor, *Proc. European Working Session on Learning EWSL-91*, Porto, pages 206-219.

Kononenko, I., Bratko, I., and Roškar E. (1984). Experiments in automatic learning of medical diagnostic rules. In *Proc. of International School for the Synthesis of Expert's Knowledge Workshop*, Bled, Slovenia, August, 1984.

Kononenko, I. and Bratko, I. (1991). Information based evaluation criterion for classifier's performance. *Machine Learning*, 6:67-80.

Kononenko, I. and Šimec, E. (1995). Induction of decision trees using ReliefF. In Della Riccia, G., Kruse, R., and Viertl, R., editors, *Proc. of ISSEK Workshop on Mathematical and Statistical Methods in Artificial Intelligence*, pages 199-220, Springer Verlag.

Kukar, M., Kononenko, I., and Silvester, T. (1996). Machine learning in prognostics of the femoral neck fracture recovery. *Artificial Intelligence in Medicine*, 8(5):431-451.

Michie, D., Spiegelhalter, D. J., and Taylor, C. C., editors, (1994). *Machine Learning, Neural and Statistical Classification*. Ellis Horwood.

Pirnat, V., Kononenko, I., Janc, T., and Bratko, I. (1989). Medical estimation of automatically induced decision rules. In *Proc. of 2nd Europ. Conf. on Artificial Intelligence in Medicine*, pages 24-36, City University, London.

Quinlan, R., Compton, P., Horn, K. A., and Lazarus L. (1987). Inductive knowledge acquisition: A case study. In Quinlan, J.R., editor, *Applications of expert systems*, Turing Institute Press and Addison-Wesley.

Ragavan, H. and Rendell, L. (1993). Lookahead feature construction for learning hard concepts. In *Proc. 10th Intern. Conf. on Machine Learning*, pages 252–259. Morgan Kaufmann.

Roškar, E., Abrams, P., Bratko, I., Kononenko, I., and Varšek A. (1986). MCUDS - An expert system for the diagnostics of lower urinary tract disorders. *Journal of Biomedical Measurements, Informatics and Control*, 1(4):201–204.

Roy, A., Govil, S., and Miranda, R. (1995). An algorithm to generate RBF-like nets for classification problems. *Neural Networks*, 8(2):179–201.

Rumelhart, D. E. and McClelland J. L., editors, (1986). *Parallel Distributed Processing, Vol. 1: Foundations*. MIT Press, Cambridge.

Schalkoff, R. (1992). *Pattern Recognition: Statistical, Structural and Neural Approaches*. John Wiley & Sons.

Šter, B., Dobnikar, A., Kranjec, I., Klemenc, M., and Gabrijel, I. (1995). Comparison of different neural and statistical methods on medical databases. Internal Report, Laboratory of Adaptive Systems, Faculty of Computer and Information Science, University of Ljubljana, Slovenia.

Šter, B. and Dobnikar, A. (1995). Neural networks in medical diagnosis: Comparison with other methods. In Bulsari, A. and Tsaptsinos, D., editors, *Proc. International Conference on Engineering Applications of Neural Networks*, London.

Weigend, A. S., Huberman, B. A., and Rumelhart, D. E. (1991). Generalization by weight-elimination with application to forecasting. In Lippmann, R. P., Moody, J. E., and Touretzky, D. S., editors, *Advances in Neural Information Processing Systems 3*, pages 875–882. Morgan-Kaufmann.

11 NOISE ELIMINATION APPLIED TO EARLY DIAGNOSIS OF RHEUMATIC DISEASES

Nada Lavrač,
Dragan Gamberger,
and Sašo Džeroski

Abstract: Machine learning methods can be used to induce diagnostic rules from patient records with known diagnoses. In a medical application it is crucial that a machine learning system is capable of detecting regularities in the data by appropriately dealing with imperfect data, i.e., data that contains various kinds of errors, either random or systematic. This chapter presents a compression-based method that is capable of detecting data which is suspected to contain errors and is therefore unsuitable for the extraction of genuine regularities. This noise elimination method is applied to a problem of early diagnosis of rheumatic diseases which is known to be difficult due to its nature and to the imperfections in the available dataset. The method is evaluated by applying the noise elimination algorithm in conjunction with the CN2 rule induction algorithm, and by comparing their performance to earlier results obtained by CN2 in this diagnostic domain.

11.1 INTRODUCTION

Machine learning methods [Michie et al., 1994] have been applied in numerous medical domains [Kononenko and Kukar, 1995]. These domains include diagnostic and prognostic problems in oncology, liver pathology, neuropsychology, gynaecology, etc. Using machine learning, improved medical diagnosis and prognosis can be achieved through automatic analysis of patient data stored in medical records, i.e., by learning from past experiences.

Machine learning assumes that a set of examples E with known classifications is given. An example is described by the values of a fixed collection of attributes A_i, $i \in \{1, \ldots, n\}$. Each attribute can either have a finite set of values (discrete) or take real numbers as values (continuous). An example e_j is a vector of attribute values, $e_j = (v_{1j}, \ldots, v_{nj})$, together with a class assignment c_j, where c_j is one of the N possible values of the class variable C. For instance, in the domain of early diagnosis of rheumatic diseases, described in Section 11.4, patient records are described by 16 anamnestic attributes. Some of these are continuous (e.g., age, duration of morning stiffness) and some are discrete (e.g., joint pain, which can be arthrotic, arthritic, or not present at all). There are eight class values, corresponding to the following diagnoses: degenerative spine diseases, degenerative joint diseases, inflammatory spine diseases, other inflammatory diseases, extraarticular rheumatism, crystal-induced synovitis, nonspecific rheumatic manifestations, and nonrheumatic diseases.

On the basis of training examples, machine learning systems either construct explicit symbolic rules that generalize the training cases (rule induction), store (some of) the training cases for reference (instance-based learning), or build non-symbolic classifiers (Bayesian classifiers and neural networks). Different machine learning methodologies are presented in [Michie et al., 1994]. In this chapter we only consider rule induction methods [Clark and Niblett, 1989].

The rules, induced from the set of training examples, can be used for the classification (diagnosis/prediction) of new cases. In medicine, such cases are new patients with an unknown diagnosis/prognosis.

In an ideal inductive learning problem, the induced hypothesis H will 'agree' with the classifications of all the training examples E. In practice, however, it frequently happens that data given to the learner contain various kinds of errors, either random or systematic. Random errors are usually referred to as *noise*. Therefore, in most real-life problems the success of machine learning very much depends on the learner's noise-handling capability, i.e., its ability of appropriately dealing with noisy data.

The problem of noise handling has been extensively studied in attribute-value learning. This problem has been approached in different ways. Noise-handling mechanisms can be incorporated in search heuristics [Mingers, 1989b] and in stopping criteria [Clark and Boswell, 1991] used in hypothesis construction. Hypotheses fulfilling stopping criteria may further be evaluated according to some quality measure, giving a preferential order of hypotheses. In addition, the induced hypotheses can be subjected to some form of post-processing, such as postpruning and simplifying of decision trees [Cestnik and Bratko, 1991, Mingers, 1989a, Quinlan, 1987]. Systems employing such techniques are called *noise-tolerant* systems since they try to avoid overfitting the possibly noisy training set. Compression measures [Muggleton et al., 1992], based on the Minimum Description Length (MDL) principle [Rissanen, 1978], provide a theoretically justified basis for grading candidate hypotheses, by integrating a measure of complexity (simplicity or understandability) and correctness (expected accuracy) into a single heuristic measure for hypothesis evaluation.

The noise-handling technique proposed in this chapter is different: it detects and eliminates noisy examples in preprocessing of the training set by using a simple compression measure, whereas a consistent and complete hypothesis can then be built from the set of remaining examples [Gamberger et al., 1996]. The separation of noise detection and hypothesis formation has the advantage that noisy examples do not influence hypothesis construction. Moreover, the explicit detection of potentially noisy examples allows us to show the examples to the expert, who can distinguish outliers from errors. A general hypothesis can then be built from error-free data (therefore better capturing the regularities of the domain), and outliers can be added to the hypothesis as exceptions to the general rule.

In order to describe the proposed approach to noise detection and elimination we assume a learning setting, described in Section 11.2, that involves a preprocessing step. The proposed approach to noise detection and elimination is presented in Section 11.3. Section 11.4 presents the problem of early diagnosis of rheumatic diseases, Section 11.5 gives the experimental setting and previous results achieved in this problem domain. Section 11.6 outlines the experimental results of applying the proposed noise-handling method in this diagnostic problem. The chapter concludes with a summary and gives directions for further research.

11.2 THE LEARNING SETTING

In our approach, we assume an inductive learning algorithm consisting of three separate steps: (1) preprocessing of the training set, (2) noise detection and elimination, and (3) hypothesis formation.

11.2.1 Preprocessing

We first consider a two-class learning problem where the training set E consists of positive and negative examples of a concept ($E = P \cup N$) and the examples $e \in E$ are tuples of truth-values of *literals* in the hypothesis language. The set of all literals is denoted by L.

Let us represent the training set E as a table where rows correspond to training examples and columns correspond to literals. An entry in the table has the value *true* when the given example satisfies the corresponding condition (literal), otherwise its value is *false*.

If the training set does not have the form of tuples of truth-values, a transformation to this form is performed during the preprocessing of the training set. The transformation procedure is based on an analysis of the values of training examples. For each attribute A_i, let v_{ix} ($x = 1..k_{ip}$) be the k_{ip} different values of the attribute that appear in the positive examples and let w_{iy} ($y = 1..k_{in}$) be the k_{in} different values appearing in the negative examples. The transformation results in a set of literals L:

- For discrete attributes A_i, literals of the form $A_i = v_{ix}$ and $A_i \neq w_{iy}$ are generated. In the case that a positive and a negative example have the same value $v_{ix} = w_{iy}$ of A_i, two literals are created: $A_i = v_{ix}$ and $A_i \neq w_{iy}$.

  For illustration, consider a problem with two attributes, A and B, and a training set of three examples, two positive examples (a_2, b_1) and (a_3, b_2) and a negative example (a_1, b_2). Then the following literals are created: $A \neq a_1$, $A = a_2$, $A = a_3$, $B = b_1$, $B = b_2$, $B \neq b_2$, and the three examples correspond to the following truth-value tuples of literals: 110101, 101010 and 000010, respectively (where 1 stands for *true* and 0 stands for *false*). The literals $A = a_1$, $A \neq a_2$, ... are not even considered since they are either *false* for all positive examples ($A = a_1$) or *true* for all negative examples ($A \neq a_2$); as such they are useless for constructing a concept description.

- Similar to [Fayyad and Irani, 1992], literals of the following two forms are created for continuous attributes A_i:

  - $A_i \leq (v_{ix}+w_{iy})/2$ are created for all neighboring value pairs (v_{ix}, w_{iy}) which satisfy the property $v_{ix} < w_{iy}$ and for which no value v_{iz} or w_{iz} of attribute A_i exists such that $v_{ix} < v_{iz} < w_{iy}$ or $v_{ix} < w_{iz} < w_{iy}$.
  - $A_i > (v_{ix} + w_{iy})/2$ are created for all neighboring pairs (w_{iy}, v_{ix}) which satisfy the property $w_{iy} < v_{ix}$ and for which no value v_{iz} or

w_{iz} exists between values v_{ix} and w_{iy} such that $w_{iy} < v_{iz} < v_{ix}$ or $w_{iy} < w_{iz} < v_{ix}$ holds.

- For integer valued attributes A_i, literals are generated as if A_i were both discrete and continuous, resulting in literals of four different forms: $A_i \leq (v_{ix} + w_{iy})/2$, $A_i > (v_{ix} + w_{iy})/2$, $A_i = v_{ix}$, and $A_i \neq w_{iy}$, depending on the training set.

In our approach, we use an implicit definition of equality for continuous attributes which allows for all values (also non-integer) in some range. This has the following advantages. First, by allowing only literals of the form $A_i \leq (v_{ix} + w_{iy})/2$ and $A_i > (v_{ix} + w_{iy})/2$ we avoid the precision problem that would have occurred if literals of the form $A_i = v_{ij}$, say $A_i = 3.143$, were allowed for continues attributes. Namely, if the system were to determine the truth-value of the literal $A_i = 3.143$ for an example which has value 3.1432 of attribute A_i, should the literal be evaluated as *true* or *false*? This decision depends on the precision applied in the comparison, but this precision is not defined. Moreover, the fact that continuous attributes do not have literals of the form $A_i = 3.143$ does not prevent testing whether A_i has the value 3.143 in the generated rule; a learner can namely build a condition as a conjunction of elementary literals, such as for instance $(A_i > 3.142) \wedge (A_i \leq 3.144)$. The advantage of constructing conditions in this form is that they have an explicitly defined precision.

11.2.2 Noise elimination for multiclass learning

The basic algorithm for detecting noisy examples, described in detail in Section 11.3, works for two-class problems where positive and negative examples of a single concept are described by literals. This section describes how to perform noise elimination for multiclass problems,

Given an example set E of a multiclass learning problem, the elimination of noisy examples is performed as follows.

1. For each of the N classes c_j, create a two-class learning problem: examples that belong to class c_j become the positive examples for learning the concept c_j and all other examples become the negative examples of this concept. Each pair (e_i, c_i) is thus mapped into a new pair (e_i, c_{ij}), where $c_{ij} = 1$ if $c_i = c_j$ and $c_{ij} = 0$ otherwise.

2. Transform each pair (e_i, c_{ij}), where e_i is described by attribute values, into a pair $(f(e_i), c_{ij})$ where $f(e_i)$ is a tuple of truth-values of literals (see above). This results in new example sets E_j, $j = 1..N$.

3. For each of the N two-class learning problems, a set of noisy examples $O'_j \subseteq E_j$ is detected by Algorithm 11.1 (see Section 11.3.3). Let $O_j = \{e_i \mid f(e_i) \in O'_j\}$.

4. Finally, the noisy examples O_j of each E_j are eliminated from the original multiclass training set E. This results in a reduced training set

$$NE = E \setminus \bigcup_{j=1..N} O_j.$$

A learning algorithm that assumes a noiseless training set can be now applied to the reduced training set NE.

11.2.3 Hypothesis formation with CN2

Given a set of classified examples, CN2 [Clark and Boswell, 1991] constructs a set of if-then rules. The condition part of a rule contains one or more attribute tests of the form $A_i = v_i$ for discrete attributes, and $A_i < v_i$ or $A_i > v_i$ for continuous attributes. The conclusion part has the form $C = c_i$, assigning a value c_i to the class variable C. We say that an example is covered by a rule if the attribute values of the example obey the conditions in the antecedent (if part) of the rule.

CN2 uses the covering approach to construct a set of rules for each possible class c_i in turn: when rules for class c_i are being constructed, examples of this class are positive, all other examples are negative. The covering approach works as follows: CN2 constructs a rule that correctly classifies some examples, removes the positive examples covered by the rule from the training set and repeats the process until no more examples remain. To construct a single rule that classifies examples into class c_i, CN2 starts with a rule with an empty antecedent (if part) and the selected class c_i as a consequent (then part). The antecedent of this rule is satisfied by all the examples in the training set, and not only those of the selected class. CN2 then progressively refines the antecedent by adding conditions to it, until only examples of class c_i satisfy the antecedent.

The choice of the condition to be added to the partially built rule depends on the number of examples of each class covered by the refined rule and the heuristic estimate of the quality of the rule. The heuristic estimate is mainly designed to estimate the performance of the rule on unseen examples in terms of classification accuracy. This is in accordance with the task of achieving high classification accuracy on unseen cases. Suppose that a rule covers p positive and n negative examples. Its accuracy can be estimated by the so-called Laplace estimate, computed as $(p+1)/(p+n+N)$, where N is the number of possible classes [Clark and Boswell, 1991].

To allow for handling imperfect data, CN2 may construct a set of rules which is imprecise, i.e., does not classify all of the examples in the training set correctly. This happens when the *significance* measure of CN2 is applied to enforce the induction of reliable rules. A rule is deemed reliable (significant) if the class distribution of the examples it covers is significantly different from the prior class distribution as given by the entire training set. This is measured by the *likelihood ratio statistic* [Clark and Boswell, 1991].

Suppose a rule covers r_i examples of class c_i, $i \in \{1, \ldots, N\}$. Let $q_i = r_i/(r_1 + \ldots + r_N)$ and let $p_i = p(c_i)$ be the prior probability of class c_i. The likelihood ratio statistic is computed as follows:

$$2(r_1 + \ldots + r_N) \sum_{i=1}^{N} q_i \, log(q_i/p_i)$$

This statistic is distributed as χ^2 with $N-1$ degrees of freedom. If its value is above a specified significance threshold, the rule is deemed significant.

The most recent version of CN2 [Džeroski et al., 1993] can measure its classification performance also in terms of the *relative information score* [Kononenko and Bratko, 1991]. The relative information score is a performance measure which is not biased by the prior class distribution. It accounts for the possibility to achieve high accuracy easily in domains with a very likely majority class by taking into account the prior probability distribution of the training examples.

Let the correct class of example e_k be c_k, its prior probability $p_k = p(c_k)$ and the probability returned by the classifier $p'_k = p'(c_k)$. The *information score* of this answer is:

$$I(e_k) = \begin{cases} -log\ p_k + log\ p'_k & p'_k \geq p_k \\ log(1-p_k) - log(1-p'_k) & p'_k < p_k \end{cases}$$

As $I(e_k)$ indicates the amount of information about the correct classification of e_k gained by the classifier's answer, it is positive if $p'_k > p_k$, negative if the answer is misleading ($p'_k < p_k$) and zero if $p'_k = p_k$.

The *relative information score* I_r of the answers of a classifier on a testing set consisting of examples $e_1, e_2, ..., e_t$ each belonging to one of the classes $c_1, c_2, ..., c_N$ can be calculated as the ratio of the average information score of the answers and the entropy of the prior distribution of the classes:

$$I_r = \frac{\frac{1}{t} \times \sum_{k=1}^{t} I(e_k)}{-\sum_{i=1}^{N} p_i \ log\ p_i}$$

11.3 NOISE DETECTION AND ELIMINATION

11.3.1 Literals and p/n pairs

We first consider a two-class learning problem where the training set E consists of tuples of truth-values of literals.

For noise detection and elimination, we need to investigate the properties of literals that hold on individual pairs of training examples, each pair consisting of a positive and a negative example.

Definition 1 *A p/n pair is a pair of two examples e_i and e_j such that $e_i \in P$ and $e_j \in N$. When appropriate, we will use the notation p_i/n_j for a p/n pair consisting of $p_i \in P$ and $n_j \in N$.*

Definition 2 *A literal $l \in L$ covers a p_i/n_j pair if the literal has value $true$ for p_i and value $false$ for n_j.*[1]

The notion of p/n pairs can be used to prove important properties of literals for building complete and consistent concept descriptions [Gamberger, 1995].

Theorem 1 *Assume that a training set E and a set of literals L are given such that a complete and consistent hypothesis H can be found. Let $L' \subseteq L$. A complete and consistent concept description H can be found using only literals from the set L' if and only if for each possible p/n pair from the training set E there exists at least one literal $l \in L'$ that covers the p/n pair.*

The proof of this statement can be found in [Gamberger et al., 1996]. It will be shown that this theorem plays a central role in noise elimination. Namely, if the set L is sufficient for constructing a complete and consistent hypothesis H from E, several such hypotheses may be found. Among these, one may prefer the simplest according to some complexity measure. Given the sets E and L, the minimal complexity of a hypothesis that uses literals from L and is complete and consistent w.r.t. E is denoted by $q(E, L)$. One possible measure of complexity of a hypothesis H is the number of different literals that appear in it: $q(E, L) = |L'|$, where L' is the smallest subset of L that allows the construction of a hypothesis H consistent and complete w.r.t. E. As Theorem 1 suggests, one can compute $q(E, L)$ without actually constructing the hypothesis H. This is crucial for our approach to noise elimination.

11.3.2 Background

Let us assume that for the given training set E and the given set of literals L a consistent and complete hypothesis H (an approximation to an unknown target theory T) can be found.[2] Let $q(E, L)$ represent the complexity of the simplest hypothesis complete and consistent with training examples in E and built of literals from L. Let us temporarily fix the set of literals L and study the complexity q only as a function of E: $q(E, L) = q(E)$.

Given the sets E and L, assume that the training set E contains enough training examples to induce/identify a correct hypothesis H.[3] If the set of examples is large enough to identify the correct hypothesis H then, by adding examples to E, the complexity of the simplest hypothesis that can be generated from the enlarged training set will not increase. Let $m = |E|$. This means that for the examples $e_{m+1}, e_{m+2}, \ldots$ that are not included in the initial training set E it holds that:

$$q(E) = q(E \cup \{e_{m+1}\}) = q(E \cup \{e_{m+1}, e_{m+2}\}) = \ldots$$

By adding to E a noisy example f that is inconsistent with the target theory T, the complexity of the hypothesis increases:

$$q(E \cup \{f\}) > q(E).$$

Theorem 2 *Suppose that the set of examples E is non-noisy and is large enough to enable a unique simplest correct hypothesis H to be generated. By adding an example to the training set, a new training set is generated $E' = E \cup \{e\}$. If e is consistent with the target theory T (e is non-noisy), then $q(E') = q(E)$. If e is inconsistent with T (e is noisy), then $q(E') > q(E)$.*

The proof of this statement can be found in [Gamberger et al., 1996], Theorem 2 presents the basis for the suggested noise elimination algorithm - see [Gamberger and Lavrač, 1997] for a theoretical study of the applicability of Occam's razor for noise elimination, including a discussion of when a training set is 'large enough' (a so-called 'saturation' requirement). Note that the theorem has some practical disadvantages. First, it makes use of the definition of a training set E that is 'large enough', i.e., $|E| > m_T$, for some minimal number of examples m_T needed to enable the construction of a complete and consistent hypothesis H that is 'correct' w.r.t. the target theory T. In practice it is hard to know whether a training set E is large enough, and a unique simplest correct hypothesis H may not exist. The consequence is that the assumptions of the theorem need not necessarily hold, which may result in imperfect noise detection. However, the assumption is that with the increase of the number of non-noisy examples in E, the conditions of the theorem will be better satisfied, thus increasing the probability of successful noise detection. On the other hand, an important advantage of the theorem is that its claims do not depend on the actual definition of the hypothesis complexity function $q(E)$. Nevertheless, the sensitivity of this function may influence the value m_T, the number of training examples necessary for the applicability of the theorem.

Now we can try to answer the following question: Does the training set E contain noise? Based on Theorem 2 we can answer the question in the following way. If it holds that

$$q(E) = q(E \setminus \{e\})$$

for all possible examples $e \in E$ then there is no noise in the dataset and the dataset is large enough for a correct hypothesis H to be induced. If this is not the case and an example e enables complexity reduction, i.e., $q(E) > q(E \setminus \{e\})$, then the example e is potentially incorrect. If there is more than one such example whose elimination leads to complexity reduction, it is advisable to eliminate the example that reduces the complexity the most. The elimination of 'potentially noisy' examples is an iterative process where one example is eliminated in each iteration until no elimination can result in further complexity reduction.

11.3.3 The noise elimination algorithm

Theorem 1 can be used as a basis for the implementation of an efficient algorithm for noise elimination which eliminates noisy examples from $E = P \cup N$, given a two-class learning problem.

Let the heuristic estimate of the complexity of the hypothesis $q(E, L)$ be defined as the minimal number of literals $|L'|$ needed to build a complete and consistent hypothesis H (see also the discussion following Theorem 1).

The basic idea of the noise elimination algorithm is to detect the minimal subset L', $L' \subseteq L$, and use it to answer the following question: 'Can any of the literals in L' be made unnecessary for building a complete and consistent hypothesis if one (or more) training example(s) are eliminated?' The practical applicability of the proposed approach follows from the observation that, in most cases, for a detected noisy example e_i a set L'_i can be found such that $L'_i \subset L'$, and L'_i covers all p/n pairs of the set $E \setminus \{e_i\}$. The noisy examples that do not have this property will not be detected by the noise elimination algorithm.

The proposed algorithm consists of the heuristic noise elimination algorithm (Algorithm 11.1), which employs the heuristic literal minimization algorithm (Algorithm 11.2).

Algorithm 11.1 computes weights of literals $l \in L'$ and selects 'potentially noisy' examples as those whose elimination will eliminate many 'heavy' literals from L'. Weights are computed as $v(l) = 1/z$, where z is the number of examples that should be eliminated in order to make l unnecessary. Thus the 'heaviest' literal l with $v(l) = 1$ is the one that is made unnecessary by the elimination of only one example.

Algorithm 11.1: Noise elimination

Given: quality function $q(E, L) = |L'|$ (number of literals in the minimal set L'), noise sensitivity parameter ε_h

Input: nonempty example set $E = P \cup N$, set of literals L

Output: example set of noiseless examples E'

initialize $E' \leftarrow E$ (set of noiseless examples)

repeat

initialize $w(e) \leftarrow 0$ for all $e \in E'$

initialize PN (a set of all p/n pairs of E')

find by heuristic search a minimal subset L' of L such that a complete and consistent hypothesis $H(E', L')$ can be built (Algorithm 11.2)

for all $l \in L'$ **do**

find the minimal subset E_l of examples from E' by whose elimination the literal l can be made unnecessary (Procedure 11.1)

compute weight $v(l) = 1/z$, where $z = |E_l|$

for all examples $e \in E_l$, compute weights $w(e) = w(e) + v(l)$

end for

select example e_s: $e_s = arg\ max\ w(e)$, where max is computed over all $e \in E'$

if $w(e_s) > \varepsilon_h$ **then** $E' \leftarrow E' \setminus \{e_s\}$

until $w(e_s) \leq \varepsilon_h$

The basic idea underlying the literal minimization algorithm (Algorithm 11.2) is based on the coverage of p/n pairs: select the minimal literal set L' from L so that all the p/n pairs are covered by L'. To do so, the idea is to compute weights of p/n pairs and construct L' from literals covering many 'heavy' p/n pairs. Weights are computed as $v(p/n) = 1/z$, where z is the number of literals that cover the p/n pair; thus the 'heaviest' p/n pair with $v(p/n) = 1$ is the one covered by one literal only. The algorithm outputs a list of literals L' which is the heuristically selected minimal literal set.

Algorithm 11.1 uses a parameter ε_h that determines the noise sensitivity of the algorithm. The parameter can be adjusted by the user in order to tune the algorithm according to the domain characteristics. Reasonable values are between 0.25 and 2. For instance, the value 1.0 guarantees the elimination of every such example by whose elimination the set L' will be reduced for

Algorithm 11.2: Minimization of literals

Input: set of literals L, set of all p/n pairs PN

Output: minimal set of literals L'

initialize $L' \leftarrow \emptyset$

initialize $PN' \leftarrow PN$ (set of p/n pairs not yet covered by any literal in L')

for all $p/n \in PN'$ compute weights $v(p/n) = 1/z$, where z is the number of literals that cover the p/n pair

while $PN' \neq \emptyset$ **do**

select p_s/n_s (a pair covered by the least number of literals):
$p_s/n_s = arg\ max\ v(p/n)$, where max is computed over all $p/n \in PN'$

for all $l \in L \setminus L'$ covering p_s/n_s compute weights $w(l) = \sum v(p/n)$, where summation is over all $p/n \in PN'$ covered by l

select literal l_s: $l_s = arg\ max\ w(l)$, where max is computed over all $l \in L \setminus L'$ covering p_s/n_s

$L' \leftarrow L' \cup \{l_s\}$

$PN' \leftarrow PN' \setminus \{p/n$ pairs covered by $l_s\}$

end while

Procedure 11.1: Minimal example set selection

Input: set of literals L' such that a complete and consistent hypothesis $H(E, L')$ can be generated, literal $l \in L'$

Output: minimal set of examples E_l that needs to be eliminated in order to make l unnecessary

construct PN_l as a set of all p_i/n_j pairs covered by l and not covered by any other literal from L'

construct P_l from positive examples p_i of PN_l

construct N_l from negative examples n_j of PN_l

if $|P_l| < |N_l|$ **then** $E_l \leftarrow P_l$ (minimal set) **else** $E_l \leftarrow N_l$ (minimal set)

at least one literal. Lower ε_h values mean greater algorithm sensitivity (i.e., elimination of more examples): lower ε_h values should be used when noise in the domain is not completely random, and when dealing with large training sets (since statistical properties of noise distribution in large training sets can have similar effects). The default values of ε_h are determined based on the number of training examples in the smaller of the two subsets of E: the set of positive examples P or the negative examples N. The default values are: 1.5

for training sets with 2–50 examples, 1.0 for 51–100 examples, 0.75 for 101–200 examples, and 0.5 for more than 200 examples.

Algorithm 11.1 calls Procedure 11.1 which, for the given subset L' and some literal $l \in L'$, determines the minimal subset of examples that must be eliminated in order to make l unnecessary when building a complete and consistent hypothesis.

11.4 EARLY DIAGNOSIS OF RHEUMATIC DISEASES

Correct diagnosis in the early stage of rheumatic disease is a difficult problem. Having passed all the investigations, many patients can not be reliably diagnosed after their first visit to the specialist. The reason is that anamnestic, clinical, laboratory and radiological data of patients with different rheumatic diseases are frequently similar. In addition, diagnosis can also be incorrect due to the subjective interpretation of data [Pirnat et al., 1989].

11.4.1 Dataset description

Data about 462 patients were collected at the University Medical Center in Ljubljana [Pirnat et al., 1989]. There are over 200 different rheumatic diseases which can be grouped into three, six, eight or twelve diagnostic classes. As suggested by a specialist, eight diagnostic classes were considered [Karalič and Pirnat, 1990]. Table 11.1 gives the names of the diagnostic classes and the numbers of patients belonging to each class.

Table 11.1 The eight diagnostic classes and the corresponding numbers of patients.

Class	Name	# patients
$A1$	degenerative spine diseases	158
$A2$	degenerative joint diseases	128
$B1$	inflammatory spine diseases	16
$B234$	other inflammatory diseases	29
C	extraarticular rheumatism	21
D	crystal-induced synovitis	24
E	nonspecific rheumatic manifestations	32
F	nonrheumatic diseases	54

To facilitate the comparison with earlier experiments in rule induction in this domain [Lavrač et al., 1993], the experiments were performed on anamnestic data, without taking into account data about patients' clinical manifestations, laboratory and radiological findings. There are sixteen anamnestic attributes: Sex, Age, Family anamnesis, Duration of present symptoms (in weeks), Duration of rheumatic diseases (in weeks), Joint pain (arthrotic, arthritic), Number of painful joints, Number of swollen joints, Spinal pain (spondylotic, spondylitic), Other pain (headache, pain in muscles, thorax, abdomen, heels), Duration of morning stiffness (in hours), Skin manifestations, Mucosal manifestations, Eye manifestations, Other manifestations, and Therapy. Some of these attributes are continuous (e.g., Age, Duration of morning stiffness) and some are discrete (e.g., Joint pain, which can be arthrotic, arthritic, or not present at all).

11.4.2 Medical background knowledge

The available patient data, described by 16 anamnestic attributes, can be augmented with additional diagnostic knowledge which can be considered as additional information by the learner. In machine learning terminology, additional expert knowledge is usually referred to as *background knowledge.*

A specialist for rheumatic diseases has provided his knowledge about typical co-occurrences of symptoms. Six typical groupings of symptoms (called Grouping 1–6) were suggested by the specialist as background knowledge [Lavrač et al., 1993, Lavrač and Džeroski, 1994]. The background knowledge is encoded in the form of functions, introducing specific function values for each characteristic combination of symptoms. All the other combinations (except the ones explicitly specified) have the same function value *irrelevant.* The characteristic combinations of attribute values are given names which are understandable to experts as they represent meaningful co-occurrences of symptoms which have their role in expert diagnosis.

The application of the system LINUS [Lavrač and Džeroski, 1994], that is capable of dealing with background knowledge, resulted in 6 new attributes to be considered by the learner.

The first grouping relates the attributes Joint pain and Duration of morning stiffness. The characteristic combinations are given in Table 11.2, all other combinations are considered insignificant or irrelevant by the expert.

Table 11.2 Characteristic combinations of values in Grouping 1.

Joint pain	Morning stiffness	Grouping 1 values
no pain	$\leq$ 1 hour	no pain & dms $\leq$ 1 hour
arthrotic	$\leq$ 1 hour	arthrotic & dms $\leq$ 1 hour
arthritic	$>$ 1 hour	arthritic & dms $>$ 1 hour

Grouping 2 relates Spinal pain and Duration of morning stiffness. The following are the characteristic combinations: no spinal pain and morning stiffness up to 1 hour, spondylotic pain and morning stiffness up to 1 hour, spondylitic pain and morning stiffness longer than 1 hour.

The third grouping relates the attributes Sex and Other pain. Indicative is the pain in the thorax or in the heels for male patients, all other combinations are nonspecific: the corresponding values of Grouping 3 are 'male & thorax' and 'male & heels'.

The fourth grouping relates Joint pain and Spinal pain. Grouping 5 relates Joint pain, Spinal pain and Number of painful joints, and the sixth grouping relates Number of swollen joints and Number of painful joints.

11.5 EXPERIMENTAL SETTING AND PREVIOUS RESULTS

The goal of our experiments is to show the utility of noise elimination in learning from noisy data. Since the ultimate test of the quality of induced rules is their performance on unseen examples, experiments were performed on ten different random partitions of the data into 70% training and 30% testing examples. In this way, ten training sets E_i and ten testing sets T_i, $i = 1..10$ were generated. These are the same training and testing sets as used in our previous experiments [Lavrač et al., 1993, Lavrač and Džeroski, 1994], from where the results of CN2 on the original datasets are taken. In these experiments, CN2 [Džeroski et al., 1993] was applied with and without its significance test noise-handling mechanism. When using the significance test in CN2, a significance level of 99% was applied. For an eight class problem, this corresponds to a threshold 18.5 for the value of the likelihood ratio statistic. The other CN2 parameters were set to their default values [Clark and Boswell, 1991]. When using Algorithm 11.1 for noise elimination, the noise sensitivity parameter ε_h had its default values: 1.5 for training sets with 2–50 examples (training sets for diagnoses $B1$, $B234$, C, D, E), 1.0 for 51–100 examples (F), 0.75 for 101–200 examples ($A1$, $A2$) and 0.5 for more than 200 examples (no such training set).

Previous experiments [Lavrač et al., 1993, Lavrač and Džeroski, 1994] show that the CN2 noise-handling mechanism improves the classification accuracy, but decreases the relative information score. These results are reproduced in Table 11.3, columns Original CN2-ST and Original CN2-NoST (ST denotes the use of Significance Test in CN2, and NoST means that No Significance Test was used).

11.6 RESULTS OF NOISE ELIMINATION

In our experiments, we tested the performance of the noise elimination algorithm by comparing the results achieved by CN2 before and after noise elimination. Noise elimination resulted in reduced datasets NE_1, ..., NE_{10}. Rules were induced by CN2 from NE_i, while the accuracy and relative information score were measured on T_i, $i = 1..10$. These results are given in columns Reduced CN2-NoST of Table 11.3.

Table 11.3 Accuracy and relative information score.

	Accuracy			Relative information score		
Partition	Original CN2-ST	Original CN2-NoST	Reduced CN2-NoST	Original CN2-ST	Original CN2-NoST	Reduced CN2-NoST
1	47.5	38.1	45.3	17.0	21.0	26.0
2	45.3	44.6	44.6	20.0	23.0	28.0
3	51.1	45.3	47.5	17.0	19.0	24.0
4	44.6	43.9	38.8	17.0	24.0	20.0
5	46.0	40.3	41.7	21.0	22.0	25.0
6	49.6	48.2	50.4	15.0	26.0	24.0
7	44.6	42.4	46.8	21.0	27.0	31.0
8	41.0	38.8	43.2	21.0	19.0	25.0
9	43.9	45.3	48.2	16.0	23.0	29.0
10	39.6	41.7	43.2	23.0	23.0	25.0
Mean	45.3	42.9	45.0	18.8	22.7	25.7

In order to observe the effect of noise elimination, the results in columns Original CN2-NoST and Reduced CN2-NoST of Table 11.3 need to be compared. On the other hand, in order to compare the noise elimination algorithm to the CN2 noise-handling mechanism using the significance test, compare the columns Original CN2-ST and Reduced CN2-NoST in Table 11.3. This is actually the most interesting comparison since, in terms of classification accuracy, CN2 with significance test (CN2-ST) is known to perform well on noisy data.

The elimination of noisy examples increases the classification accuracy from 42.9% to 45.0%. This increase is statistically significant at the 96% level according to the one-tailed paired t-test. This result is in favor of our expectation that the elimination of noisy examples is useful for concept learning. The effect of noise-handling by the noise elimination algorithm (accuracy 45.0%) is comparable to the effect of the significance test (accuracy 45.3% achieved by CN2-ST); the difference in performance is not significant.

In terms of the relative information score, substantial improvements are achieved by applying the noise elimination algorithm. The relative information score significantly increases (from 22.7% to 25.7%) after the elimination of noisy examples. Particularly favorable is the comparison between the noise elimination and the significance test used as the CN2 noise-handling mechanism: there is an almost 7 % difference in favor of noise elimination, i.e., an increase from 18.8% to 25.7%.

11.7 SUMMARY AND FURTHER WORK

This chapter presents a method for noise detection and elimination for inductive learning and its application to the problem of early diagnosis of rheumatic diseases. The latter is indeed a difficult problem, as reflected by the relatively low classification accuracy results achieved by various learning algorithms [Cestnik and Bratko, 1991, Pirnat et al., 1989, Karalič and Pirnat, 1990, Lavrač et al., 1993, Lavrač and Džeroski, 1994].

The results achieved in this study show the adequacy of the elimination of noisy examples as a noise-handling mechanism. On the reduced datasets, obtained by applying our noise elimination procedure, the CN2 learning algorithm without its noise-handling mechanism (significance test) yielded accuracies comparable to those of CN2 with its noise-handling mechanism (significance test) on the original datasets. More importantly, noise elimination resulted in significantly better relative information scores, thus improving the overall performance. These relative information scores are the best scores achieved with CN2 in this domain [Lavrač et al., 1993, Lavrač and Džeroski, 1994].

Further experimental evaluation of the noise elimination approach is planned, in particular on the medical datasets from the Irvine machine learning dataset repository.

Acknowledgments

This research was financially supported by the Ministry of Science and Technology of Slovenia, the Ministry of Science of Croatia, and the ESPRIT Project 20237 Inductive Logic Programming 2. The authors are grateful to the specialists of the University Medical Center in Ljubljana who helped collecting the data, especially to Vladimir Pirnat. Aram Karalič and Igor Kononenko prepared the data in a form appropriate for the experiments.

Notes

1. In the standard machine learning terminology we may reformulate the definition of coverage of p/n pairs as follows: literal l covers a p_i/n_j pair if l covers the positive example p_i and does not cover the negative example n_j.

2. This means that there are no contradictions in the training set, i.e., examples with same truth-values of literals belonging to two different classes. As a consequence of Theorem 1, no complete and consistent hypothesis H can be built from a training set that contains contradictions.

3. Correctness of H means that H is complete and consistent for all, including unseen, examples of the unknown target theory T. In other words this means that H represents the same concept as T.

References

Cestnik, B. and Bratko, I. (1991). On estimating probabilities in tree pruning. In *Proc. 5th European Working Session on Learning*, pages 138–150. Springer Verlag.

Clark, P. and Niblett, T. (1989). The CN2 induction algorithm. *Machine Learning*, 3(4):261–283.

Clark, P. and Boswell, R. (1991). Rule induction with CN2: Some recent improvements. In *Proc. 5th European Working Session on Learning*, pages 151–163. Springer Verlag.

Džeroski, S., Cestnik, B., and Petrovski, I. (1993). Using the m-estimate in rule induction. *Journal of Computing and Information Technology*, 1:37–46.

Fayyad, U.M. and Irani, K.B. (1992). On the handling of continous-valued attributes in decision tree generation. *Machine Learning*, 8:87–102.

Gamberger, D. (1995). A minimization approach to propositional inductive learning. In *Proc. 8th European Conference on Machine Learning*, pages 151–160. Springer Verlag.

Gamberger, D., Lavrač, N., and Džeroski, S. (1996). Noise elimination in inductive concept learning: A case study in medical diagnosis. In *Proc. 7th International Workshop on Algorithmic Learning Theory*, pages 199–212. Springer Verlag.

Gamberger, D. and Lavrač, N. (1997). Conditions for Occam's razor applicability and noise elimination. In *Proc. 9th European Conference on Machine Learning*, pages 108–123. Springer Verlag.

Karalič, A. and Pirnat, V. (1990). Machine learning in rheumatology. *Sistemica* 1(2):113–123.

Kononenko, I. and Bratko, I. (1991). Information–based evaluation criterion for classifier's performance. *Machine Learning*, 6(1):67–80.

Kononenko, I. and Kukar, M. (1995). Machine learning for medical diagnosis. In *Proc. Computer-Aided Data Analysis in Medicine*, IJS Scientific Publishing, IJS-SP-95-1, Ljubljana.

Lavrač, N., Džeroski, S., Pirnat, V., and Križman, V. (1993). The utility of background knowledge in learning medical diagnostic rules. *Applied Artificial Intelligence*, 7:273–293.

Lavrač, N. and Džeroski, S. (1994). *Inductive Logic Programming: Techniques and Applications.* Ellis Horwood, Chichester.

Lavrač, N., Gamberger, D., and Džeroski, S. (1995). An Approach to Dimensionality Reduction in Learning from Deductive Databases. In *Proc. 5th International Workshop on Inductive Logic Programming*. Katholieke Universiteit Leuven, 1995.

Lavrač, N., Džeroski, S., and Bratko, I. (1996). Handling imperfect data in inductive logic programming. In De Raedt, L., editor, *Advances in Inductive Logic Programming*. pages 48–64, IOS Press, Amsterdam.

Michie, D., Spiegelhalter, D.J., and Taylor, C.C., editors (1994). *Machine Learning, Neural and Statistical Classification*. Ellis Horwood, Chichester.

Mingers, J. (1989a). An empirical comparison of pruning methods for decision tree induction. *Machine Learning*, 4(2):227–243.

Mingers, J. (1989b). An empirical comparison of selection measures for decision-tree induction. *Machine Learning*, 3(4):319–342.

Muggleton, S.H., Srinivasan, A., and Bain, M. (1992). Compression, significance and accuracy. In *Proceedings of the Ninth International Conference on Machine Learning*, pages 338–347. Morgan Kaufmann.

Pirnat, V., Kononenko, I., Janc, T., and Bratko, I. (1989). Medical analysis of automatically induced rules. In *Proc. 2nd European Conference on Artificial Intelligence in Medicine*, pages 24–36. Springer Verlag.

Rissanen, J. (1978). Modeling by shortest data description. *Automatica*, 14:465–471.

Quinlan, J.R. (1987). Simplifying decision trees. *International Journal of Man-Machine Studies*, 27(3):221–234.

12 DITERPENE STRUCTURE ELUCIDATION FROM ^{13}C NMR-SPECTRA WITH MACHINE LEARNING

Sašo Džeroski,
Steffen Schulze-Kremer,
Karsten R. Heidtke,
Karsten Siems,
and Dietrich Wettschereck

Abstract: Diterpenes are organic compounds of low molecular weight with a skeleton of 20 carbon atoms. They are of significant chemical and commercial interest because of their use as lead compounds in the search for new pharmaceutical effectors. The interpretation of diterpene ^{13}C NMR-spectra normally requires specialists with detailed spectroscopic knowledge and substantial experience in natural products chemistry, more specifically knowledge on peak patterns and chemical structures. Given a database of peak patterns for diterpenes with known structure, we apply machine learning approaches to discover correlations between peak patterns and chemical structure. Backpropagation neural networks, nearest neighbor classification and decision tree induction are applied, as well as approaches from the field of inductive logic programming. Performance close to the one of domain experts is achieved, which suffices for practical use.

12.1 INTRODUCTION

Structure elucidation of compounds isolated from plants, fungi, bacteria or other organisms is a common problem in natural product chemistry. There are many useful spectroscopic methods of getting information about chemical structures, mainly nuclear magnetic resonance (NMR) and mass spectroscopy. The interpretation of these spectra normally requires specialists with detailed spectroscopic knowledge and substantial experience in natural products chemistry. NMR-spectroscopy is the best method for complete structure elucidation (including stereochemistry) of non-crystalline samples.

For structure elucidation of secondary natural products (not proteins) only ^{1}H NMR- and ^{13}C NMR-spectroscopy, including combined methods such as 2D NMR-spectroscopy, are important because hydrogen and carbon are the most abundant atoms in natural products. In structure elucidation of peptides and proteins ^{15}N NMR is sometimes helpful [Abraham and Loftus, 1978]. ^{1}H NMR- and ^{13}C NMR-spectroscopy are quite different: in a ^{13}C NMR-spectrum every carbon atom occurs as a separate signal in most cases, while in ^{1}H NMR-spectra many signals overlap and are therefore difficult to interpret [Schulze-Kremer, 1995]. Because of the simpler nature of ^{13}C NMR-data as compared to ^{1}H NMR-data, the former are easier to handle and therefore remain the preferred basis for automatic structure elucidation [Gray, 1981].

Diterpenes are one of a few fundamental classes of natural products with about 5000 members known [CDROM, 1995]. The skeleton of every diterpene contains 20 carbon atoms. Sometimes there are additional groups linked to the diterpene skeleton by an oxygen atom with the possible effect of increasing the carbon atom count to more than 20 per diterpene. About 200 different diterpene skeletons are known so far, but some of them are only represented by one member compound. Most of the diterpenes belong to one of 20 common skeleton types.

The problem of structure elucidation of diterpenes requires knowledge about biosynthesis, the way in which biological organisms synthesize natural products. Not every combination of carbons, protons and oxygens that is feasible from a chemical point of view actually occurs in nature, as biosynthesis in biological organisms is limited to a characteristic subset of chemical reactions that constrain the structure space. Structure elucidation of diterpenes can be separated into three main stages:

1. identification of residues (ester and/or glycosides),

2. identification of the diterpene skeleton, and

3. arrangement of the residues on the skeleton.

This work deals with the second stage, the identification of the skeleton. A skeleton is a unique connection of carbon atoms each with a specific atom number and, normalized to a pure skeleton molecule without residues, a certain multiplicity. The latter is the number of hydrogens directly connected to a particular carbon atom: `s` stands for singulet, which means there is no proton (i.e., hydrogen) connected to the carbon; `d` stands for a doublet with one proton connected to the carbon; `t` stands for a triplet with two protons and `q` for a quartet with three protons bound to the carbon atom.

The task we address is to identify the skeleton (type) of diterpenoid compounds, given their ^{13}C NMR-spectra that include the multiplicities and the frequencies of the skeleton atoms. To this end, we apply machine learning techniques on a database containing ^{13}C NMR-spectra and structural information on diterpenes with known structure (and skeleton type).

The chapter is organized as follows: Section 12.2 describes the database, the preprocessing of the data, and the methodology used for data analysis, which includes backpropagation neural networks, nearest neighbor classification, and decision tree induction. Section 12.3 describes the application of propositional methods to analyze the data that include atom numbers. Section 12.4 describes the application of propositional and first-order learning methods to analyze the data without atom numbers. Section 12.5 summarizes and compares the results of all approaches, discusses their significance for the application area, and suggests topics for further work.

12.2 DATA ANALYSIS WITH MACHINE LEARNING

12.2.1 The database

AnalytiCon GmbH, a company that performs research, development, and quality control in biotechnology and pharmacy, maintains a database[1] of diterpenoid compounds. The relational database contains information on 1503 diterpenes with known structure, stored in three relations - `atom`, `bond`, and `nmr`.

The relation `atom` specifies to which element an atom in a given compound belongs. The relation `bond` specifies which atoms are bound and in what way in a given compound. The `nmr` relation stores the measured ^{13}C NMR-spectra. For each of the 20 carbon atoms in a diterpene skeleton, it contains the atom number, its multiplicity and frequency. For each compound, the skeleton which it represents is also specified within the database. The relation schema is `nmr(MoleculeID,SkeletonType,AtomID,AtomNumber,Multiplicity,Frequency)`. The fact `nmr(v1,52,v1_1,1,t,39.00)` thus describes atom `v1_1` of molecule `v1`: the latter belongs to the skeleton type Labdan (52).

Twenty-three different skeleton groups are represented in the set of 1503 available compounds. Out of these, only sixteen are present with more than one instance. The correspondence between the chemical names and the codes used in the database is given in Table 12.1, together with the number of instances of each skeleton type. Only skeleton types with more than one instance are listed. For example, c52 corresponds to the skeleton type Labdan, most common among the 1503 diterpenes in the database (448 instances).

Table 12.1 The classes, their chemical names and numbers of instances in the database.

Code	Chemical name	#	Code	Chemical name	#
c2	Trachyloban	9	c33	Erythoxilan	9
c3	Kauran	353	c36	Spongian	10
c4	Beyeran	72	c47	Cassan	12
c5	Atisiran	33	c52	Labdan	448
c15	Ericacan	2	c54	Clerodan	356
c18	Gibban	13	c71	Portulan	5
c22	Pimaran	155	c79	5,10-seco-Clerodan	4
c28	6,7-seco-Kauran	9	c80	8,9-seco-Labdan	6

12.2.2 Preprocessing

Every substituent or residue connected to a carbon atom exerts a characteristic shift on the resonance frequency signal of the carbon atom and sometimes also changes its multiplicity. Simple rules based on expert knowledge can be used to take this effect into account. They transform the raw, measured, NMR-multiplicities into the so-called reduced multiplicities, which carry more information about the skeleton types. These rules are given in Table 12.2. They leave the measured frequencies unchanged.

Consider, for example, the fact `nmr(v1,52,v1_8,8,s,148.60)`, describing atom `v1_8` of molecule `v1`. The third rule of Table 12.2 applies, thus changing the atom description to `red(v1,52,v1_8,8,d,148.60)`.

12.2.3 The problems

The task we address is to discover knowledge for solving the problem of diterpene structure elucidation. More precisely, given the multiplicities and frequencies for the 20 skeleton atoms of a diterpenoid compound, the task is to assign the compound to the appropriate skeleton type. Two data analysis problems can be identified here, depending on whether or not atom number information is available.

Table 12.2 Rules for generating reduced multiplicities (RedM) from observed multiplicities (ObsM).

```
IF ObsM = s AND Frequency in [ 64.5, 95 ] THEN RedM = d
IF ObsM = s AND Frequency in [ 96, 114 ]  THEN RedM = t
IF ObsM = s AND Frequency in [ 115, 165 ] THEN RedM = d
IF ObsM = s AND Frequency in [ 165, 188 ] THEN RedM = q
IF ObsM = s AND Frequency in [ 188, inf ] THEN RedM = t
IF ObsM = d AND Frequency in [ 64.5, 95 ] THEN RedM = t
IF ObsM = d AND Frequency in [ 105, 180 ] THEN RedM = t
IF ObsM = d AND Frequency in [ 96, 104 ]  THEN RedM = q
IF ObsM = d AND Frequency in [ 180, inf ] THEN RedM = q
IF ObsM = t AND Frequency in [ 59, 90 ]   THEN RedM = q
IF ObsM = t AND Frequency in [ 90, inf ]  THEN RedM = q
```

If atom number information is available, a propositional learning problem is easily formulated where the attributes are (a subset of) the multiplicities and frequencies of each of the skeleton atoms. Propositional machine learning approaches were applied to this problem: one from the area of artificial neural networks, one from statistical pattern recognition, and one from symbolic machine learning [Michie et al., 1994]. The details are given in Section 12.3.

Without atom number information, there is no obvious propositional representation of the problem and more careful representation engineering (feature construction) or the use of more powerful techniques, such as inductive logic programming (ILP) [Lavrač and Džeroski, 1994], seem necessary. Both approaches were explored. The details are given in Section 12.4.

For the first problem, data analysis was performed on both the original (observed) data and the data with reduced multiplicities. For the second problem, only the data with reduced multiplicities were analyzed.

12.2.4 The methodology

For each learning problem, each of the learning systems was first applied to the entire data set comprising information on all 1503 diterpenes. The classification accuracy was recorded and the symbolic rules learned were shown to the expert, where available.

A ten-fold cross-validation was then performed. The set of 1503 diterpenes was randomly split into ten sets of roughly equal size (7 sets of 150 examples and 3 sets of 151 example). Training was performed on the union of 9 sets and testing on the remaining one. The same partitions were used for all machine learning tools and all problems. The average classification accuracy over the ten partitions was recorded.

12.3 LEARNING WITH ATOM NUMBERS

When atom numbers are available, an attribute-value learning problem can be formulated, where the class is the skeleton type and the attributes are the multiplicities and frequencies of each of the 20 skeleton atoms. For instance, attribute `A1M` is the multiplicity of atom number 1, and `A7F` is the frequency of atom number 7. There are thus 40 attributes, twenty discrete (multiplicities) and 20 continuous (frequencies). As suggested by the domain expert, a version of the problem was also considered where only the multiplicities were used as attributes. Twenty-three different skeleton groups are represented in the set of 1503 compounds: there are thus 23 possible class values.

For each of the machine learning methods specified below, four series of experiments were performed, with the following sets of attributes: observed multiplicities and frequencies, reduced multiplicities and frequencies, observed multiplicities only and reduced multiplicities only.

Three different machine learning approaches were used to address the above problem. These are suited for solving classification problems and come from the areas of artificial neural networks, statistical pattern recognition, and symbolic machine learning [Michie et al., 1994]. The approaches used are backpropagation networks [Freeman and Skapura, 1991], nearest neighbor classification [Cover and Hart, 1968], and decision tree induction [Quinlan, 1986]. In particular, the shareware standard backpropagation network simulator of Tveter [Tveter, 1995] was used, and its results confirmed through a comparison with experiments on the same data performed using the public domain neural network package SNNS [SNNS, 1995]. The k-nearest neighbor pattern classifier as implemented by Wettschereck [Wettschereck, 1994] was used. Finally, the C4.5 program [Quinlan, 1993] for decision tree induction was used. A detailed description of the parameter settings used for each tool are given in the following sections.

The results of the three approaches on each of the four problems are summarized in Table 12.3. The accuracies on unseen cases and the accuracies on the training cases (in brackets) are listed.

12.3.1 Backpropagation networks

The networks we experimented with had 23 output nodes, representing the 23 types of diterpene skeletons. Input and output nodes were fully interconnected. Weights were initialized at random with values between -400 and 400. A thousand iterations of weights adjustment were performed.

Two different network architectures were experimented with. In the first (100-23), the signal from each skeleton atom (identified by the atom number `i`) was represented with five neurons, one of which carries the frequency `AiF`

Table 12.3 Classification accuracy on unseen cases (and on training cases) when learning from data on classified ^{13}C NMR-spectra with assigned atom numbers.

	Backpropagation	Nearest neighbor	C4.5
Observed	89.6% (98.3%)	96.7% (100%)	96.4% (99.0%)
Reduced	95.5% (99.5%)	99.3% (100%)	97.6% (99.3%)
Observed - No Frequencies	83.9% (88.8%)	94.4% (100%)	93.1% (96.2%)
Reduced - No Frequencies	97.1% (99.1%)	98.8% (100%)	98.4% (99.1%)

as a floating point number. The other four neurons are used to represent the multiplicity `AiM` in binary coding. One neuron is used for each of the four possible values `s`, `d`, `t`, and `q`. Exactly one of these neurons has the value 1 (corresponding to the actual value of `AiM`), while the others have value 0. Altogether 100 input neurons were thus used.

In the second architecture (80-23), 80 input nodes were used, four per skeleton atom. The four neurons correspond to the possible multiplicity values. However, instead of feeding 1 to the neuron corresponding to the actual value of `AiM`, this neuron is fed the frequency `AiF` as a floating point number. When no frequencies are used, the binary coding mentioned above is applied and the neuron is fed a 1 instead of `AiF`.

The second architecture performed much better than the first one in terms of learning progress and classification accuracy achieved (the parameter settings for both architectures were 0.2 for the learning rate and 0.5 for the momentum (0.2, 0.5)), both for the observed (nmr) and the reduced (red) data set. The second architecture was thus chosen for further experiments. With the second architecture already chosen, the setting (0.5, 0.9) yielded still better performance in terms of learning progress, so that the results reported in Table 12.3 were obtained by the second architecture with this setting.

Through all experiments, the so-called reduced data set yielded significantly better performance than the raw, observed data set. This difference in performance becomes particularly drastic when only multiplicities and no frequency data are used. While the reduced data set yields slightly better performance without frequency information than with it (1.6% on unseen cases), the observed data set yields much lower performance (5.7% on unseen cases) without frequency information. In summary, the backpropagation networks achieve a high degree of discrimination among the diterpene skeleton classes (97.1% on unseen cases for the reduced data set without frequency information). As preprocessing greatly improves performance, we can conclude that the rules used for preprocessing contain chemical knowledge useful for diterpene structure elucidation.

12.3.2 *Nearest neighbor classification*

The nearest neighbor (NN) algorithm treats attributes as dimensions of a Euclidean space and examples as points in this space. In the training phase, the classified examples are stored without any processing. When classifying a new instance, the Euclidean distance between that instance and all training examples is calculated and the class of the closest training example is assigned to the new instance.

The more general k-NN method takes the k nearest training examples and determines the class of the new instance by majority vote. The votes of each of the k nearest neighbors are weighted by their respective proximity to the new instance. An optimal value of k is determined automatically from the training set by using leave-one-out cross-validation. Finally, the contribution of each attribute to the distance may be weighted by the mutual information between that attribute and the class. These so-called feature weights can also be determined automatically on the training set. For our experiments, we used the k-NN algorithm as implemented by Wettschereck [Wettschereck, 1994].

The value $k = 1$ turned out to be the best in all cases. Feature weighting based on mutual information actually decreased the performance. The results shown are thus results of the basic NN algorithm, without feature weighting.

As the NN algorithm stores all training examples, its accuracy is 100% given the entire data set. Very high accuracy is achieved also on unseen cases (99.3% for the reduced data sets with frequency information). Performance on the reduced data sets is better than performance on the observed data sets, just as for the backpropagation networks. Unlike backpropagation networks, the NN algorithm performs consistently better (on both observed and reduced data sets) with frequency information. Although only a slight improvement is achieved, this indicates that frequency information is not completely irrelevant and that the NN algorithm is able to make effective use of all the information given.

12.3.3 *Decision tree induction*

The paradigm of decision tree induction is among the most well known and understood machine learning paradigms and algorithms in this paradigm are often applied to practical problems. For our diterpene structure elucidation problems, we applied the C4.5 algorithm [Quinlan, 1993]. In all experiments, we used the default parameter settings for C4.5, with one exception: groups of discrete attributes' values are also considered along branches, instead of single values only (as done by default). This produces smaller and thus more

```
A10M = q: c52 (0.0)
A10M in {d,t}:
|   A5F > 84.7 : c79 (4.0)                                  **1**
|   A5F <= 84.7 :
|   |   A13M = s: c33 (9.0)                                 **2**
|   |   A13M = t: c54 (0.0)
|   |   A13M in {d,q}:
|   |   |   A9M = d: c15 (3.0/1.0)
|   |   |   A9M in {q,t}: c54 (0.0)
|   |   |   A9M = s:
|   |   |   |   A5M = d: c60 (1.0)
|   |   |   |   A5M = s: c54 (356.0)                        **3**
|   |   |   |   A5M = t: c71 (5.0)
|   |   |   |   A5M = q: c54 (0.0)
```

Figure 12.1 Decision tree induced by C4.5 from the entire data set using the frequencies and the reduced multiplicities only. Only the left branch is shown here, the right branch is shown in the second part of the figure.

understandable trees at no cost in terms of accuracy. The accuracies achieved by C4.5 on the four different problems of diterpene structure elucidation are given in the rightmost column of Table 12.3.

The preprocessed, reduced, data sets yield better performance, as was the case for the backpropagation networks and the nearest neighbor classifier. Like the backpropagation networks, and unlike the nearest neighbor classifier, C4.5 performs best on the reduced data sets with no frequency information. High classification accuracy is achieved (98.4% on unseen cases).

Unlike the backpropagation networks and the nearest neighbor classifier, C4.5 produces an explicit symbolic description of the discovered knowledge in the form of a decision tree. Figure 12.1 shows the decision tree induced by C4.5 from the entire reduced data set with frequency information. The tree precisely captures the regularities that exist in the data (as it is over 99% accurate).

This tree was shown to the expert, who found it understandable and commented that the tree is almost as simple as possible. The most important multiplicities are used appropriately in the tree. Several specific comments were made, a selection of which we list below. The nodes/leaves of the tree that are commented on are indicated by a number between asterisks (e.g., `**1**`) and referred to by the number. The numbers in brackets denote the number of examples covered by the corresponding leaf. The marking (10.0), for instance, that leaf 5 covers 10 examples of class c47 (skeleton type Cassan). The marking (154.0/1.0) means that leaf 7 covers 154 examples, of which one does not belong to class c22 (skeleton type Pimaran).

```
A10M = s:
|   A16M in {d,s}:
|   |   A12M in {q,s}: c3 (0.0)
|   |   A12M = d:
|   |   |   A1F <= 35.1 : c8 (3.0/2.0)
|   |   |   A1F > 35.1 :
|   |   |   |   A16M = d: c5 (33.0)
|   |   |   |   A16M = s: c2 (10.0/1.0)
|   |   |   |   A16M in {q,t}: c5 (0.0)
|   |   A12M = t:                                          **4**
|   |   |   A7M in {d,s,t}:
|   |   |   |   A13M in {d,t}: c3 (352.0)
|   |   |   |   A13M = s: c4 (8.0)
|   |   |   |   A13M = q: c3 (0.0)
|   |   |   A7M = q:
|   |   |   |   A6M = d: c18 (12.0)
|   |   |   |   A6M in {q,t}: c28 (10.0/1.0)
|   |   |   |   A6M = s: c18 (0.0)
|   A16M in {q,t}:
|   |   A13M in {d,q,t}:
|   |   |   A12M = d: c47 (10.0)                           **5**
|   |   |   A12M in {q,s}: c52 (0.0)
|   |   |   A12M = t:                                      **6**
|   |   |   |   A9F > 181.2 : c80 (4.0)
|   |   |   |   A9F <= 181.2 :
|   |   |   |   |   A8F <= 36.5 : c36 (11.0/1.0)
|   |   |   |   |   A8F > 36.5 :
|   |   |   |   |   |   A8M = t: c80 (3.0/1.0)
|   |   |   |   |   |   A8M = q: c52 (0.0)
|   |   |   |   |   |   A8M in {d,s}:
|   |   |   |   |   |   |   A12F <= 196.2 : c52 (443.0/1.0)
|   |   |   |   |   |   |   A12F > 196.2 : c47 (3.0/1.0)
|   |   A13M = s:
|   |   |   A8M = q: c22 (0.0)
|   |   |   A8M in {d,t}:
|   |   |   |   A14M = d: c52 (2.0)
|   |   |   |   A14M = t: c22 (154.0/1.0)                  **7**
|   |   |   |   A14M in {q,s}: c22 (0.0)
|   |   |   A8M = s:
|   |   |   |   A8F <= 60.3 : c4 (65.0/1.0)
|   |   |   |   A8F > 60.3 : c22 (2.0)                     **8**
```

Figure 12.1 (continued)

The rule `IF A10M in {d, t} AND A5F > 84.7 THEN c79` corresponds to leaf 1. It predicts the skeleton type 5,10-seco-Clerodan and was judged as good, but exceptions exist, according to the expert. These exceptions, however, belong to the skeleton type Haliman, which was not present in the training examples. A similar comment was made on leaf 2, corresponding to the rule `IF A10M in {d, t} AND A5F <= 84.7 AND A13M = s THEN c33`. This rule predicts the skeleton type Erythoxilan and has exceptions of the skeleton type Rosane.

Commenting on leaf 3, which correctly classifies all 356 diterpenes that belong to the skeleton type Clerodan (`c54`), the expert noted that atom number 5 (of the 20 skeleton atoms) is the most diagnostic carbon for Clerodans. The subtree rooted at node 4 was also judged as good – this subtree includes a leaf that classifies correctly 352 of the 353 Kaurans (`c3`). Leaf 5 characterizes a special type of Cassans (`c47`) where a phenolic OH substituent is present at carbon number 12. Leaf 7 gives a natural characterization of Pimarans (`c22`), but also covers one diterpene that does not belong to this skeleton type. Leaf 8 is necessary for the two exceptions to leaf 7, for which the preprocessing rules for reducing multiplicities are not so good.

The subtree rooted at node 6 is based mainly on frequencies. The expert thought that was not necessary and suggested that multiplicities should be sufficient to distinguish among the different types of diterpenes skeletons. Trees were thus induced, which use multiplicities only and are, in the expert's opinion, much better. Multiplicity-only trees perform better on unseen cases, confirming the expert's opinion.

12.4 LEARNING WITHOUT ATOM NUMBERS

While the accuracies reported above are very high and the problem may seem solved, the propositional formulation specified in Section 12.3 crucially depends on the atom number information. The assignment of atom numbers is a very difficult and important part of the classification process, and classification rules that do not rely on atom number assignments need to be derived for practical purposes. Without atom number information, there is no obvious propositional representation of the problem and more careful representation engineering (feature construction) or the use of more powerful techniques, such as inductive logic programming (ILP) [Lavrač and Džeroski, 1994], seem necessary. In this section, we explore both approaches.

The three propositional approaches from above (backpropagation networks, the nearest neighbor classifier, and the C4.5 decision tree inducer) were applied to the propositional formulations. For the ILP problems, the systems FOIL [Quinlan, 1990] and RIBL [Emde and Wettschereck, 1996] were used.

In the ILP formulations, there are 23 target relations `classC(MoleculeID)`, where `C` ranges over the possible classes. For example, the target relation `class52(MoleculeID)` corresponds to the skeleton type Labdan, most common among the 1503 diterpenes in the database (448 instances). Two different background predicates were used that will be described below.

12.4.1 Applying FOIL

Using multiplicities and frequencies. Given that much better results were obtained using the reduced multiplicities in earlier experiments, we decided to use only these (and not the observed multiplicities) for our experiments with ILP. After one takes the atom number information away, the background relation `red` can be simplified to `red(MoleculeID,Multiplicity,Frequency)`. A particular fact of this relation states that the ^{13}C NMR-spectrum of a given molecule contains a peak of a given multiplicity and frequency. For example, the fact `red(v1,t,39.00)` states that the ^{13}C NMR-spectrum of molecule `v1` has a peak at frequency 39.00 with multiplicity `t` (a triplet).

The background relation `red` is nondeterminate, i.e., there are 20 tuples for each molecule that correspond to the 20 skeleton atoms. This prevents the use of ILP systems like GOLEM [Muggleton and Feng, 1990] or DINUS [Lavrač and Džeroski, 1994]. While PROGOL [Muggleton, 1995] would be applicable, preliminary experiments showed that it has prohibitive time complexity if longer rules/clauses are needed. Therefore, we used FOIL [Quinlan, 1990], in particular FOIL6.4. Except for a variable depth limit of one, all other settings were left in their default state.

We first used FOIL to induce rules on the entire data set, and then performed ten-fold cross validation on the same partitions of training examples as used for the propositional case (Section 12.3). For each experiment, FOIL was run 23 times, i.e., once for each target relation. The rules from the 23 runs were then taken together to produce a rule set. Before classification, the rules from the rule set were checked against the training set to record the number of examples of each class that they cover, as well as to note the majority class in the training set. This information is then used when classifying new examples, e.g., when testing the accuracy of the rule set.

For classification, we implemented a procedure analogous to that of CN2 [Clark and Boswell, 1991]: when an example is classified, all clauses that cover it are taken into account. The distributions of examples of each class are summed for all rules that match and the majority class is assigned to the example. If no rule matches, the majority class (from the training set) is assigned.

Given the relation `red(MoleculeID,Multiplicity,Frequency)`, FOIL induced 90 rules from the entire data set, comprising 607 literals in their bodies.

At first sight, the rules are quite specific, covering relatively few examples. Also, many examples are left uncovered. Thus, even on the training set, these rules only achieve 51.6% accuracy. The ten-fold cross-validation yields 46.5% accuracy on unseen cases as the average over the ten runs. It seems that the background knowledge is sufficient to distinguish among the different classes (the rules typically cover examples of one class only), but FOIL induces too specific rules. The most general rule `class52(A) :- red(A,d,B), B=<73.7, red(A,C,D), D>38.5, D=<44.6, B>73.2` covers 43 examples of class 52.

Using multiplicities only. According to a domain expert, the multiplicities should suffice for correct classification, at least when atom numbers are available. If we remove the `Frequency` argument from the relation `red`, all the information left about a particular molecule is captured by the number of atoms which have multiplicity `s`, `d`, `t`, and `q`, respectively. We store this information in the `prop(MoleculeID,SAtoms,DAtoms,TAtoms,QAtoms)` relation. For our molecule `v1`, we have the fact `prop(v1,2,4,8,6)`.

Given the entire data set, the 23 target relations and the background relation `prop`, FOIL induced 17 rules with 52 literals in the bodies. Same settings were applied in FOIL as for the experiments with `red`. The rules induced in this case are much more general than the ones obtained with `red`. The most general rule `class52(A) :- prop(A,B,C,D,E), E>5, C>3, D>7, B>1` covers 429 examples (of which 355 of class 52, 72 of class 54). Many rules cover examples of several classes. The background knowledge is insufficient to completely distinguish among the different classes and FOIL is forced to induce overly general rules. This, however, has a positive effect on accuracy as compared to the experiments with `red`. Using `prop`, FOIL achieves 69.0% accuracy on the entire data sets, and 70.1% accuracy on unseen cases (for ten-fold cross-validation).

At this point, note that we have in fact applied FOIL to a propositional problem. Namely, from the nondeterminate representation with the `red` relation, we have constructed a four-feature representation of each molecule.

Combining engineered features and a relational representation. Having introduced the four new features with the `prop` relation, which seem to capture some general properties of the molecules, we repeated the experiment with the nondeterminate relational representation. This time FOIL was given both the relation `red` and the relation `prop`. The same settings of FOIL were applied as in the previous two cases.

Given the entire data set, the 23 target relations and the background relations `red` and `prop`, FOIL induced 68 rules with 401 literals in the bodies. The rules were more general than those induced using `red` only, but were more specific than the rules induced using `prop` only. In most cases, each rule covers examples of one class only. The most general rule `class52(A) :- prop(A,B,C,D,E), E>5, C>3, D>7, B>1, red(A,d,F), F>54.8, F=<72.3` covers 227 examples of the correct class. The induced rules achieve 83.2% accuracy on the entire data set and 78.3% accuracy on unseen cases (ten-fold cross-validation). Combining the engineered features with the relational representation thus has a positive effect.

12.4.2 Comparing FOIL to propositional approaches

C4.5 using multiplicities only. As mentioned above, the relation `prop` defines a propositional version of our classification problem. We therefore applied a propositional learner, C4.5 [Quinlan, 1993], to this problem. The same experimental setting (tree induced on whole data set first, then ten-fold cross-validation) and the default settings of C4.5 were used.

The induced tree achieves 80.4% accuracy on the entire data set. The leaves of the tree typically contain examples of several different classes, confirming the suspicion that the four features do not suffice for completely correct classification. The classification accuracy on unseen cases as measured by ten-fold cross-validation (same folds as above) is 78.5%, which is almost the same as the accuracy achieved by FOIL using both `red` and `prop`.

Nearest neighbor using multiplicities only. We also applied nearest neighbor classification [Cover and Hart, 1968, Wettschereck, 1994] to the propositional problem defined by the relation `prop`. The same experimental setting (cross-validation folds) was used. Training on the entire data set gives 100% accuracy.

Cross-validation on the number of neighbors used in classification was tried out, as well as two different forms of feature weighting, but the basic nearest neighbor method performed best. The classification accuracy on unseen cases (average over the ten folds) is 79.0%, which is almost the same as the accuracy of C4.5 and the accuracy achieved by FOIL using both `red` and `prop`.

Backpropagation networks. Various network architectures were explored to see how in comparison backpropagation networks would perform at the classification of skeletons based on unassigned ^{13}C NMR-data. This was done independently of the above experimental setup, but using the same partitions for cross-validation.

A standard backpropagation network [Tveter, 1995, SNNS, 1995] with 960 input neurons, no hidden units and 23 output units was trained with the same input data as for the ILP experiments. We divided the 960 input neurons into four equally large sets of 240 nodes, one each for singulets, doublets, triplets

Table 12.4 Classification accuracy on unseen cases when learning from classified ^{13}C NMR-spectra without assigned atom numbers.

	FOIL	RIBL	Backprop.	Nearest neigh.	C4.5
Background red	46.5%	86.5%	NA	NA	NA
Background prop	70.1%	79.0%	79.9%	79.0%	78.5%
Background red+prop	78.3%	91.2%	NA	NA	NA

and quadruplets. The best representation was to have for each multiplicity 24 frequency intervals (0 – 10, 11 – 20, ..., 231 – 240) with 10 nodes each and to feed the value of 1 for each frequency in the spectrum into the next unoccupied input neuron of the appropriate interval. All remaining input nodes are assigned zeros. Thus, the artificial neural net sees a discretized distribution of multiplicity signals.

During cross-validation, accuracy on the training set (average for the 10 runs) reached 97.9%, while accuracy on unseen cases reached 79.9%. Other network variations, e.g., providing the actual frequency value to the appropriate neuron instead of 1 or using a 4 x 15 architecture that receives the sorted frequencies for each multiplicity as input did not produce better results.

12.4.3 Applying RIBL

RIBL (relational instance-based learning) [Emde and Wettschereck, 1996] generalizes the nearest neighbor method to a relational representation. RIBL first constructs cases by putting together all facts that relate to (in this case) a single molecule. Training cases are stored for further reference. When a new molecule has to be classified, RIBL calculates the similarities between it and each of the training cases, then assigns it the class of the nearest training case.

The similarity measure used in RIBL is a generalization of similarity measures used in propositional instance-based learners. In fact, given a propositional problem, RIBL becomes the classical nearest neighbor method and has the same performance as the latter. This is a very desirable property for a relational learner.

We used the same formulations and experimental methodology as for FOIL. When there are no identical cases classified differently, RIBL achieves 100% accuracy given the entire data set for both training and testing. To estimate the accuracy on unseen cases, ten-fold cross validation was performed.

Table 12.4 gives the accuracies on unseen cases achieved by FOIL and RIBL on the three different formulations of the problem, as well as the accuracies achieved by backpropagation, nearest neighbor and C4.5 on the propositional formulation(s). Note that the backpropagation networks used a different propositional formulation from the other approaches (as discussed above). Given only the `red` relation, RIBL achieved 86.5% classification accuracy (average over the ten partitions) on unseen cases. This is an increase of 40% over the accuracy achieved by FOIL. Note that propositional approaches are not applicable to this formulation of the problem.

Given only the `prop` relation, RIBL behaves identically to the nearest neighbor method, yielding 79.0% accuracy on unseen cases, a performance equivalent to that of C4.5 and the backpropagation networks. When provided with both the `red` and the `prop` relations, RIBL achieves 91.2% accuracy on unseen cases. Using the engineered features improves RIBL's performance by roughly 5%, pushing further the best result achieved at classifying diterpene NMR-spectra without assigned atom numbers. Again, propositional approaches are not applicable to this formulation of the problem.

12.5 DISCUSSION

The problem of diterpene structure elucidation from ^{13}C NMR-spectra was addressed with several machine learning approaches. Chemical background knowledge was used to preprocess the raw measurements, thus greatly improving the performance of the machine learning tools used.

Three propositional approaches (backpropagation networks, the nearest neighbor classifier, and the C4.5 decision tree learner) were applied to the problem of classifying ^{13}C NMR-spectra in the presence of atom number information.

All three tools achieved very high accuracy in assigning skeleton types to diterpenes with known skeletal atoms, atom numbers, multiplicities and frequencies. Accuracies between 97% and 99% on unseen cases were achieved on the preprocessed (reduced) data sets. Overall, the nearest neighbor classifier performed slightly better than the decision trees, while these in turn performed slightly better than the backpropagation networks. On the reduced data sets, the omission of frequency information causes at most a slight decrease in the performance, thus confirming the expert opinion that multiplicities alone should be sufficient for the task.

In comparison to the backpropagation networks and the nearest neighbor classifier, C4.5 has the advantage of producing an explicit symbolic description of the discovered knowledge in the form of a decision tree. The decision trees induced from the reduced data sets were inspected by a domain expert and were found to be understandable and to contain valuable domain knowledge. Given the accuracy on unseen cases, this means the trees can be used to solve the problem addressed, which currently requires expert labor.

For practical purposes, ^{13}C NMR-spectra of diterpenes without assigned atom numbers have to be classified. This is a problem that is not directly transformable to a propositional form and calls for either representation engineering or the use of inductive logic programming. We explored both approaches separately and in combination. Adding the engineered features to the natural relational representation improved the performance of both ILP systems used.

Using the engineered features only, propositional approaches (in particular C4.5, nearest neighbor and neural networks) achieve around 79% accuracy on unseen cases. This is roughly 20% less than the accuracies achieved when classifying ^{13}C NMR-spectra of diterpenes with assigned atom numbers.

Using FOIL on the natural relational representation yields unsatisfactory results. Combining the relational representation with the engineered features greatly improves FOIL's performance. However, given only the engineered features, FOIL performs much worse than C4.5, so that the best performance of FOIL (combining the relational representation and the engineered features) is comparable to that of C4.5. The reason for FOIL's poor performance is that it induces overly specific rules as indicated by their coverage and confirmed by expert comments. However, the rules found by FOIL are short, indicating that the problem lies in the search heuristic that prefers short rules with small coverage, despite the fact that longer rules with higher coverage exist.

From the above it is clear that a desirable property of relational learning systems is the following: given a propositional problem, a relational learning system should perform comparably to propositional systems. RIBL, which extends the nearest neighbor approach to a relational framework has this property. Given the engineered features only, it achieves 79% accuracy on unseen cases. Given the relational representation only, RIBL performs much better than FOIL (86% vs. 46% accuracy on unseen cases). Finally, combining the relational representation and the engineered features it achieves 91% accuracy on unseen cases, 11% better than the best propositional result of 80% (backpropagation networks with 960 features).

The 91% accuracy achieved by RIBL is in the range of the accuracies with which experts classify diterpenes into skeleton types given ^{13}C NMR-spectra only. Actually, that number can only be estimated since it is expensive to have an expert carry out a statistically significant number of structure predictions without using other additional information that often becomes available from heterogeneous sources (such as literature, and ^{1}H NMR-spectra). This basically means that ^{13}C NMR is not completely sufficient for classifying diterpenes and that great improvements of classification accuracy are not to be expected.

The main direction for further work is to provide classification accuracy at the level already achieved in conjunction with satisfactory explanation. RIBL can offer only the nearest neighbor used to classify a given instance as an explanation of that classification, but no general knowledge can be offered for inspection by domain experts. Newer versions of RIBL (based on Aha's IB3 [Aha et al., 1991]), which store only a fraction of the training cases, may offer a small number of prototypes as explanations. Alternatively, one might apply mFOIL [Džeroski, 1993, Lavrač and Džeroski, 1994] and use the m-estimate to guide the search towards more general rules (larger m in the estimate of the accuracy prefers rules that cover more examples). It would also be interesting to apply the ILP system ICL [De Raedt and Van Laer, 1995] to this problem.

Acknowledgments

The research described in this chapter was conducted while Sašo Džeroski was an ERCIM (European Research Consortium for Informatics and Mathematics) fellow at GMD (German National Research Center for Information Technology, Sankt Augustin) and ICS-FORTH (Institute of Computer Science, Foundation of Research and Technology-Hellas, Heraklion, Greece). It was supported in part by the ESPRIT IV LTR Project 20237 Inductive Logic Programming 2.

Notes

1. The database is maintained using ISIS (Integrated Scientific Information System), a product of MDL Information Systems, Inc., on IBM PCs under MS Windows.

References

Aha, D., Kibler, D., and Albert, M. (1991). Instance-based learning algorithms. *Machine Learning*, 6:37–66.

Abraham, R.J. and Loftus, P. (1978). *Proton and Carbon 13 NMR-Spectroscopy, An Integrated Approach.* Heyden, London.

(1995). *Natural products on CD-ROM.* Chapman and Hall, London.

Clark, P. and Boswell, R. (1991). Rule induction with CN2: Some recent improvements. In *Proc. Fifth European Working Session on Learning*, pages 151–163, Springer Verlag.

Cover, T.M. and Hart, P.E. (1968). Nearest neighbor pattern classification. *IEEE Transactions on Information Theory*, 13:21–27.

De Raedt, L. and Van Laer, V. (1995). Inductive constraint logic. In *Proc. Sixth International Workshop on Algorithmic Learning Theory*, pages 80–94, Springer Verlag.

Džeroski, S. (1993). Handling imperfect data in inductive logic programming. In *Proc. Fourth Scandinavian Conference on Artificial Intelligence*, pages 111–125, IOS Press, Amsterdam.

Emde, W., Wettschereck, D. (1996). Relational instance-based learning. In *Proc. Thirteenth International Conference on Machine Learning*, pages 122–130, Morgan Kaufmann, San Mateo, CA.

Freeman, J.A. and Skapura, D.M. (1991). *Neural Networks - Algorithms, Applications and Programming Techniques.* Addison-Wesley, Wokingham.

Gray, N.A.B. (1982). *Progress in NMR-Spectroscopy, Vol. 15*, pages 201–248.

Lavrač, N. and Džeroski, S. (1994). *Inductive Logic Programming: Techniques and Applications.* Ellis Horwood, Chichester.

Michie, D., Spiegelhalter, D.J., and Taylor, C.C., editors. (1994). *Machine Learning, Neural and Statistical Classification.* Ellis Horwood, Chichester.

Muggleton, S. (1995). Inverse entailment and PROGOL. *New Generation Computing*, 13:245–286.

Muggleton, S. and Feng, C. (1990). Efficient induction of logic programs. In *Proc. First Conference on Algorithmic Learning Theory*, pages 368–381, Ohmsha, Tokyo.

Quinlan, J.R. (1986). Induction of decision trees. *Machine Learning* 1(1):81–106.

Quinlan, J.R. (1990). Learning logical definitions from relations. *Machine Learning*, 5(3):239–266.

Quinlan, J.R. (1993). *C4.5: Programs for Machine Learning.* Morgan Kaufmann, San Mateo, CA.

Schulze-Kremer, S. (1995). *Molecular Bioinformatics - Algorithms and Applications.* de Gruyter, Berlin.

(1995). *Stuttgart Neural Network Simulator.* Computer code available from the University of Stuttgart, Germany, via anonymous ftp `ftp://ftp.informatik.uni-stuttgart.de/pub/SNNS`.

Tveter, D. R. (1995). *Fast-Backpropagation.* Computer code available from the author. Address: 5228 N Nashville Ave, Chicago, Illinois, 60656, `drt@chinet.chi.il.us`.

Wettschereck, D. (1994). A study of distance-based machine learning algorithms. PhD Thesis, Department of Computer Science, Oregon State University, Corvallis, OR.

13 USING INDUCTIVE LOGIC PROGRAMMING TO LEARN RULES THAT IDENTIFY GLAUCOMATOUS EYES

Fumio Mizoguchi,
Hayato Ohwada,
Makiko Daidoji,
and Shiroaki Shirato

Abstract: This chapter examines the applicability and performance of Inductive Logic Programming (ILP) in learning classification rules for a medical domain. The domain is glaucoma diagnosis where ocular fundus images are used to identify glaucomatous eyes. An ILP system called GKS was developed, not only to deal with low-level measurement data such as images but also produce diagnostic rules that are readable and comprehensive for interactions with medical experts. Since such rules are directly used as diagnostic rules, the present method provides automatic construction of a knowledge base from an expert's accumulated diagnostic experience. A variety of experiments are conducted to clarify the performance of classification based on the induced rules. The resulting performance is comparable with human-level classification. This indicates that an ILP-based method can be used as a highly-valuable medical decision tool.

13.1 INTRODUCTION

The present study focuses on an inductive learning approach to glaucoma diagnosis. The motivation for this study comes from collaborative research between Rutgers University, the University of Tokyo (Dept. of Ophthalmology) and the Science University of Tokyo which began in 1978. The aim of the research was to compare the difference between the CASNET system and medical doctors' clinical decisions [Weiss et al., 1978]. The next year, based on this experience, we developed a glaucoma consultation system using a general expert system shell [Mizoguchi et al., 1979]. We then moved to a logic programming approach to designing logic-oriented expert systems [Mizoguchi et al., 1984]. Furthermore, we developed a new qualitative model of intraocular pressure which describes causal processes of glaucoma [Ohwada and Mizoguchi, 1988]. This provided a means to explain how glaucomatous damage was caused.

Although such experience leads to high-level glaucoma consultation systems, we have a fundamental problem for medical consultation. This is a kind of instruction or data entry problem. Expert physicians obtain findings and symptoms from the interaction with patients and acquire measurement data through instruments. They then interpret measurement data and produce somewhat qualitative information from the data. Thus, the input to a consultation system depends on experts' interpretation of measurement data, and consultation systems for specific applications need experts who can make clinical decisions. The ultimate goal of the present study is to develop consultation systems that can deal with measurement data directly.

As measurement data, we focus on images and provide a method for learning from images, because an image is the primary measurement data. Current medical technology allows us to acquire useful quantitative parameters using very expensive instruments. However, some experts suspect the reliability of such parameters. In contrast, images can be obtained with relatively low cost systems. Also, it is hard to obtain clinical parameters from images because an image is a distributed two-dimensional data set. In clinical decisions, real number parameters are easy to use, but an image is not. Thus, a machine learning approach to extracting decision rules from images is important. Since such rules are induced from an expert's accumulated diagnostic experience, they can be used directly for diagnosis.

In this chapter, we provide an empirical study of an inductive logic programming (ILP) method through the application of ocular fundus images classification for glaucoma diagnosis. An ILP system called GKS (GaKuShu which means "learning" in Japanese) was developed to deal with low-level measurement data including image, and to produce diagnostic rules that are readable and comprehensive for interactions with medical experts. This compre-

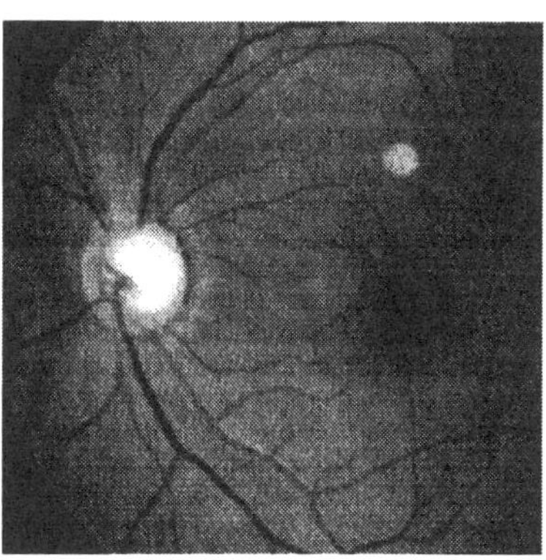

Figure 13.1 Ocular fundus image.

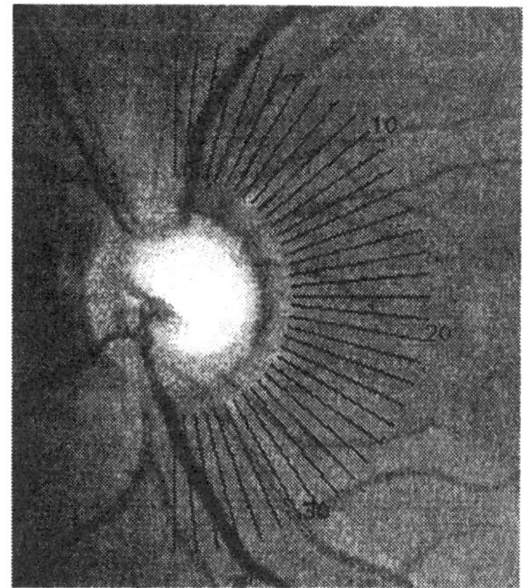

Figure 13.2 Image segmentation.

hensiveness is important because most experts tend to interpret and modify the machine-produced rules in comparison with their own decision rules. ILP provides a reasonable method for this requirement where produced rules are expressed in a first-order formalism, yielding knowledge-level descriptions for diagnosis [Muggleton, 1991].

The chapter is organized as follows. Section 13.2 describes the learning task in the present study. Section 13.3 shows our learning method based on GKS. Section 13.4 shows our experiment on learning from ocular fundus images and its result using GKS. In Section 13.5, the resultant performance of GKS is presented. Finally, Section 13.6 concludes the discussion.

13.2 LEARNING TASK

Since glaucoma causes vision loss, early detection of optic nerve damage and assessment of its progression are key clinical issues. Ocular fundus images are important clues for glaucoma diagnosis. Such images involve specific optic nerve parameters (e.g., rim-disc ratio and neuroretinal rim area). Medical experts must use measurement data obtained from image analysis in order to improve the accuracy of clinical evaluation.

Figure 13.1 shows an ocular fundus image of a glaucomatous eye. A physician decides whether the image shows glaucomatous damage or not with a classification accuracy of 95%. In contrast, the accuracy of young doctors acting as an assistant is about 60%. However, after being trained how to identify glaucomatous image by an expert, the accuracy increases to about 80%. This

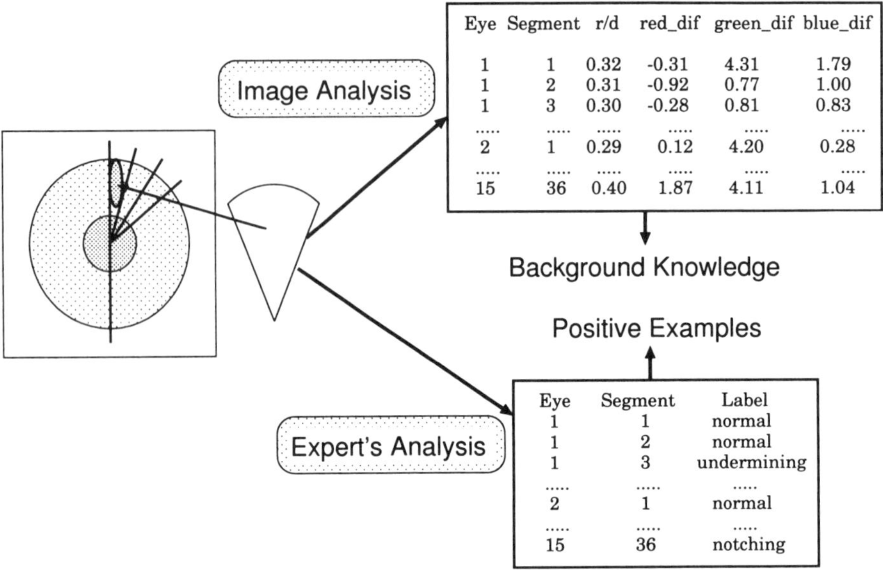

Figure 13.3 Relationship between image analysis and expert's analysis.

implies that clinical experience plays an important role in improving the performance of classification. We therefore seek to show the applicability of ILP to classifying images.

Figure 13.2 shows the basic idea of learning from images. In general, the abnormality of a glaucomatous image is partial, and we divide the original image into several segments. In the figure, the image is circularly divided. This segmentation reflects an expert's heuristics in image analysis.

The learning task in the present study is to automatically construct diagnostic rules from image analysis and expert's analysis. Image analysis produces a set of numerical data such as optic-nerve parameters (e.g., rim-disc ratio) and RGB color information; an expert's analysis provides a set of expert interpretations. Figure 13.3 shows the relationship between image analysis and an expert's analysis. Each segment for which an expert's analysis indicates a normal or specific abnormality (e.g., undermining and notching that leads to optic-nerve damage) is analyzed.

In this setting, numerical data becomes background knowledge, and labeling becomes a set of positive and negative examples. Although this setting can be simply captured within the decision tree learning system C4.5 [Quinlan, 1992], we are concerned with the relationship between abnormal segments. For example, the following statement should be produced:

(1) If a certain segment is abnormal, then adjacent segments are also abnormal.

This statement contains the target predicate to be learned in both the left- and right-hand sides of induced rules, and represent interrelations between abnormal segments. From a clinical point of view, such relationships may indicate a structural description of the underlying optic nerve damage.

The learning target is the expert's evaluation rules for abnormal segments, and is described as follows:

`class(Image,Segment,normal)`, stating that the expert's evaluation about segment `Segment` in image `Image` is normal.

`class(Image,Segment,undermining)`, stating that the expert's evaluation about segment `Segment` in image `Image` is undermining, which is a specific abnormality of ocular damage.

Image analysis provides background knowledge as shown below.

`rd(Image,Segment,RealNumber)`, stating that the rim-disc ratio of segment `Segment` in image `Image` is `RealNumber`.

`color(Image,Segment,Color,RealNumber)`, stating that color information of segment `Segment` in image `Image` is `RealNumber`.

Also, topological relationships between segments are included in the background knowledge as follows:

`clockwise(Segment,Adjacent,Distance)`, stating that the clockwise adjacent segment of segment `Segment` is `Adjacent` where the distance between the segments is `Distance`.

`counterclockwise(Segment,Adjacent,Distance)`, stating that the counterclockwise adjacent segment of segment `Segment` is `Adjacent` where the distance between the segments is `Distance`.

This background knowledge can be viewed as initial background knowledge in the sequential learning method mentioned in the next section. Once a rule is produced, it is added to the background knowledge for the next learning phase. To differentiate produced rules from the learning target, the rules are described as follows:

`class_confirmed(Image,Segment,Class)`, stating that the evaluation of segment `Segment` in image `Image` is `Class`

In this setting, statement (1) can be described as follows:

```
class(Image,Segment,undermining) :-
                        clockwise(Segment,Adjacent,1),
                        class_confirmed(Image,Adjacent,undermining).
```

where the symbol `:-` denotes "if" and the statement means that `Segment` of `Image` is classified as undermining if the conditions in the right-hand side are satisfied. This is a distinctive feature of our ILP approach to learning classification rules.

13.3 LEARNING METHOD

This section outlines our ILP system GKS, which can be regarded as a constraint-based generalization of ILP because it allows users to produce a constraint logic program whose domain is real numbers and linear constraints [Jaffar et al., 1987].

While several ILP systems have been developed (e.g., FOIL [Quinlan and Cameron-Jones, 1993] and Progol [Muggleton, 1995]), GKS combines "bottom-up" and "top-down" search. In a "top-down" search, GKS starts with a most general clause and adds literals until a certain condition is satisfied. The search strategy is characterized by an objective function and constraints. An objective function indicates "goodness" of a hypothesis. Intuitively, a good hypothesis covers as many positive examples as possible and as few negative examples as possible. In addition, a simpler hypothesis is more preferable based on a compression measure such as the Minimum Description Length principle. As an objective function, Progol adopted a linear combination of the number of positive and negative examples covered. Since these numbers are inversely proportional, the function does not satisfy the monotonicity property of a hypothesis search. If a new literal is added and the resulting clause is specialized, it is impossible to generally say whether the function increases.

To guarantee monotonicity, GKS supports the objective function of the number of uncovered positive examples (p) and the rule length (l) and treats negative examples as constraints. More specifically, GKS search is formulated as follows:

$$\begin{array}{rl} Objective function & Minimizing \quad f(p,l) \\ Constraint & \quad g(n) \leq Err \end{array}$$

where function f is linearly combined with respect to p and l. Parameter Err indicates the permissible ratio of negative examples covered.

A "bottom-up" search is employed for learning from numerical data. Progol selects one example and produces a bottom clause with respect to this example. The bottom clause is the most specific for the Herbrand Universe. However, it is not the most specific for other domains such as real numbers. Suppose that we have a geometric point in two dimensions. In this case, most specific constraints construct four segments. If we have more than one point, more specific constraints can be generated.

GKS first focuses on one example in the order found in the source file, and produces a hypothesis (h_1) using a top-down search. Adding a new exam-

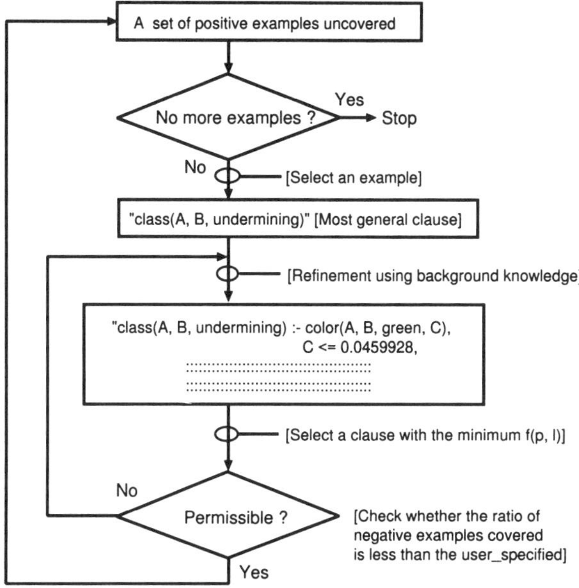

Figure 13.4 GKS search procedure.

ple, GKS then repeatedly produces another hypothesis (h_2) using a top-down search. If $f(p, l)$ of h_2 is less than that of h_1, this cycle repeats, adding other examples. Otherwise, GKS returns h_1 as the best hypothesis.

Figure 13.4 shows how top-down and bottom-up searches are combined. The outer loop corresponds to the bottom-up search, handling a set of examples sequentially. The inner loop provides a top-down search to produce a most preferable hypothesis under a set of given examples. The stop criteria of the outer loop is whether all the positive examples are covered. For the inner loop, search is terminated when the ratio of negative examples covered is less than the user-specified ratio.

Figure 13.5 shows how the GKS system works. The left window includes mode and type description, background knowledge, and positive and negative examples. The left arrow (<=) indicates the target predicate, and the right arrow (=>) specifies background knowledge. GKS is implemented in standard Prolog languages.

Input data includes an expert's evaluation of the state of a segment. Here, the first argument `Image` of the predicate `class` is an image ID number, the second is the segment number, and the third indicates the abnormal or normal state. The symbol `+` means input mode, and `#` means ground term, which in

```
mizo-can:/LearnGla/1st more glaucoma1.db

% Mode & Type

<= class(+image, +segment, undermining).
=> rd(+image, +segment, -real).
=> color(+image, +segment, #, -real).

% Background Knowledge

class(1, 4, undermining).
class(1, 5, undermining).
class(1, 6, undermining).
class(1, 7, undermining).
class(1, 8, undermining).
class(1, 9, undermining).
class(1, 10, undermining).
class(2, 13, undermining).
class(2, 14, undermining).
class(2, 15, undermining).
class(2, 16, undermining).
```

```
mizo-can:LearnGla/1st gks glaucoma1 -c -err 0.05
% {Pos=14/80, Neg=17/353, comp=0.127}
class(A, B, undermining) :-
        color(A, B, green, C),
        rd(A, B, D),
        C >= 0.192927957,
        D =< 0.286746.

% {Pos=48/80, Neg=15/353, comp=0.558}
class(A, B, undermining) :-
        rd(A, B, D),
        C >= 0.224052.

% {Pos=50/80, Neg=17/353, comp=0.577}
class(A, B, undermining) :-
        color(A, B, blue, C),
        color(A, B, red, D),
        rd(A, B, E),
        D >= -0.500916,
        E =< 0.244362,
        C =< 0.0514370203.
```

Figure 13.5 Input and output of GKS.

cludes no variables. Such notation is similar to a Progol mode declaration. The predicate `rd` means rim-disc ratio which is an important optic-nerve parameter. The predicate `color` specifies color information, and the fourth argument takes as output a real number, which may be constrained by inequalities.

The right window displays the invocation of GKS, specifying the command `gks` with a filename and options. The `-c` option is for learning rules with constraints, and `-err` means the permissible ratio of negative examples covered. Learned rules are displayed with the ratios of positive (`Pos`) and negative (`Neg`) examples covered and with their $f(p, l)$ (`comp`).

In addition to learning constrained rules, GKS provides a sequential learning method. This is used to generate relational rules between abnormalities that have already been detected by the previously obtained rules. Given the initial background knowledge B_1 and positive examples, the first learning phase generates a clause that covers a subset of positive examples with respect to B_1. The second learning phase adds this clause h_1 into B_1 as background knowledge B_2, then generates a clause h_2 that covers a subset of the residual positive examples with respect to B_2.

The learning target for glaucoma diagnosis is the abnormality of a given segment, and learned rules are expected to represent the structural relationships between such abnormalities. Thus, in the first learning phase, GKS finds the relationship between the abnormality and measurement data of a specific segment. GKS may then generate relational rules between abnormalities that have already been detected by the previously obtained rules.

Note that sequential learning is very similar to the work on predicting the protein secondary structure in [Muggleton et al., 1992], where the ILP system GOLEM repeatedly generalizes the three levels of rules. While GOLEM gen-

```
mizo-can:/LearnGla/1st more glaucoma2.db

% Mode & Type
<= class(+image, +segment, undermining).
=> rd(+image, +segment, -real).
=> color(+image, +segment, #, -real).
=> clockwise(+segment, -adjacent, #).
=> counterclockwise(+segment, -adjacent, #).
=> class_confirmed(+image, #, undermining).
=> class_confirmed(+image, +adjacent, undermining).

% Background Knowledge
class_confirmed(A, B, undermining) :-
        color(A, B, blue, C),C =< 0.0514370203,
        color(A, B, red, D),D >= -0.500916,
        rd(A, B, E),E =< 0.244362.

class(1, 4, undermining).
class(1, 5, undermining).
class(1, 6, undermining).
```

Figure 13.6 Input for sequential learning.

```
mizo-can:LearnGla/1st gks glaucoma2 -c -err 0.05

% {Pos=64/80, Neg=14/353, comp=0.760}
class(A, B, undermining) :-
        class_confirmed(A, 11, undermining),
        rd(A, B, C),
        C =< 0.286746.

% {Pos=42/80, Neg=17/353, comp=0.477}
class(A, B, undermining) :-
        class_confirmed(A, 22, undermining),
        rd(A, B, C),
        C =< 0.240727.

% {Pos=35/80, Neg=14/353, comp=0.398}
class(A, B, undermining) :-
        undermining1(A, 6, undermining),
        color(A, B, red, C),
        rd(A, B, D),
        C >= -0.151857018,
        D =< 0.299482.
```

Figure 13.7 Some learned rules.

erated all rules at each level, GKS selects the best rule from a set of induced rules.

Figure 13.6 shows a typical input for sequential learning. The predicate clockwise (counterclockwise) represents topological relationships between segments. Its third argument indicates the distance between the target segment and the adjacent segment. The meaning of the predicate `class_confirmed` is the same as the class predicate, but this is used to identify abnormalities detected by learned rules. In Figure 13.7, such a predicate appears in the body of a hypothesis.

13.4 EXPERIMENT

This section shows how sequential learning is applied to classifying ocular fundus images and gives experimental results. A set of examples was taken from 15 pictures and each picture was divided into 36 segments. One of the authors, a specialist for glaucoma diagnosis, categorized 540 examples into normal and three types of ocular damage; "undermining" is a typical one. There were 433 examples of either normal or undermining segments. A set of examples and initial background knowledge is shown in Table 13.1. Each argument in a predicate has a type and a mode where `+` and `-` mean input and output variables, `class` is the classification predicate and `\+` denotes negation. Argument description `-real` is special in that the output variable takes a real number and its value is constrained by a set of linear constraints.

Since sequential learning increments background knowledge, relational predicates for segments are added as shown in Table 13.2. Argument description `#` specifies ground (variable-free) instantiation. For instance, the third argument

Table 13.1 Examples and initial background knowledge.

Positive and negative examples	Number of clauses
class(+image, +segment, undermining)	80
\+ class(+image, +segment, undermining)	353
Background knowledge	**Number of clauses**
rd(+image, +segment, -real)	433
color(+image, +segment, red, -real)	433
color(+image, +segment, green, -real)	433
color(+image, +segment, blue, -real)	433

Table 13.2 Background knowledge for sequential learning.

Background knowledge	Number of clauses
rd(+image, +segment, -real)	433
color(+image, +segment, red, -real)	433
color(+image, +segment, green, -real)	433
color(+image, +segment, blue, -real)	433
clockwise(+segment, -adjacent, #)	420
counterclockwise(+segment, -adjacent, #)	420
class_confirmed(+image, #, undermining)	???
class_confirmed(+image, +adjacent, undermining)	???

in predicate `clockwise` must be instantiated to ground terms. The number of clauses for predicate `class_confirmed` is unknown, because rules for this predicate may be incrementally added.

We introduce here a variety of performance measures that are taken from [Weiss et al., 1990] and are shown in the appendix. Although the predictive accuracy is widely used in the ILP community, we also pay attention to "sensitivity" which means how much true hypotheses are covered by induced rules. For example, medical diagnosis needs high sensitivity, i.e., very few false negatives. However, accuracy and sensitivity may move in opposite directions. Increasing sensitivity tends to cover more negative examples; thus accuracy becomes lower.

GKS allows users to specify the permissible ratio of negative examples covered. Induced rules depend on this ratio, and we investigate what ratio is reasonable with regard to the sensitivity and accuracy.

Figure 13.8 shows the result of the normal learning mode using the initial background knowledge mentioned above. We set 5 to 15% permissible ratios. This figure indicates a general trend in which learning for greater ratios yields higher sensitivity but lower predictive accuracy. In the extreme case (15%),

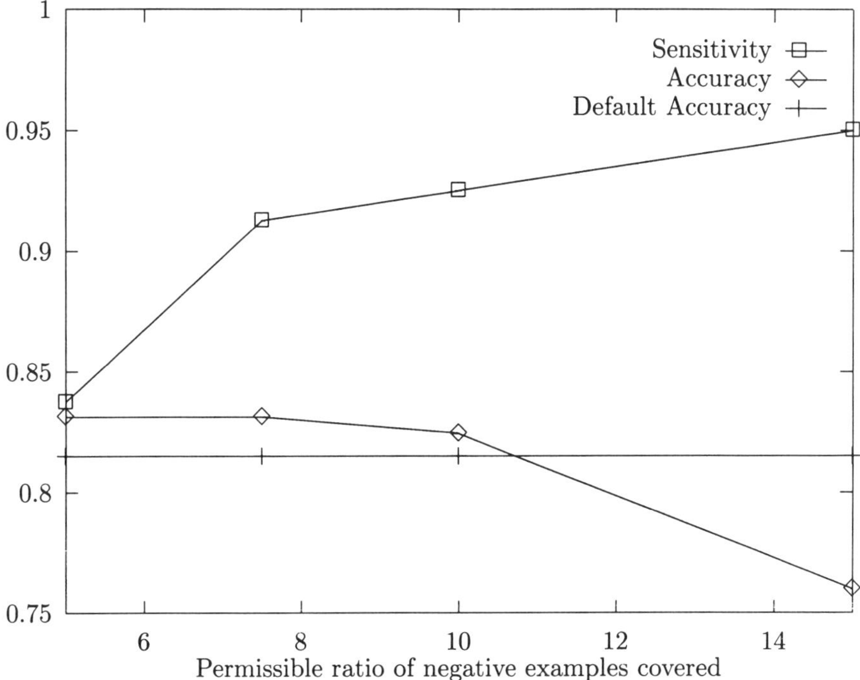

Figure 13.8 Performance vs. different permissible ratios.

the accuracy is less than the default accuracy. This result suggests that 5 and 10% ratios are reasonable for testing the performance of sequential learning.

For a 5% ratio, GKS produced seven clauses as shown in the appendix. The 8th iteration is immaterial, because no more rules were produced. The rule produced in the first learning phase is as follows:

```
% {Pos=50/80, Neg=17/353}
class(A, B, undermining) :-
        color(A, B, blue, C), C =< 0.0514370203,
        color(A, B, red, D), D >= -0.500916,
        rd(A, B, E), E =< 0.244362.
```

where `Pos` and `Neg` are the ratios of positive and negative examples covered by the rule. This rules means that for all `A`(eye) and `B`(segment), `B` of `A` is classified as **`undermining`** if the RGB information of `B` satisfies the associated inequalities. Each real number in the right-hand side of an inequality is found within a positive example using the GKS algorithm.

In the second learning phase, GKS produces the following rule:

```
% {Pos=64/80, Neg=14/353}
class(A, B, undermining) :-
        class_confirmed(A, 11, undermining),
        rd(A, B, C), C =< 0.286746.
```

where predicate `class_confirmed` is a renamed version of the clause obtained in previous learning. This rule means that `B` of `A` is classified as `undermining` if segment `11` of `A` is classified as `undermining` and the rim-disc ratio of `B` is less than `0.286746`. Note that the second argument of the condition is not a variable (in this case, 11). This means that a particular abnormal segment leads to abnormalities of other segments. Such a rule can be interpreted as an "absolute" relationship between abnormal segments.

In contrast, the rule produced in the third learning phase is of the "relative" form shown below.

```
% {Pos=52/80, Neg=15/353}
class(A, B, undermining) :-
        clockwise(B, C, 1),
        class_confirmed(A, C, undermining).
```

The rule says that if a certain segment is undermining, adjacent segments are also undermining. The rule implies a structural relationship between abnormal segments, yielding a high-level description for glaucoma diagnosis.

13.5 PERFORMANCE

Performance results of sequential learning are listed in Table 1.1, which includes some performance measures shown in the appendix (Table A1), and all the measures are obtained by 10-fold cross-validation. This table includes positive predictive value (Predictive(+)), indicating how often a decision is correct when a test result is positive.

The table illustrates the advantage of sequential learning over normal learning and C4.5. Two typical permissible ratios (5% and 10%) are chosen as reasonable settings. Taking a training set of examples, sequential learning repeatedly generates a set of rules from this training set and incremental background knowledge. The performance measures are calculated by applying the produced rules to the residual examples.

The figure shows that sequential learning increases both the sensitivity and accuracy of induced rules. This indicates that hierarchically structured hypotheses provide a high-performance classifier. This is due to the expressive power of the first-order clausal form in the ILP-based approach.

Table 13.3 Performance of sequential learning and C4.5.

		Sensitivity	Accuracy	Predictive(+)
Permissible ratio = 5 %	Normal learning	87.5	84.8	56.6
	Sequential learning	93.8	87.7	62.0
Permissible ratio = 10 %	Normal learning	91.3	77.4	45.3
	Sequential learning	96.3	84.5	55.8
C4.5		86.5	74.1	86.4

We now summarize the lessons from this experiment. First, performance is as good as human-level classification, and its accuracy (85%) is high. Second, learned rules are comprehensive; this is the advantage of the ILP approach. In the medical area, statistical methods have been used, but such methods can not provide insight for classification rules. The expert's decision process is quite different from such a method, but the ILP method reduces the gap between machine-produced rules and expert's rules. Third, sequential learning increases both performance and readability.

13.6 CONCLUSION

This chapter demonstrates how to apply an ILP method to classifying ocular fundus images for glaucoma diagnosis. The motivation was the difficulty of automatically acquiring diagnostic rules from measurement data such as images. We adopted a constraint-based generalization, which allows producing clauses with numerical constraints. GKS is designed and implemented to handle measurement data directly. Furthermore, we introduced sequential learning, which is a kind of incremental learning where learned hypotheses are progressively added into background knowledge. Such hypotheses take the form of high-level descriptions because relationships between abnormalities can be represented in this form. We also showed the performance result of sequential learning which increases both the sensitivity and accuracy of the learned hypotheses. The result indicates the great advantage and potential of the ILP approach in learning from measurement data.

Future work includes showing the advantage of first-order learning. We have to use a first-order formalism to construct relevant background knowledge. Also, we must compare our approach with expert's decision rules and refine the machine-produced rules by interacting with experts. Data selection and performance evaluation have to be re-examined to obtain "true" performance.

References

Jaffar, J. and Lassez, J. L. (1987). Constraint logic programming. *Proc. of the 14th ACM Principles of Programming Language Conference*, pages 111–119.

Kitazawa, Y., Shirato, S., Mizoguchi, F. (1981). A new computer-aided glaucoma consultation system (G4-Expert), *Royal Society of Medicine International Congress and Symposium Series*, 44:161-168.

Mizoguchi, F., Maruyama, K., Kitazawa, Y. and Kulikowski, C. A. (1979). A case study of EXPERT formalism: An approach to a design of medical consultation system through EXPERT formalism, *Proc. of IJCAI*, pages 583–585.

Mizoguchi, F., Ohwada, H. and Katayama, Y. (1984). LOOKS: Knowledge representation system for designing expert systems, *Proc. of International Conference on Fifth Generation Computer Systems*, pages 606–612.

Mizoguchi, F. and Ohwada, H. (1995). Constrained relative least general generalization for inducing constraint logic programs. *New Generation Computing*, 13(3,4):335-368.

Muggleton, S. (1991) Inductive logic programming. *New Generation Computing*, 8(4):295-318.

Muggleton, S., King, R. and Sternberg, M. (1992). Protein secondary structure prediction using logic-based machine learning. *Protein Engineering*, 5(7):647-657.

Muggleton, S. (1995). Inverse entailment and Progol. *New Generation Computing*, 13(3,4):245-286.

Ohwada, H. and Mizoguchi, F. (1988). An examination of applicability of FGHC: The experience of designing a qualitative reasoning system. *Proc. of the International Conference on Fifth Generation Computer Systems*, pages 1193–1200.

Quinlan., J. R. (1992). *C4.5: Programs for machine learning.* Morgan Kaufmann, San Mateo, California.

Quinlan, J. R. and Cameron-Jones, R. M. (1993). FOIL: A midterm report, *Proc. of European Conference on Machine Learning*, pages 3-20, Springer Verlag.

Weiss, S. M., Kulikowski, C. A., Mizoguchi, F. and Kitazawa, T. (1978). A computer-based comparison of Japanese and American decision-making, *Proc. of International Conference on Cybernetics and Society*, pages 1–3.

Weiss, S. M., Galen, R. S. and Tadepalli, P. (1990). Maximizing the predictive value of production rules. *Artificial Intelligence*, 45:47-71.

Appendix: Performance measures

Table 13.A.1 Performance measures.

	Rule Positive(R^+)	Rule Negative(R^-)
Hypothesis Positive(H^+)	True Positive(TP)	False Negative(FN)
Hypothesis Negative(H^-)	False Positive(FP)	True Negative(TN)

$$\begin{aligned}
\text{Sensitivity} &= TP/H^+ \\
\text{Specificity} &= TN/H^- \\
\text{Predictive value}(+) &= TP/R^+ \\
\text{Accuracy} &= (TP+TN)/((H^+)+(H^-))
\end{aligned}$$

Appendix: Induced rules

```
% 1st %
% {Pos=50/80, Neg=17/353}
class(A, B, undermining) :-
        color(A, B, blue, C), C =< 0.0514370203,
        color(A, B, red, D), D >= -0.500916,
        rd(A, B, E), E =< 0.244362.

% 2nd %
% {Pos=64/80, Neg=14/353}
class(A, B, undermining) :-
        class_confirmed(A, 11, undermining),
        rd(A, B, C), C =< 0.286746.

% 3rd %
% {Pos=52/80, Neg=15/353}
class(A, B, undermining) :-
       clockwise(B, C, 1),
       class_confirmed(A, C, undermining).

% 4th %
% {Pos=42/80, Neg=17/353}
class(A, B, undermining) :-
        class_confirmed(A, 22, undermining),
        rd(A, B, C), C =< 0.240727.
```

```
% 5th %
% {Pos=34/80, Neg=13/353}
class(A, B, undermining) :-
        class_confirmed(A, 6, undermining),
        color(A, B, red, C), C >= -0.151857018,
        rd(A, B, D), D =< 0.29496.

% 6th %
% {Pos=23/80, Neg=8/353}
class(A, B, undermining) :-
        color(A, B, blue, C), C =< -0.909224,
        rd(A, B, D), D =< 0.279323.

% 7th %
% {Pos=10/80, Neg=3/353}
class(A, B, undermining) :-
        color(A, B, green, C), C >= 1.46823204,
        rd(A, B, D), D =< 0.302881.
```

14 CARCINOGENESIS PREDICTIONS USING INDUCTIVE LOGIC PROGRAMMING

Ashwin Srinivasan,
Ross D. King,
Stephen H. Muggleton,
and Michael J. E. Sternberg

Abstract: Obtaining accurate structural alerts for the causes of chemical cancers is a problem of great scientific and humanitarian value. This chapter builds on our earlier research that demonstrated the use of Inductive Logic Programming (ILP) for predictions for the related problem of mutagenic activity amongst nitroaromatic molecules. Here we are concerned with predicting carcinogenic activity in rodent bioassays using data from the U.S. National Toxicology Program conducted by the National Institute of Environmental Health Sciences. The 330 chemicals used here are significantly more diverse than the mutagenesis study, and form the basis for obtaining Structure-Activity Relationships (SARs) relating molecular structure to cancerous activity in rodents. We describe the use of the ILP system Progol to obtain SARs from this data. The rules obtained from Progol are comparable in accuracy to those from expert chemists, and more accurate than most state-of-the-art toxicity prediction methods. The rules can also be interpreted to give clues about the biological and chemical mechanisms of cancerogenesis, and make use of those learned by Progol for mutagenesis. Finally, we present details of, and predictions for, an ongoing international blind trial aimed specifically at comparing prediction methods.

14.1 INTRODUCTION

The task of obtaining the molecular mechanisms for biological toxicity has been a prominent area of application for Inductive Logic Programming (ILP) systems. Recently, this has seen the use of an ILP program to the task of predicting the mutagenic activity of a restricted class of molecules [King et al., 1996, Srinivasan et al., 1994]. The results reported, while interesting, were preliminary for the following reasons. Firstly, the data pertain to a relatively homogeneous class of compounds — although, in themselves, they were more diverse than those analyzed previously by ILP [King et al., 1992]. Secondly, while some comparative studies were performed [Srinivasan et al., 1996b], they were not against state-of-the-art methods designed specifically for toxicity prediction. Finally, a single success is clearly not sufficient grounds for claiming general applicability of a technique. In this chapter we remedy each of these shortcomings. In the course of doing so, we present an important new problem where any scientific discoveries made by ILP programs will be measured against international competition in true blind trials.

The chapter is organized as follows. Section 14.2 describes the problem of carcinogenesis prediction of rodent bioassays. These assays are conducted as part of the National Toxicology Program (NTP) by the U.S. National Institute for Environmental Health Sciences (NIEHS). A prominent feature associated with the NTP is the NIEHS Predictive Toxicology Evaluation — or PTE — project [Bristol et al., 1996]. The PTE project identifies a "test" set of chemicals from those currently undergoing tests for carcinogenicity within the NTP. Predictions on this test set are collected and then compared against the true activity observed in rodents, once such data are available. The description of these blind trials, including details of a trial scheduled for completion in 1998, is described in Section 14.3. Section 14.4 provides an informal introduction to ILP and the system Progol [Muggleton, 1995]. Section 14.5 reviews our earlier work on the use of Progol to obtain structural alerts for mutagenic activity. These alerts form part of the "background knowledge" for the carcinogenicity prediction problem addressed here. Section 14.6 describes the use of Progol to extract molecular descriptions for cancerous activity. These are used to compare against state-of-the-art predictions on an earlier trial in the PTE project (Section 14.6.3). Predictions of the activity of chemicals in the ongoing PTE trial are also in Section 14.6.3. Section 14.7 concludes this chapter.

14.2 THE CARCINOGENESIS PROBLEM AND THE NTP DATA BASE

Prevention of environmentally-induced cancers is a health issue of unquestionable importance. Almost every sphere of human activity in an industrialized society faces potential chemical hazards of some form. In [Huff et al., 1991], it is estimated that nearly 100,000 chemicals are in use in large amounts every day. A further 500–1000 are added every year. Only a small fraction of these chemicals have been evaluated for toxic effects like carcinogenicity. The U.S. National Toxicology Program (NTP) contributes to this enterprise by conducting standardized chemical bioassays — exposure of rodents to a range of chemicals — to help identify substances that may have carcinogenic effects on humans. However, obtaining empirical evidence from such bioassays is expensive and usually too slow to cope with the number of chemicals that can result in adverse effects on human exposure. This has resulted in an urgent need for models that propose molecular mechanisms for carcinogenesis. It is envisaged that such models would (a) generate reliable toxicity predictions for all kinds of chemicals; (b) enable low cost identification of hazardous chemicals; and (c) refine and reduce the reliance on the use of large number of laboratory animals [Bristol et al., 1996]. Pattern-recognition methods can "...help identify, characterize, and understand the various mechanisms or modes of action that determine the type and level of response observed when biological systems are exposed to chemicals" [Bristol et al., 1996].

Tests conducted by the NTP have so far resulted in a data base of more than 300 compounds that have been shown to be carcinogenic or otherwise in rodents. Amongst other criteria, the chemicals have been selected on the basis of their carcinogenic potential — for example, positive mutagenicity tests — and on evidence of substantial human exposure [Huff et al., 1991]. Using rat and mouse strains (of both genders) as predictive surrogates for humans, levels of evidence of carcinogenicity are obtained from the incidence of tumors on long-term (two years) exposure to the chemicals. The NTP assigns the following levels of evidence: CE, clear evidence; SE, some evidence; E, equivocal evidence; and NE, no evidence. Precise definitions for determining these levels can be found in [Huff et al., 1991], and a complete listing of all chemicals tested is available at the NTP Home Page: *http://ntpserver.niehs.nih.gov/*.

The diversity of these compounds present a general problem to many conventional SAR techniques. Most of these, such as the regression-based techniques under the broad category called Hansch Analysis [Kubini, 1993], can only be applied to model compounds that have similar mechanisms of action. This "congeneric" assumption does not hold for the chemicals in the NTP data base, thus limiting the applicability of such methods. The Predictive Toxicology Evaluation project undertaken by the NIEHS aims to obtain an unbiased comparison of prediction methods by specifying compounds for blind trials. One such trial, PTE-1, is now complete. Complete results of NTP tests for compounds in the second trial, PTE-2, will be available by mid 1998.

14.3 THE BLIND TRIALS PTE-1 AND PTE-2

The PTE project [Bristol et al., 1996] is concerned with predictions of overall cancerous activity of a pre-specified set of compounds. This overall activity is either "POS" if the level of activity is CE or SE, or "NEG". The PTE project identifies a set of compounds either scheduled for, or currently undergoing, NTP tests. Information concerning the bioassays is disseminated with the view of encouraging the use of state-of-the-art toxicity prediction schemes. Once the true results of biological activity are available, the project collects a set of leading predictors and publishes their results. The first of these trials, termed PTE-1 is now complete, and results for 39 chemicals are available in [Bahler and Bristol, 1993a].[1]

A second round of toxicology evaluation — PTE-2 — consisting of 30 compounds (of which 5 are inorganic) is currently in progress. True biological activity for 13 of these have been determined at the time of writing of this chapter. A complete description of chemicals in PTE-2, along with a schedule of dates is available in [Bristol et al., 1996]. The remaining activity levels should be determined by 1998. In this work, we use Progol to obtain structural alerts from chemicals in the NTP data base. In the first instance, predictions from these alerts will be compared against other predictions available for PTE-1. This will be followed by predictions for compounds in PTE-2.

14.4 INDUCTIVE LOGIC PROGRAMMING AND PROGOL

The formation of a theory to explain a set of observations is central to science. Computer-based methods to assist in this process include statistical techniques, such as regression, neural networks, and programs that construct theories inductively in a formal logic. It is this last category that describes Inductive Logic Programming (ILP) [Muggleton, 1991]. Given a set of observations and background knowledge, in the form of logic programs — usually written as Prolog statements — an ILP system attempts to construct explanations for the observations. The explanations are in the same language as that describing the observations and background knowledge, namely logic programs.

Logic, with its symbolic formalism, provides an easily comprehended representation for scientific theories. In contrast statistical techniques and neural networks use representations which generally are hard to comprehend and provide less insight into underlying general principles. Most symbolic machine learning algorithms employ simple propositional logic representations which are prohibitively bulky for many scientific and engineering domains. This contrasts with ILP systems which use the rich representation of a subset of first-order predicate calculus (FOPC). Thus, a hypothesis such as "Every drug that contains a bonded pair of aromatic rings is mutagenic." can be expressed straightforwardly as a logic program within an ILP system. A system employing a propositional logic would need precoding of the feature "contains a bonded pair of aromatic rings".

The ILP system Progol [Muggleton, 1995] is provided with a set of "positive" and (optionally) "negative" examples, together with background knowledge B about the problem. The aim is to generate a hypothesis, expressed as a set of rules, which explains all the positive examples in terms of the background knowledge whilst remaining consistent with the negative examples. Progol 1) randomly selects a positive example e_i; 2) uses "inverse implication" to construct the most specific hypothesis $\bot(B, e_i)$ which explains e_i in terms of B; 3) finds a rule D_i which generalizes $\bot(B, e_i)$ and which maximally compresses a set of entailed examples E_i; and 4) adds D_i to the hypothesis H and repeats from 1) with examples not covered so far until no more compression is possible. Compression is here defined as the difference, in numbers of descriptors, between E_i and D_i. Compression formalizes the reduction of information provided by the rule in describing the data. Figure 14.1 illustrates the reduced, finite, search space of Progol. The reduction in the search space is such that, unlike most machine learning algorithms, it is generally feasible to find the optimal rule in reasonable time. In the previous system Golem [Muggleton and Feng, 1990] efficiency was gained at the expense of expressiveness of representation. Golem's two restrictions of tabulated background knowledge and determinate rules have been relaxed in Progol without noticeable loss of speed.

14.5 STRUCTURE ACTIVITY RELATIONSHIPS FOR MUTAGENICITY USING PROGOL

The construction of new scientific knowledge from real-world data remains an active focus for machine learning. One such problem is the Structure Activity Relationships (SAR) of chemical compounds. This forms the basis of rational drug design. One widely used method of SAR stems from the work of Hansch and co-workers [Kubini, 1993] who developed the use of regression-like methods to predict activity from molecular properties such as hydrophobicity, sigma effect, molar reflectivity and LUMO (the energy of the Lowest Unoccupied Molecular Orbital). This and many other approaches are limited in their representation of molecular connectivity and structure. In our earlier work on drug design [King et al., 1992] the use of the language constraints within the Golem system made it impossible to explicitly encode connectivity information. Effectively, this constraint required that each atom was bonded to at most one other atom. Progol's use of first-order predicate calculus, without determinate restrictions, allows encoding of arbitrary atomic and bond connectivities and properties, thus thus offering a new approach for SAR.

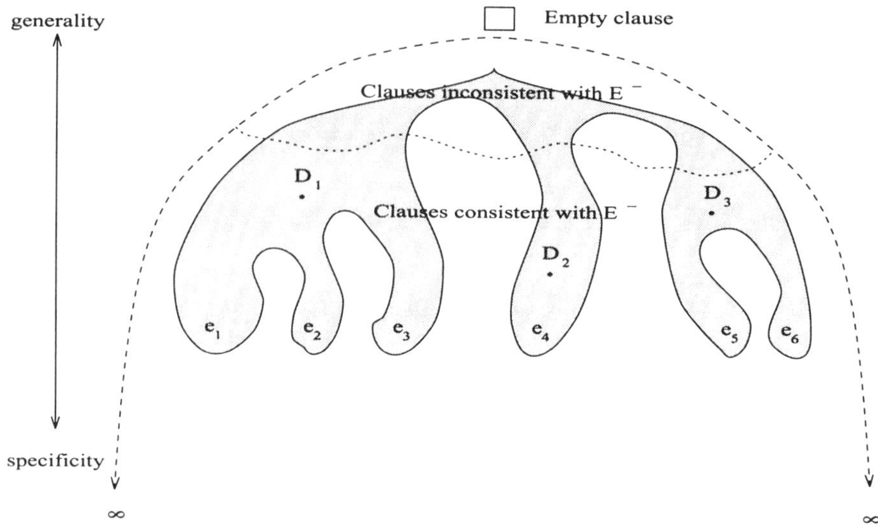

Figure 14.1 The space of clauses (rules) searched by logic-based learning algorithms. The space enclosed by the parabolic broken line contains all clauses that can potentially be included in a theory. Clauses near the top are usually too general, that is, are inconsistent with the negative examples. Clauses become progressively more specific as one proceeds downwards. For example, given a set of positive examples, $E^+ = e_1 \wedge e_2 \wedge \ldots e_6$ and negative examples E^-, the shaded area shows the part of the space searched by Progol. In this space, the clauses D_i represent clauses that maximally compress the examples 'under' them in the search space. Usually, while other logic-based algorithms search the entire space under the empty clause, Progol ensures that it only searches those parts in the grey space.

Progol has been applied to the problem of identifying Ames test mutagenicity within a series of heteroaromatic nitro compounds. Hansch and coworkers have studied 230 compounds using classical regression [Debnath et al., 1991]. For 188 of these compounds, they successfully obtain a regression using hydrophobicity, LUMO and two hand-crafted structural indicator (Boolean) variables. However the remaining 42 compounds could not be successfully modeled by regression and no structural principles were proposed. Progol was applied to this mutagenicity data using the split of the data suggested by Hansch and coworkers. For the discrimination task attempted compounds whose mutagenic activity in log revertants/nmol is > 0 are taken to be highly mutagenic. All compounds were represented relationally in terms of atoms, bond and their partial charge. This information was automatically generated by the modeling program QUANTA^{TM}, and amounts to $\approx$ 18300 facts for the entire set of 230 compounds. For the 188 compounds found to be amenable to regression, the additional Hansch attributes of LUMO and hydrophobicity were also provided.

Details of the results obtained using Progol are described in [King et al., 1996]. In summary, Progol's theory for the 188 compounds matches the accuracy of both the regression analysis of Hansch and coworkers, and a more recent effort using neural networks [Villemin et al., 1993]. Progol's theory is easier to comprehend and was generated automatically, without access to any structural indicator variables hand-crafted by experts. For the 42 "outlier" compounds Progol derived a single rule with an estimated accuracy of 88% (this is significant at $P < 0.001$). In contrast, linear regression and linear discrimination on the parameters used by Hansch and coworkers yield theories with accuracies estimated at 69% and 62% which are no better than random guesses supplied with the default accuracy of 69%. Progol's rule provides the chemical insight that the presence of a five-membered aromatic carbon ring with a nitrogen atom linked by a single bond followed by a double bond indicates mutagenicity. To our knowledge, this is a new structural alert for mutagenicity.

The problem of predicting carcinogenesis addressed here builds on this work since mutagenic chemicals have often been found to be carcinogenic [Debnath et al., 1991]. To this end, we use all structural descriptions with Progol for the 188 nitroaromatic compounds. These rules include those found with different amounts of background information — starting from the very sparse atom/bond information, and proceeding up to the 3-dimensional structural descriptions of the compounds. Complete listings of these rules are available in [Srinivasan et al., 1996a].

14.6 CARCINOGENESIS PREDICTIONS USING PROGOL

The experiment described here has the following aims.

1. Use the ILP system Progol to obtain rules for carcinogenicity from data that does not include compounds in PTE-1 and PTE-2.

2. Predict carcinogenic activity of compounds in PTE-1, and compare against other state-of-the-art toxicity prediction methods.

3. Predict carcinogenic activity of compounds in PTE-2.

14.6.1 Materials

Data. Table 14.1 shows the distribution of compounds in the NTP data base having an overall activity of $POS(+)$ or $NEG(-)$.

Table 14.1 Class distribution of compounds. Complete details of PTE-2 will be available by 1998.

Compounds	+	−	Total
PTE-1	20	19	39
PTE-2	≥7	≥6	30
Rest	162	136	298

Background knowledge. The following background knowledge is available for each category of compounds listed in Table 14.1. Complete Prolog descriptions are available via anonymous ftp to *ftp.comlab.ox.ac.uk*, directory *pub/Packages/ILP/Datasets*.

Atom-bond description. These are ground facts representing the atom and bond structures of the compounds. The representation first introduced in [Srinivasan et al., 1994] is retained. These are Prolog translations of the output of the molecular modeling package QUANTA. Bond information consist of facts of the form *bond(compound,atom1,atom2,bondtype)* stating that *compound* has a bond of *bondtype* between the atoms *atom1* and *atom2*. Atomic structure consists of facts of the form *atm(compound, atom,element,atomtype,charge)*, stating that in *compound*, *atom* has element *element* of *atomtype* and partial charge *charge*.

Generic structural groups. This represents generic structural groups (methyl groups, benzene rings etc.) that can be defined directly using the atom and bond description of the compounds. Here we use definitions for 29 different structural groups, which expands on the 12 definitions used in [Srinivasan et al., 1996b]. We pre-compute these structural groups for efficiency. An example fact that results is in the form *methyl(compound, atom_list)*, which states that the list of atoms *atom_list* in *compound* form a methyl group. Connectivity amongst groups is defined using these lists of atoms.

Genotoxicity. These are results of short-term assays used to detect and characterize chemicals that may pose genetic risks. These assays include the *Salmonella* assay, in-vivo tests for the induction of micro-nuclei in rat and mouse bone marrow etc. A full report available at the NTP Home Page lists the results from such tests in one of 12 types. Results are usually + or − indicating positive or negative response. These results are encoded into Prolog facts of the form *has_property(compound,type,result)*, which states that the *compound* in genetic toxicology *type* returned *result*. Here *result* is one of p (positive) or n (negative). In cases where more than 1 set of results are available for a given type, we have adopted the position of returning the majority result. When positive and negative results are returned in equal numbers, then no result is recorded for that test.

Mutagenicity. Progol rules from the earlier experiments on obtaining structural rules for mutagenesis are included [King et al., 1996, Srinivasan et al., 1996a].

Structural indicators. We have been able to encode some of the structural alerts used in [Ashby and Tennant, 1991]. At the time of writing this chapter, the NTP proposes to make available nearly 80 additional structural attributes for the chemicals. Unfortunately, this is not yet in place for reuse in experiments here.

Prediction methods. The ILP system used here is P-Progol (Version 2.3). This is a Prolog implementation of the Progol algorithm [Muggleton, 1995], and we will refer to this simply as Progol in the rest of this chapter. P-Progol is available via anonymous ftp to *ftp.comlab.ox.ac.uk*, directory *pub/Packages/ILP*. The other toxicity prediction methods compared against Progol's PTE-1 predictions are: Ashby [Tennant et al., 1990], RASH [Jones and Easterly, 1991], TIPT [Bahler and Bristol, 1993b], Benigni [Benigni, 1995], DEREK [Sanderson and Earnshaw, 1991], Bakale [Bakale and McCreary, 1992], TOPKAT [Enslein et al., 1990], CASE [Rosenkranz and Klopman, 1990], and COMPACT [Lewis et al., 1990]. We take the PTE-1 predictions of each these algorithms as reported in [Bahler and Bristol, 1993a].

14.6.2 Method

The task is to obtain a theory for carcinogenesis using the 298 chemicals under the "Rest" category in Table 14.1. This theory is then to be used to predict the classes of compounds in PTE-1 and PTE-2. Progol constructs theories within the language and statistical constraints provided by the user. In domains such as the one considered here, it is difficult to know beforehand any reasonable set of constraints to provide. Further, it is not evident that the theory returned by default settings within the program is the best possible. Consequently, we adopt the following three-stage procedure.

Stage 1: Parameter identification. Identify 1 or more critical parameters for Progol. Changing these should result in significant changes in the theory returned by Progol.

Stage 2: Model selection. This proceeds as follows.

1. Randomly select a small subset of the 298 chemicals to act as a "validation" set. The remaining chemicals form the "training" set for Progol.
2. Systematically vary the critical parameters. For each setting obtain a theory from the training set, and record its accuracy on the validation set.
3. Return the theory with the highest accuracy on the validation set.

Stage 3: Model evaluation. The predictions for PTE-1 and PTE-2 by the theory returned from Stage 2 are recorded. For other toxicity prediction methods, the probability that Progol classifies PTE-1 compounds in the same proportion as that method is obtained using McNemar's Test (see below).

For a given set of background predicate definitions, theories returned by Progol are usually affected by the following parameters: (1) c, bounding the number of literals in any hypothesized clause; (2) *noise*, bounding the minimum acceptable training set accuracy for a clause; and (3) *nodes*, bounding the number of clauses searched. Initial experimentation (Stage 1) suggested that the most sensitive parameter for Progol was *noise*. The experiments here consider theories arising from 4 settings corresponding *noise* values 0.35, 0.30, 0.25, and 0.20. For the data here, the size of the validation set is taken to be 30% of the 298 chemicals — that is, 89 compounds. Of these 49 are labeled + and the remaining 40 are labeled −. This leaves 209 compounds for training. Of these 113 are + and the remaining 96 are −.

We also note one other detail concerning the procedure for obtaining a final theory. The Prolog implementation used here can obtain clauses using two different search strategies. The first is as in [Muggleton, 1995], and results in redundant examples being removed after an acceptable clause is found. A second strategy retains these examples, which gives correct estimates for the accuracy of the clause found. Clauses obtained in this fashion can have significant overlap in the examples they make redundant. The preferred final theory is then the subset of these clauses that has maximal compression (within acceptable resource limits).[2]

McNemar's test. McNemar's test for changes is used to compare algorithms. For a pair of algorithms, this is done by a cross-comparison of the compounds correctly and incorrectly classified as shown in Table 14.2.

The null hypothesis is that the proportion of examples correctly classified by both algorithms is the same. If there is no significant difference in the

Table 14.2 Cross-comparison of the predictions of a pair of algorithms $A_{1,2}$ n_1 is the number of compounds whose class is correctly predicted by both algorithms. Similarly for the entries $n_{2,3,4}$.

		Predicted (A_1)		
		Correct	Incorrect	
Predicted (A_2)	Correct	n_1	n_2	n_a
	Incorrect	n_3	n_4	n_b
		n_c	n_d	N

performance of the two algorithms, half of the n_2+n_3 cases whose classifications disagree should be classified correctly by A_1 and A_2 respectively. Because of small numbers, we directly estimate the probability of a chance classification using the binomial distribution, with probability of success at 0.5. In effect, this is likened to probability of obtaining at least n_2 (or n_3, if greater) heads in a sequence of $n_2 + n_3$ tosses of a fair coin.

It is evident that repeated cross-comparisons will yield occasions when Progol's performance will apparently seem better than its adversary. For repeated comparisons of a given pair of algorithms on different random samples of data, it is possible to apply a correction (known as the Bonferroni adjustment) for this problem. The situation of repeated comparisons of different pairs of algorithms on a given set of data (as is here) does not, on the surface, appear to be amenable to the same correction. However, adopting the spirit of the correction, we advocate caution in quantitative interpretations of the binomial probabilities obtained.

14.6.3 Results and discussion

Table 14.3 tabulates the accuracies on the validation set for each of the parameter settings explored. These results lead to the choice of 0.30 as the preferred setting for minimum noise for acceptable clauses.

Figure 14.2 shows an English translation of the theory with highest validation accuracy in Table 14.3. Each disjunct in Figure 14.2 represents a rule followed by Progol. Rules 1-3 are based on biological tests. Additional comments on the rules follow.

Rule 1. The result of the Ames biological test for mutagenicity. The effectiveness of the Ames test is widely recognized, but it is gratifying that Progol identifies it as the most important.

Table 14.3 Validation set accuracies at the model selection stage. "Noise" values provide a lower bound on the training set accuracy for a clause hypothesized by Progol. "Validation accuracy" is the corresponding accuracy on the validation set of the theory obtained from Progol at that noise level.

Noise	Validation accuracy
0.35	0.63
0.30	0.70
0.25	0.63
0.20	0.65

Rule 2. This rule is a test based on using whole (not cell culture) Drosopha. Like the Ames test it tests for mutagenicity.

Rule 3. This rule is puzzling as it would be expected that a positive test for chromosome aberration would be a test for carcinogenesis, not a negative test. More specialized variants of this rule were obtained in other theories obtained in Stage 1 of the experimental methodology, suggesting absence of chromosal aberrations does have some role to play, reasons for which requires investigation.

Rule 4. Aromatic compounds are often carcinogens and the low partial charge indicates relative reactivity. The use of a precise number for partial charge is an artifact of using the information from QUANTA, resulting from a particular molecular substructure around the aromatic carbon.

Rule 5. Amine groups are recognized by Ashby [Tennant et al., 1990] as indicators of cancerogenesis. This rule is a more accurate specification of this rule.

Rule 6. Aromatic hydrogen with a very high partial charge (often chlorinated aromatics). Such aromatics are relatively unreactive (perhaps giving time to diffuse to DNA).

Rule 7. The high partial charge on the hydroxyl oxygen suggests that the group is relatively unreactive. The significance of the aromatic (or resonant) hydrogen is unclear.

Rule 8. Compounds with bromine have been widely recognized as carcinogens [Tennant et al., 1990].

Rule 9. A tetrahedral carbon with low partial charge. The Progol rules for mutagenicity are shown to have utility outside of their original application

Compound A is carcinogenic if:

(1) it tests positive in the Salmonella assay; or
(2) it tests positive for sex-linked recessive lethal mutation in Drosphila; or
(3) it tests negative for chromosome aberration (an in-vivo cytogenetic assay); or
(4) it has a carbon in a six-membered aromatic ring with a partial charge of -0.13; or
(5) it has a primary amine group and no secondary or tertiary amines; or
(6) it has an aromatic (or resonant) hydrogen with partial charge $\geq$ 0.168; or
(7) it has an hydroxy oxygen with a partial charge $\geq$ -0.616 and an aromatic (or resonant) hydrogen; or
(8) it has a bromine; or
(9) it has a tetrahedral carbon with a partial charge $\leq$ -0.144 and tests positive on Progol's mutagenicity rules.

Figure 14.2 Progol's theory for carcinogenesis.

domain. This is interesting as it displays perhaps the first reuse of ILP-constructed knowledge between different scientific problems.

Predicting PTE-1. Table 14.4 tabulates the accuracies of the different toxicity prediction methods on the compounds in PTE-1. This shows Progol to be comparable to the top 3 state-of-the-art toxicity predictors.

This result should be seen in the following perspective. The only method apparently more accurate than Progol is that of Ashby, which involves the participation of human experts and a large degree of subjective evaluation. All the methods with accuracy close to Progol (Ashby, RASH, and TIPT) have access to biological data that was not available to Progol (information form short-term — 13 week — rodent tests). It should also be noted that all the methods compared with Progol were specifically developed for chemical structure activity and toxicity prediction. Some recent information available to us suggest that results are also comparable to those obtained by a mixture of ILP and regression with additional biological information.[3]

Predicting PTE-2. Table 14.5 tabulates the predictions made by the theory in Figure 14.2 for compounds in PTE-2. The results to date show that Progol has currently predicted $8/13 \approx 62\%$ of the compounds correctly. Progol is currently ranked equal first for accuracy. The accuracy of Progol is again

Table 14.4 Comparative accuracies on PTE-1. Here P represents the binomial probability that Progol and the corresponding toxicity prediction method classify the same proportion of examples correctly. The "Default" method predicts all compounds to be carcinogenic. Methods marked with a † have access to short-term in-vivo rodent tests that were unavailable to other methods. Ashby and RASH also involve some subjective evaluation to decide on structural alerts.

Method	Type	Accuracy	P
Ashby†	Chemist	0.77	0.29
Progol	ILP	0.72	1.00
RASH†	Biological potency analysis	0.72	0.39
TIPT†	Propositional ML	0.67	0.11
Bakale	Chemical reactivity analysis	0.63	0.09
Benigni	Expert-guided regression	0.62	0.02
DEREK	Expert system	0.57	0.02
TOPKAT	Statistical discrimination	0.54	0.03
CASE	Statistical correlation analysis	0.54	< 0.01
COMPACT	Molecular modeling	0.54	0.01
Default	Majority class	0.51	0.01

comparable to Ashby (7/13) and RASH (8/13) (no predictions are available as for TIPT). The lower accuracy of Progol (and the other participating methods) in PTE-2 compared with PTE-1 probably reflects the different distribution of compounds in PTE-2 compared to PTE-1 and training data. For example: the percentage of compounds with positive a Ames test in PTE-2 is only 16% compared to an average 42% for PTE-1 and the training data. The changing distribution has been previously noted in [Tennant et al., 1990] and probably reflects a different testing strategy by the NIEHS.

14.7 CONCLUSIONS

The carcinogenesis prediction trials conducted by the NIEHS offer ILP systems a unique opportunity to participate in true scientific discovery. The prediction of chemical cancerogenesis is both an important medical problem and a fascinating research area. This chapter provides initial performance benchmarks that we hope will act as an incentive for participation by other ILP systems in the field. Progol has achieved accuracy as good or better that current state-of-the-art methods of toxicity prediction. Results from other studies [Srinivasan et al., 1996a] suggest that addition of further relevant background knowledge

Table 14.5 Progol predictions for PTE-2. The first column are the compound identifiers in the NTP database. The column headed "Actual" are tentative classifications from the NTP. Here the entry T.B.A. means "to be announced" — confirmed classifications will be available by July, 1998. The 5 compounds marked with a † are inorganic compounds.

Compound Id.	Name	Actual	Progol
6533-68-2	Scopolamine hydrobroamide	-	-
76-57-3	Codeine	-	-
147-47-7	1,2-Dihydro-2,2,4-trimethyquinoline	+	-
75-52-8	Nitromethane	-	-
109-99-9	Tetrahydrofuran	+	+
1948-33-0	t-Butylhydroquinone	-	+
100-41-4	Ethylbenzene	+	-
126-99-8	Chloroprene	+	+
8003-22-3	D&C Yellow No. 11	+	-
78-84-2	Isobutyraldehyde	-	-
127-00-4	1-Chloro-2-Propanol	T.B.A.	+
11-42-2	Diethanolamine	T.B.A.	-
77-09-8	Phenolphthalein	+	-
110-86-1	Pyridine	T.B.A.	+
1300-72-7	Xylenesulfonic acid, Na	-	-
98-00-0	Furfuryl alcohol	T.B.A.	+
125-33-7	Primaclone	+	+
111-76-2	Ethylene glycol monobutyl ether	T.B.A.	-
115-11-7	Isobutene	T.B.A.	-
93-15-2	Methyleugenol	T.B.A.	-
434-07-1	Oxymetholone	T.B.A.	-
84-65-1	Anthraquinone	T.B.A.	+
518-82-1	Emodin	T.B.A.	+
5392-40-5	Citral	T.B.A.	-
104-55-2	Cinnamaldehyde	T.B.A.	-
10026-24-1 †	Cobalt sulfate heptahydrate	T.B.A.	+
1313-27-5 †	Molybdenum trioxide	T.B.A.	-
1303-00-0 †	Gallium arsenide	T.B.A.	-
7632-00-0 †	Sodium nitrite	T.B.A.	+
1314-62-1 †	Vanadium pentozide	T.B.A.	-

should improve the Progol's prediction accuracy even further. In addition, Progol has produced nine rules that can be biologically and chemically interpreted and may help to provide a better understanding of the mechanisms of cancerogenesis.

The results for the prediction of carcinogenesis, taken together with the previous applications of predicting mutagenicity in nitro-aromatic compounds, and the inhibition of angiogenesis by suramin analogues [King et al., 1993], show that ILP can play an important role in understanding cancer related compounds.

Acknowledgments

This research was supported partly by the Esprit Basic Research Action Project ILP II, the SERC project project 'Experimental Application and Development of ILP' and an SERC Advanced Research Fellowship held by Stephen Muggleton. Stephen Muggleton is a Research Fellow of Wolfson College Oxford. R.D. King was at Imperial Cancer Research Fund during the course of much of the early work on this problem. We would also like to thank Professor Donald Michie and David Page for interesting and useful discussions concerning the use of ILP for predicting biological activity.

Notes

1. A preliminary effort by Progol in presented in [King and Srinivasan, 1996]. The results in this paper subsume these early results as a number of toxicology indicators were unavailable to us at that time. Further details are in Section 14.6.
2. This subset is currently obtained by a companion program to P-Progol called T-Reduce (Version 1.0). Compression of a set of clauses is defined analogous to the measure in [Muggleton, 1995], namely, $P - N - L$ where P is the positive examples covered by the theory, N is the negative examples covered by the theory, and L is the number of clauses in the theory. T-Reduce is available on request from the first author.
3. Personal communication from S. Kramer to the second author.

References

Ashby, J. and Tennant, R. (1991). Definitive relationships among chemical structure, carcinogenicity and mutagenicity for 301 chemicals tested by the U.S. NTP. *Mutation Research*, 257:229–306.

Bahler, D. and Bristol, D. (1993a). The induction of rules for predicting chemical carcinogenesis in rodents. In Hunter, L., Searls, D., and Shavlick, J., editors, *Intelligent Systems for Molecular Biology-93*, pages 29–37. MA:AAI/MIT, Cambridge, MA.

Bahler, D. and Bristol, D. (1993b). The induction of rules for predicting chemical carcinogenesis. In *Proceedings of the 26th Hawaii International Conference on System Sciences*, Los Alamitos. IEEE Computer Society Press.

Bakale, G. and McCreary, R. (1992). Prospective ke screening of potential carcinogens being tested in rodent bioassays by the US National Toxicology Program. *Mutagenesis*, 7:91–94.

Benigni, R. (1995). Predicting chemical carcinogenesis in rodents: the state of the art in the light of a comparative exercise. *Mutation Research*, 334:103–113.

Bristol, D., Wachsman, J., and Greenwell, A. (1996). The NIEHS Predictive-Toxicology Evaluation Project. *Environmental Health Perspectives*, pages 1001–1010. Supplement 3.

Debnath, A., de Compadre, R. L., Debnath, G., Schusterman, A., and Hansch, C. (1991). Structure-Activity Relationship of Mutagenic Aromatic and Heteroaromatic Nitro compounds. Correlation with molecular orbital energies and hydrophobicity. *Journal of Medicinal Chemistry*, 34(2):786 – 797.

Enslein, K., Blake, B., and Borgstedt, H. (1990). Predicition of probability of carcinogenecity for a set of ntp bioassays. *Mutagenesis*, 5:305–306.

Huff, J., Haseman, J., and Rall, D. (1991). Scientific concepts, value and significance of chemical carcinogenesis studies. *Ann Rev Pharmacol Toxicol*, 31:621–652.

Jones, T. and Easterly, C. (1991). On the rodent bioassays currently being conducted on 44 chemicals: a RASH analysis to predict test results from the National Toxicology Program. *Mutagenesis*, 6:507–514.

King, R. D. and Srinivasan, A. (1996) Prediction of rodent carcinogenicity bioassays from molecular structure using inductive logic programming. *Environmental Health Perspectives*, 104(5):1031–1040.

King, R., Muggleton, S., Srinivasan, A., Feng, C., Lewis, R., and Sternberg, M. (1993). Drug design using inductive logic programming. In *Proceedings of the 26th Hawaii International Conference on System Sciences*, Los Alamitos. IEEE Computer Society Press.

King, R., Muggleton, S., Srinivasan, A., and Sternberg, M. (1996). Structure-activity relationships derived by machine learning: The use of atoms and their bond connectivities to predict mutagenicity by inductive logic programming. *Proc. of the National Academy of Sciences*, 93:438–442.

King, R., Muggleton, S., and Sternberg, M. (1992). Drug design by machine learning: The use of inductive logic programming to model the structure-activity relationships of trimethoprim analogues binding to dihydrofolate reductase. *Proc. of the National Academy of Sciences*, 89(23):11322–11326.

Kubini, H. (1993). *QSAR: Hansch Analysis and Related Approaches*. VCH, New York.

Lewis, D., Ionnides, C., and Parke, D. (1990). A prospective toxicity evaluation (COMPACT) on 40 chemicals currently being tested by the National Toxicology Program. *Mutagenesis*, 5:433–436.

Muggleton, S. (1991) Inductive logic programming. *New Generation Computing*, 8(4):295–318.

Muggleton, S. (1995). Inverse Entailment and Progol. *New Gen. Comput.*, 13:245–286.

Muggleton, S. and Feng, C. (1990). Efficient induction of logic programs. In *Proceedings of the First Conference on Algorithmic Learning Theory*, Tokyo. Ohmsha.

Rosenkranz, H. and Klopman, G. (1990). Predicition of the carcinogenecity in rodents of chemicals currently being tested by the US National Toxicology Program. *Mutagenesis*, 5:425–432.

Sanderson, D. and Earnshaw, C. (1991). Computer prediction of possible toxic action from chemical structure. *Human Exp Toxicol*, 10:261–273.

Srinivasan, A., King, R. D., and Muggleton, S. (1996a). The role of background knowledge: using a problem from chemistry to examine the performance of an ILP program. Submitted to: *Machine Learning*.

Srinivasan, A., Muggleton, S., King, R., and Sternberg, M. (1994). Mutagenesis: ILP experiments in a non-determinate biological domain. In Wrobel, S., editor, *Proceedings of the Fourth International Inductive Logic Programming Workshop*. Gesellschaft fur Mathematik und Datenverarbeitung MBH. GMD-Studien Nr 237.

Srinivasan, A., Muggleton, S., King, R., and Sternberg, M. (1996b). Theories for mutagenicity: A study of first-order and feature based induction. *Artificial Intelligence*, 85:277–299.

Tennant, R., Spalding, J., Stasiewicz, S., and Ashby, J. (1990). Prediction of the outcome of rodent carcinogenicity bioassays currently being conducted on 44 chemicals by the National Toxicology Program. *Mutagenesis*, 5:3–14.

Villemin, D., Cherqaoui, D., and Cense, J. (1993). Neural network studies: quantitative structure-activity relationship of mutagenic aromatic nitro compounds. *J. Chim. Phys*, 90:1505–1519.

15 CONCEPT DISCOVERY BY DECISION TABLE DECOMPOSITION AND ITS APPLICATION IN NEUROPHYSIOLOGY

Blaž Zupan,
John A. Halter,
and Marko Bohanec

Abstract: This chapter presents a "divide-and-conquer" data analysis method that, given a concept described by a decision table, develops its description in terms of intermediate concepts described by smaller and more manageable decision tables. The method is based on decision table decomposition, a machine learning approach that decomposes a given decision table into an equivalent hierarchy of decision tables. The decomposition aims to discover the decision tables that are overall less complex than the initial one, potentially easier to interpret, and introduce new and meaningful intermediate concepts. The chapter introduces the decomposition method and, through decomposition-based data analysis of two neurophysiological datasets, shows that the decomposition can discover physiologically meaningful concept hierarchies and construct interpretable decision tables which reveal relevant physiological principles.

15.1 INTRODUCTION

When dealing with a complex problem, the approach most often applied is that of "divide-and-conquer", i.e., decompose a problem to less complex and more manageable subproblems. This strategy seems to have an obvious parallel in data analysis. In inductive learning this principle is a foundation for *structured induction* (a term introduced by Donald Michie): instead of learning a single complex classification rule for a target concept given by examples, define a concept hierarchy and learn the rules for each of the concepts. Originally A. Shapiro used structured induction for the classification of a fairly complex chess endgame and demonstrated that the complexity and comprehensibility ("brain-compatibility") of the obtained solution was superior to the unstructured one [Shapiro, 1987].

The major drawback of the structured induction method is a manual development of the concept hierarchy and the selection of examples to induce the classification rules for each of the concepts in the hierarchy. Typically this is a tiresome process that requires active availability of a domain expert over long periods of time. In this chapter we propose a decomposition method that aims to automate both the process of derivation of a concept hierarchy and decomposition of the original dataset to datasets that describe each concept. The method is based on function decomposition, an approach originally developed for the design of digital circuits [Ashenhurst, 1952]. The method iteratively applies a *single decomposition step*, whose goal is to decompose a function $y = F(X)$ into $y = G(A, H(B))$, where X is a set of input attributes $x_1, \ldots, x_n$, and y is the class variable. A and B are subsets of input attributes such that $A \cup B = X$. F, G and H are functions represented as *decision tables*, i.e., possibly incomplete sets of instances in the form of attribute-value vectors with assigned classes. The functions G and H are developed in the decomposition process and are not predefined in any way. Such decomposition also discovers a new intermediate concept $c = H(B)$. Since the decomposition can be applied recursively on H and G, the result is in general a *hierarchy* of decision tables.

Especially in medicine, the comprehensibility of data may be the key issue when using a computer-based tool for data analysis. The proposed decomposition method aims at enhancing the data interpretability by (1) decomposing the original dataset to smaller sets that can be analyzed separately, (2) using the user predefined or decomposition-discovered interpretable and physiologically significant intermediate concepts which are not explicitly present in the data, and by (3) structuring the data by means of a hierarchy of intermediate concepts.

The chapter is organized as follows. The next section reviews the related work on decision table decomposition with the emphasis on its use for machine learning. The proposed decomposition algorithm is presented in Section 15.3. Since the decomposition requires decision tables with nominal attributes and classes, this section also discusses the discretization and the interval logic approach that enables the use of continuous attributes and classes. The use of decomposition-based data analysis is illustrated in Section 15.4 on two neurophysiological datasets. Section 15.5 gives a summary of the proposed method and its experimental evaluation.

15.2 RELATED WORK

The decomposition approach to machine learning was used by A. Samuel, one of the pioneers of artificial intelligence. He proposed a method based on a signature table system [Samuel, 1967] and successfully used it as an evaluation mechanism for checkers playing programs. This approach was later improved by [Biermann et al., 1982]. Their method, however, did not address the problem of deriving the structure of concepts and was mainly limited to cases where the training examples completely covered the attribute space.

Within machine learning, there are other approaches that are based on problem decomposition, but where the problem is decomposed by the expert and not induced by a machine. A well-known example is structured induction, developed by [Shapiro, 1987]. His approach is based on a manual decomposition of the problem. For every intermediate concept either a special set of training examples is used or an expert is consulted to build a corresponding decision tree. In comparison with standard decision tree induction techniques, Shapiro's approach exhibits about the same classification accuracy with the increased transparency and lower complexity of the developed models. [Michie, 1995] emphasizes the important role that structured induction will have in the future development of machine learning and lists several real problems that were solved in this way.

A decomposition approach that could both discover the structure of concepts and derive the corresponding functions was for the purpose of switching circuit design defined by Ashenhurst [Ashenhurst, 1952]. His decomposition method was essentially the same as that of Biermann, except that it was used to decompose a truth table of a specific Boolean function to be then realized with standard binary gates. Most of the other related work of those times is reported and reprinted in [Curtis, 1962]. This decomposition method was recently substantially improved by the research groups of M. A. Perkowski, T. Luba, and T. D. Ross. [Perkowski, 1995] reports on the decomposition approach for incompletely specified switching functions. [Luba, 1995] proposes a method for the decomposition of multi-valued switching functions in which each multi-valued variable is encoded by a set of Boolean variables. These authors identify the potential usefulness of function decomposition for machine learning, and indicate that the decomposition approach to switching circuit design may be referred to as knowledge discovery [Goldman et al., 1995], since functions not previously foreseen can be discovered and useful features not present at original dataset can be constructed. From the viewpoint of machine learning, however, the main drawbacks of existing methods are that they are mostly limited to Boolean functions and incapable of dealing with noise.

According to a comprehensive survey of decomposition methods by [Perkowski, 1995], there has not been much work on decomposition methods that handle continuous-valued data sets. Recently, [Demšar et al., 1997] adapted the method to be used in scientific discovery of real-valued functions, but their approach cannot handle nominal attributes and can discover only a limited set of predefined functions.

In machine learning, feature discovery is referred to as *constructive induction* [Michalski, 1986]. Perhaps closest to the function decomposition method are the constructive induction systems that use a set of existing attributes and a set of constructive operators to derive new attributes. Examples of such systems are presented in [Pfahringer, 1994, Ragavan and Rendell, 1993]. In first-order learning of relational concept descriptions, constructive induction is referred to as *predicate invention*. An overview of recent achievements in this area can be found in [Stahl, 1991].

The work presented here is based on our own decomposition algorithm [Zupan et al., 1997] inspired by the approach of [Curtis, 1962] and [Perkowski, 1995], and extended to handle nominal attributes and classes, thus being appropriate to deal with machine learning tasks, performing a form of constructive induction and induction of concept hierarchies.

To our knowledge there has been no work reported on the use of decomposition to analyze medical data. However, in some early medical expert system shells such as MYCIN [Buchanan and Shortliffe, 1984] there have been attempts to construct some intermediate states which were neither final solutions nor primary data. These were used as states in the inference process aimed at increasing the comprehensibility and accuracy of the system [Fu and Buchanan, 1985].

15.3 DECISION TABLE DECOMPOSITION

This section introduces the decomposition approach to the analysis of medical data. In the core of the method is the Ashenhurst-Curtis decomposition of decision tables, extended to handle nominal attributes and classes. This method is introduced first by an example. Then, unsupervised and supervised approaches to decomposition are proposed. The basic decomposition algorithm requires nominal-valued data. In case of continuous attributes and/or classes, we show how to preprocess the data by discretization and interval logic.

15.3.1 *Decision table decomposition - An example*

Suppose we are given a *decision table* $y = F(X) = F(x_1, x_2, x_3)$ (Table 15.1) with three attributes x_1, x_2, and x_3, and class variable (target concept) y, and we want to decompose it to decision tables G and H, such that $y = G(x_1, c)$ and $c = H(x_2, x_3)$. For this decomposition, the initial set of attributes X is partitioned to a *bound set* $\{x_2, x_3\}$ used with H and a *free set* $\{x_1\}$ used with G. The decomposition requires the introduction of a new attribute c which depends only on the variables in the bound set.

Table 15.1 A small decision table.

x_1	x_2	x_3	y
low	low	low	low
low	low	high	low
low	med	low	low
low	med	high	med
low	high	low	low
low	high	high	high
med	med	low	med
med	high	low	med
med	high	high	high
high	low	low	high
high	high	low	high

To derive G and H from F, we first need to represent the decision table by a *partition matrix* (Figure 15.1). This uses all the possible combinations of attribute values of the bound set as column labels, and of the free set as row labels. Each decision table instance is then represented by the corresponding element of the partition matrix.

Each column in a partition matrix specifies the behavior of the function F when the attributes in the bound set are constant. Two elements of a partition matrix are *compatible* if they are the same or at least one of them is unknown (denoted by "-"). Two columns are compatible if all of their elements are pair-wise compatible; these columns are considered to represent the same behavior of the function F.

The problem is now to assign labels to the columns of the partition matrix so that only groups of mutually compatible columns get the same label. Columns with the same label exhibit the same behavior with respect to F and can use a single value of the new concept c. Label assignment involves the construction of a *column incompatibility graph*, where columns of the partition matrix are nodes and two nodes are connected if they are incompatible. Column labels are

x_1 \ x_2, x_3	low, low	low, high	med, low	med, high	high, low	high, high
low	low	low	low	med	low	high
med	-	-	med	-	med	high
high	high	-	-	-	high	-
c	1	1	1	2	1	3
c_{interp}	low	low	low	med	low	high

Figure 15.1 A partition matrix with uninterpreted (c) and interpreted (c_{interp}) column labels for the decision table from Table 15.1, free set $\{x_1\}$, and bound set $\{x_2, x_3\}$ together with its corresponding incompatibility graph.

then assigned by coloring the incompatibility graph [Perkowski, 1995]. For our example, the incompatibility graph with one of the possible optimal colorings is given in Figure 15.1.

For better comprehensibility, we interpret the column labels "1" as `low`, "2" as `med`, and "3" as `high`. These labels and the partition matrix straightforwardly determine the function $c = H(x_2, x_3)$. To determine the function $G(x_1, c)$, we lookup the annotated partition matrix for all the possible combinations of x_1 and c. The final result of the decomposition is represented as a hierarchy of two decision tables in Figure 15.2. If we further examine the discovered functions G and H we can see that $G \equiv \text{MAX}$ and $H \equiv \text{MIN}$.

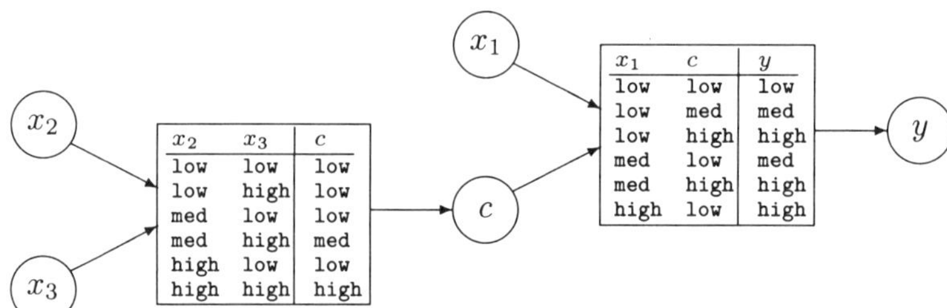

x_2	x_3	c
low	low	low
low	high	low
med	low	low
med	high	med
high	low	low
high	high	high

x_1	c	y
low	low	low
low	med	med
low	high	high
med	low	med
med	high	high
high	low	high

Figure 15.2 The result of decomposing the decision table from Table 15.1. The interpretation of decision tables yields $c = \text{MIN}(x_2, x_3)$ and $y = \text{MAX}(x_1, c)$.

15.3.2 Unsupervised decomposition

Unsupervised decomposition (Algorithm 15.1) aims to discover a hierarchy of concepts with the decision tables that are overall less complex than the initial one. Since an exhaustive search for an optimal hierarchy of decision tables is prohibitively complex, the decomposition uses a suboptimal iterative algorithm.

Input: An initial decision table $c_0 = T_0(x_1, \ldots, x_n)$ describing a single concept
A maximum number b of attributes in bound set B
Output: Its hierarchical decomposition
initialize $\mathcal{T} \leftarrow \{T_0\}$
initialize $j \leftarrow 1$
while $\mathcal{T} \neq \emptyset$
  arbitrarily select decision table $T_i \in \mathcal{T}$, where $c_i = T_i(x_1, \ldots, x_m)$
  $\mathcal{T} \leftarrow \mathcal{T} \setminus T_i$
  select best $A_{best}|B_{best} = \arg\min_{A|B} \nu(A|B)$,
    where $A|B$ are all possible partitions of $X = < x_1, \ldots, x_m >$
    such that $A \cup B = X$, $A \cap B = \emptyset$, and $||B|| \leq b$
  if T_i is decomposable using $A_{best}|B_{best}$ **then**
    decompose T_i to T_i' and T_j, such that $c_i = T_i'(A_{best}, c_j)$ and $c_j = T_j(B_{best})$
    $T_i \leftarrow T_i'$
    if $||A_{best}|| > 1$ **then** $\mathcal{T} \leftarrow \mathcal{T} \cup \{T_i\}$ **end if**
    if $||B_{best}|| > 2$ **then** $\mathcal{T} \leftarrow \mathcal{T} \cup \{T_j\}$ **end if**
    $j \leftarrow j + 1$
  end if
end while

Algorithm 15.1 Unsupervised decomposition algorithm.

In each step the algorithm tries to decompose a single decision table of the evolving structure. It evaluates all candidate disjoint partitions of the attributes and selects the best one. The candidate partitions are all possible partitions with bound sets of at least two but no more than b attributes, where b is a user defined constant. This step requires a so-called *partition selection measure* which needs to be minimized. A possible measure is the number of values of the new concept c derived through coloring of the incompatibility graph. If A and B are the free and bound sets, and | denotes a partition, this number is called the *column multiplicity* and is denoted by $\nu(A|B)$. In the above example, we have shown that $\nu(x_1|x_2, x_3) = 3$. Similarly, one can derive $\nu(x_2|x_1, x_3) = 4$ and $\nu(x_3|x_1, x_2) = 5$. According to ν, the unsupervised decomposition selects the partition $x_1|x_2, x_3$.

The decision table T_i is decomposed only if the two resulting decision tables T_i' and T_j are of lower complexity. In general, the decision table $c_i = T_i(x_1, \ldots, x_n)$ can represent $N(T_i) = ||c_i||^{(\prod_{j=1}^{n} ||x_j||)}$ functions, and the number of bits needed to encode each such function is therefore:

$$\Theta(T_i) = \log_2 N(T_i) = \log_2 ||c_i|| \prod_{j=1}^{n} ||x_j||$$

where $||x_j||$ and $||c_i||$ denote the cardinality of the set of values used by attribute x_j and c_i, respectively. $\Theta(T_i)$ thus expresses the complexity of decision table T_i. We define the decision table T_i to be decomposable to T_i' and T_j using the attribute partition $A|B$ if $\Theta(A|B) < \Theta(T_i)$, where $\Theta(A|B) = \Theta(T_i') + \Theta(T_j)$.

15.3.3 Supervised decomposition

Although the structure and associated decision tables discovered by unsupervised decomposition may be optimal with respect to some complexity measure, the essential drawback of the approach is that the user may prefer a different structure, i.e., a different dependency of concepts and attributes. Such structure may use intermediate concepts of higher complexity than those discovered by unsupervised decomposition, but these concepts may be more comprehensible and easier to interpret.

Both arguments are related to "brain compatibility" as introduced by Shapiro [Shapiro, 1987]. Decomposition methods should not only address the complexity, but rather provide methods to assist the user in the discovery of the structure and underlying principles of the domain. We therefore require the supervised decomposition to support the following operations:

- Given a user-defined hierarchical structure of concepts, derive the associated decision tables.
- Allow the user to control the decomposition process by selecting the decision table to decompose next.
- Given a decision table, allow the user to select a partition for decomposition by providing a list of partitions and their associated partition selection measures.

15.3.4 Decomposition with continuous attributes and classes

The decomposition presented so far requires a decision table that uses nominal attributes and classes. However, a common data representation for medical domains is that some attributes and even the class may be continuous. To allow for the decomposition of such domains, we discretize the continuously-valued attributes and class, and from the original dataset construct the discretized decision table. The discretization attempts to minimize the classification error of the discretized decision table with respect to the original dataset.

Discretization for a nominal class problem. Let us first suppose that the domain has a nominal-valued class and that several attributes are continuous. Let a discretization in the form of disjoint intervals be given for every continuous attribute. Every such interval is labeled and corresponds to a single nominal value of the attribute. The discretized decision table is then constructed from the original dataset such that for every combination of nominal values of attributes all corresponding non-discretized data instances are found. If any such instances exist, the most frequent class of these instances is determined and a corresponding entry to the discretized decision table is added.

The above procedure assumes that the discretization intervals are given. The appropriateness of these intervals can be estimated with the number of correctly classified original data instances where the constructed discretized decision table is used as a classifier. To minimize this error, the construction of discretized decision table is coupled with a genetic algorithm: the chromosomes encode the intervals, and the fitness of each chromosome is the classification accuracy of the discretized decision table that is derived using the intervals encoded by the chromosome. We use a standard genetic algorithm with the mutation and crossover operators as provided in the PGApack genetic algorithm library [Levine, 1995]. The limitation of the current implementation is that the number of intervals of an attribute has to be given by the user.

Discretization for a continuous class problem. We employ a similar approach to the discretization for the case of a continuously-valued class variable. In this case the class value needs to be discretized as well. Given the discretization for continuous attributes and class, the entries of discretized decision table are derived similarly as in the case of nominal class.

The discretized decision table can be used to predict the continuous value of the class for any of the instances of the original dataset. This is done using the *interval logic.* The prediction of a continuous value of class using the attribute and class intervals and discretized decision table starts by computing the interval coefficients. For each continuous attribute i and its continuous value q_i the corresponding interval (l_i, h_i) is determined, such that $l_i \leq q_i < h_i$. The *interval coefficient* k_i defines a relative position of q_i within the interval and is determined as $k_i = (q_i - l_i)/(h_i - l_i)$. By definition, interval coefficients have values between 0 and 1. Using the discretized decision table, the nominal value of the class is derived, i.e., the interval (l_y, h_y) is found to which the class value belongs to. Class' interval coefficient k_y is computed as the average of the k_i's of continuous attributes and then used to estimate the continuous value of the class variable as $y' = l_y + k_y(h_y - l_y)$.

For example, let the attributes $x_1, x_2, x_3 \in [0, 1]$ and class $y \in [0, 1]$ have the intervals given in Figure 15.3. Suppose that the original dataset was discretized

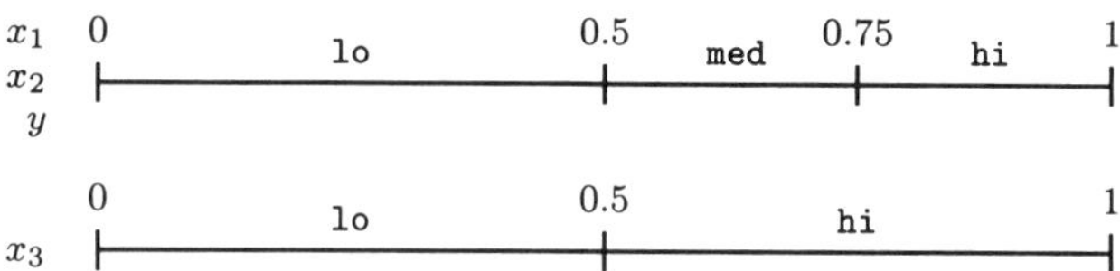

Figure 15.3 Intervals for input properties x_1, x_2, x_3 and output property y.

to the decision table of Table 15.1. Let $x_1 = 0.25$, $x_2 = 0.8$, and $x_3 = 0.75$ be the attribute values of some instance from the original dataset and $y = 0.80$ be its corresponding class value. Then, the discretized value of x_1 is `low` and its interval coefficient is $k_1 = (0.25 - 0)/(0.5 - 0) = 0.5$. Similarly, $x_2 =$ `high` with $k_2 = (0.8 - 0.75)/(1 - 0.75) = 0.2$ and $x_3 =$ `high` with $k_3 = (0.75 - 0.5)/(1 - 0.5) = 0.5$. From the discretized decision table we derive the discretized value of y, which is $y(\texttt{low}, \texttt{high}, \texttt{high}) = \texttt{high}$. The interval coefficient of y is k_y and is computed as an average of k_1, k_2, and k_3: $k_y = (0.5 + 0.2 + 0.5)/3 = 0.4$. Finally, the estimated quantitative value of y is $y' = 0.75 + k_y(1 - 0.75) = 0.85$. The estimated value $y' = 0.85$ and the value originally defined by a data instance $y = 0.85$ can then be used to compute the approximation error of the discretized decision table.

The discretization aims to derive the intervals and construct the decision table which, once used to predict the continuous class values of original instances, maximizes the prediction accuracy. Again, we couple the discretization with a genetic algorithm that uses the chromosomes that encode the intervals for attributes and classes. Such a genetic algorithm attempts to find the discretization which, when used to construct the discretized decision table, minimizes the prediction error which is defined as:

$$\varepsilon = \sum_i \left(\left| \frac{\mathrm{MAX}(y_i, y_i')}{\mathrm{MIN}(y_i, y_i')} \right| - 1 \right)$$

Here, y_i denotes a class value for the i-th instance of the original dataset and y_i' the value estimated using the discretized decision table. This error measure was proposed in [Zupan et al., 1995] and aims to minimize the errors when predicting class values that are either close to 0 or close to the maximum class value. Such cases frequently occur in realistic neurophysiological modeling, as is the case with the first example that is described later in this chapter.

15.3.5 Implementation

The described decomposition and discretization methods are implemented as part of the Hierarchy Induction Tool HINT [Zupan et al., 1997], a system for learning concept hierarchies from examples by decision table decomposition. HINT is written in C and uses the PGApack genetic algorithm library [Levine, 1995] and the Geomview 3D visualization tool [Phillips, 1994]. HINT runs on a variety of UNIX platforms, including HP/UX, SunOS and IRIS.

Although the decision tables discovered by the decomposition are smaller and have less attributes than the initial one, various tools are still required for interpretation. For this purpose, we use visualization and value-reordering tools developed for decision support systems DEX and DECMAK [Bohanec and Rajkovič, 1990, Bohanec et al., 1983] and the tools embedded within HINT.

15.4 ANALYSIS OF NEUROPHYSIOLOGICAL DATA

This section demonstrates how the proposed decomposition method can be used to analyze neurophysiological data. The data was obtained by using a physiologically realistic model of the myelinated axon of a neuron developed at Baylor College of Medicine in Houston. The model is given in the form of a system of multiple cross-coupled parabolic partial differential equations that are solved by an implicit numerical integration method. The model is used to predict the functional implications of neuronal structural and biophysical properties [Halter et al., 1995] and has recently been employed to guide laboratory experiments and a study of patophysiological significance of abnormal myelination.

An analysis of two separate datasets is presented. The first experiment, which studies the influence of sodium ionic channel properties on the sodium current, shows how a predefined concept structure can lead to the derivation of easy-to-understand principles encoded with a decomposed decision table. The second, more complex experiment, shows how the decomposition can be used to discover a physiologically relevant and interpretable concept hierarchy.

In both cases, the datasets include continuous attributes. While the class of the first domain is quantitative, the second domain has a categorical class.

15.4.1 Influence of sodium ionic channel properties on sodium current

The problem addressed here is to observe the influence of sodium ionic channel properties (steady-state activation `av` and inactivation `iv` voltage relations) and the influence of sodium permeability (`naperm`) on the peak sodium current (`ina`) in a nodal segment of the neuronal myelinated nerve fiber. For this problem, the expert (J. A. Halter) defined a concept hierarchy, given in Figure 15.4, that uses one intermediate concept (`nach`).

The problem is to discover how `iv` and `av` influence `nach`, and how `naperm` and `nach` influence `ina`. To derive these principles, the neuronal model was used to arbitrarily sample the attribute space with 100 data items. Quantitative

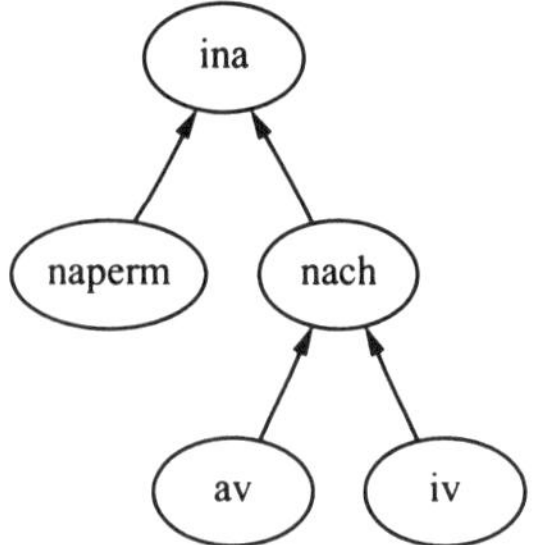

Figure 15.4 Expert defined concept hierarchy for the peak sodium current.

attributes were expressed as the offsets to corresponding parameters of the normal mammalian myelinated axon (for the values and units see [Halter and Clark, 1991]). For each data item they were selected arbitrarily from ranges [0.5,1.5] for `naperm`, [-10,10] for `av`, and [-20,20] for `iv`. The simulation results show that there is high non-linearity because of two different states of the neuron: firing and non-firing. High values of `ina` appear when the neuron fires and values close to 0 when the neuron does not fire.

We have first used the interval logic interpretation and derived corresponding intervals with the use of a genetic algorithm. The number of intervals was set to three for both attributes and class. The approximation error depended slightly on the setting of parameters of the genetic algorithm and was usually around 20 to 30. Examples with `ina` close to 0 contributed the most to this error. The intervals derived from the data (Figure 15.5) were used to construct the discretized decision table, which was then decomposed to tables for `nach` and `ina` (Table 15.2).

Table 15.2 Decision tables for `nach` and `ina`.

iv	av	nach
low	low	med
low	med	low
low	high	xlow
med	low	high
med	med	high
med	high	high
high	low	high
high	med	high
high	high	high

naperm	nach	ina
low	xlow	low
low	low	low
low	med	med
low	high	high
med	xlow	low
med	low	low
med	med	med
med	high	high
high	xlow	low
high	low	high
high	med	high
high	high	high

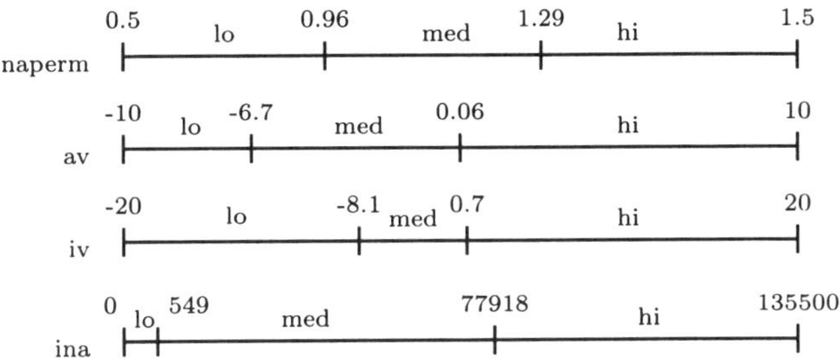

Figure 15.5 Intervals for attributes and class for the study of sodium channel properties.

By interpreting the decomposed decision tables, `ina` was found to monotonically increase with `nach`, and, importantly and to no surprise, `nach` increases with `iv` and decreases with `av`. Because of the monotonic dependence of `ina` on `nach`, `ina` increases with `iv` and decreases with `av`. These discovered principles qualitatively match with a known physiological effect of the activation and inactivation voltage on the peak sodium current [Halter et al., 1995].

We have also tried to use different numbers of intervals and, as expected, found that by increasing this number we can reduce the approximation error. But more importantly, the principles discovered were qualitatively the same. The problem with a high number of intervals is that the data becomes too sparse to cover a sufficient number of combinations of attributes in the initial decision table. Namely, sparse initial decision tables often exhibit redundancies of its attributes discovered by decomposition which need not indicate "real" irrelevance of attributes. Moreover, such decision tables are larger and harder to analyze. If the user's bias is transparency, fewer intervals should be used. In our case, three intervals were sufficient.

15.4.2 Study of conduction-block of partially demyelinated fiber

In this example, we used supervised decomposition to analyze the data used to study the influence of six nerve fiber properties (Table 15.3) to the conduction of action potential. For this study, just a part of the nerve fiber (several internodes) was demyelinated and the corresponding change of several properties was studied. The attributes and class are listed in Table 15.3. The table gives also the range of the values for `aff` and `nl`, and the ranges of orders of magnitude into which `k_conc`, `na_conc`, `scm`, and `leak` were scaled from their normal values. The dataset was generated using a realistic nerve-fiber model and consisted of 3000 random samples.

Table 15.3 Class and attributes for conduction-block domain.

block	class, indicating nerve fiber conduction [yes, no]
aff	number of affected internodes, [1, 6]
nl	number of myelin layers in the internode, [0, 100]
k_conc	concentration of K^+ channel density in the internode, [−2, 2]
na_conc	concentration of Na^+ channel density in the internode, [−2, 2]
scm	specific conductivity of the myelin in the internode, [−2, 2]
leak	nodal leakage through all the nodes of the fiber, [−2, 2]

From the dataset an initial decision table with 2543 items was derived where each of the attributes was discretized using 5 intervals. When used to classify the items in the dataset, the decision table was found to misclassify only 7 items (0.23%).

The decomposition algorithm checked all the possible partitions and the first one found was aff, nl, scm | k_conc, na_conc, leak with $\nu = 12$. This partition was clearly the best one for decomposition, and to illustrate this, Table 15.4 lists ν for all partitions with the cardinality of the bound set equal to 3.

This decomposition yielded the structure block $= T_0(\texttt{aff}, \texttt{nl}, \texttt{scm}, \texttt{c1})$ and c1 $= T_1(\texttt{na\_conc}, \texttt{k\_conc}, \texttt{leak})$. The two decision tables T_0 and T_1 were separately checked for decomposition. For T_0, decomposition with the measure $\nu(\texttt{aff}, \texttt{c1} \mid \texttt{nl}, \texttt{scm}) = 16$ was found yielding $c_2 = T_2(\texttt{nl}, \texttt{scm})$. The resulting decision table block $= T_0'(\texttt{aff}, \texttt{c1}, \texttt{c2})$ was further decomposed using the partition $\nu(\texttt{aff} \mid \texttt{c1}, \texttt{c2}) = 13$. T_1 could also be decomposed, but since all decompositions yielded the intermediate concepts with 25 values or higher, it was decided to stop the decomposition at this point.

The discovered concept hierarchy is presented in Figure 15.6. When interpreted by the domain expert (J. A. Halter), it was found that the discovered intermediate concepts are physiologically interpretable and constitute useful intermediate biophysical properties. Intermediate concept c2, for example, depends on nl and scm, the properties of the myelin sheath, which are indeed coupled within the realistic model through model-specific function $f(\texttt{nl}, \texttt{scm})$. c1 couples na_conc, k_conc, and leak, the axonal properties and the combined current source/sink capacity of the axon which is the driving force for all propagated action potentials.

The initial decision table had 2543 items, while after the decomposition the discovered concepts c1, c2, c3, and the output concept block are described by significantly simpler decision tables with 125, 25, 184, and 65 items, respectively. For this reason and due to the fact that they represent physiologically

Table 15.4 Initial decision table partitions and their column multiplicity for the conduction-block domain.

Free set	Bound set	ν
aff, nl, scm	k_conc, na_conc, leak	12
nl, scm, leak	aff, k_conc, na_conc	15
k_conc, na_conc, leak	aff, nl, scm	16
nl, na_conc, scm	aff, k_conc, leak	16
k_conc, na_conc, scm	aff, nl, leak	17
k_conc, scm, leak	aff, nl, na_conc	17
aff, nl, leak	k_conc, na_conc, scm	17
nl, k_conc, scm	aff, na_conc, leak	17
na_conc, scm, leak	aff, nl, k_conc	18
aff, scm, leak	nl, k_conc, na_conc	18
aff, na_conc, scm	nl, k_conc, leak	18
aff, k_conc, leak	nl, na_conc, scm	18
aff, k_conc, scm	nl, na_conc, leak	18
aff, k_conc, na_conc	nl, scm, leak	18
aff, nl, na_conc	k_conc, scm, leak	18
aff, nl, k_conc	na_conc, scm, leak	18
nl, k_conc, na_conc	aff, scm, leak	19
aff, na_conc, leak	nl, k_conc, scm	19
nl, na_conc, leak	aff, k_conc, scm	20
nl, k_conc, leak	aff, na_conc, scm	20

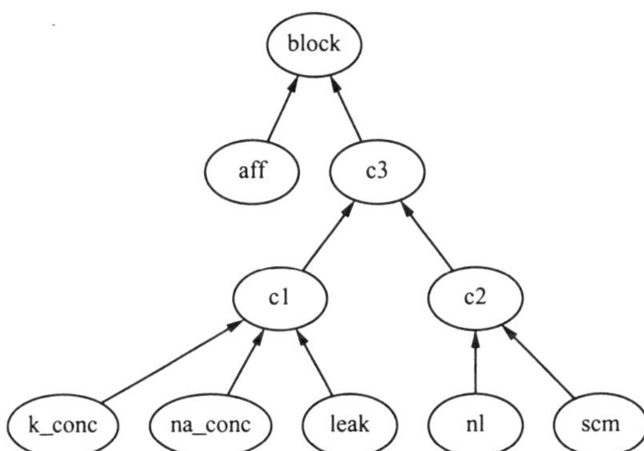

Figure 15.6 The discovered concept hierarchy for the conduction-block domain.

relevant properties, they were easier to interpret than the non-decomposed decision table. For example, it was found that `c2` exhibits monotonic dependency with `nl` and `scm`. Furthermore, `c1` represents a principle known in physiology: for a conduction of the nerve fiber, an increase of `leak` will require an increase of `na_conc`.

15.5 SUMMARY

This chapter presents a novel "divide-and-conquer" approach to assist in medical data analysis. The method is based on decision table decomposition, which, given the initial decision table, iteratively decomposes it to smaller and less complex decision tables thus resulting in a hierarchy of decision tables. In the decomposition process, new intermediate concepts are discovered. Such hierarchy can be given in advance, or can be discovered with or without the user's supervision.

The decision table decomposition was applied to two neurophysiological datasets. For the domain that studies the nerve fiber sodium current, the structure was given in advance and it was shown that the decomposition yielded decision tables that were relatively easy to interpret. The real test for the method was the second domain, where a conduction-block of the nerve fiber was studied. In this domain the decomposition discovered an interpretable hierarchy of concepts, which reveal the underlying neurophysiological principles.

Both datasets result from the simulation of a physiologically-realistic model of the myelinated axon that was developed at Baylor College of Medicine in Houston and is used to predict the functional implications of neuronal structural and biophysical properties. The model is currently used to assist the planning of the laboratory experiments in a study of the patophysiological significance of abnormal myelination. The idea we are pursuing is to embed both the realistic model and methods presented in this chapter in a framework to be efficiently used in the exploration of properties and principles in neurobiology as well as in other physiological systems.

To our knowledge, the decision table decomposition is a method that has not yet been exploited as a machine learning or knowledge discovery tool. However, preliminary experiments in non-trivial domains like the conduction-block strongly encourage further research and development.

Acknowledgments

Support for this work was provided by the Ministry of Science and Technology of Slovenia (Zupan and Bohanec), the W.M. Keck Center for Computational Biology, the Whitaker Foundation (Halter), and the Developmental Support from Information Technology Program at Baylor College of Medicine (Halter and Zupan).

References

Ashenhurst, R. L. (1952). The decomposition of switching functions. Technical report, Bell Laboratories BL-1(11), pages 541–602.

Biermann, A. W., Fairfield, J., and Beres, T. (1982). Signature table systems and learning. *IEEE Trans. Syst. Man Cybern.*, 12(5):635–648.

Bohanec, M., Bratko, I., and Rajkovič, V. (1983). An expert system for decision making. In Sol, H. G., editor, *Processes and Tools for Decision Support.* North-Holland.

Bohanec, M. and Rajkovič, V. (1990). DEX: An expert system shell for decision support. *Sistemica*, 1(1):145–157.

Buchanan, G. and Shortliffe, E. H., editors (1984). *Rule-Based Expert Systems: The MYCIN Experiments of the Stanford Heuristic Programming Project.* Addison-Wesley, Reading, Mass.

Curtis, H. A. (1962). *A New Approach to the Design of Switching Functions.* Van Nostrand, Princeton, N.J.

Demšar, J., Zupan, B., Bohanec, M., and Bratko, I. (1997). Constructing intermediate concepts by decomposition of real functions. In *Proc. European Conference on Machine Learning, ECML-96*, pages 93–107. Springer Verlag.

Fu, L.-M. and Buchanan, B. G. (1985). Learning intermediate concepts in constructing a hierarchical knowledge base. In *Proc. of International Joint Conference on Artificial Intelligence IJCAI-85*, pages 659–666, Los Angeles, CA.

Goldman, J. A., Ross, T. D., and Gadd, D. A. (1995) Pattern Theoretic Learning. In *AAAI Spring Symposium Series: Systematic Methods of Scientific Discovery.*

Halter, J. A., Carp, J. S., and Wolpaw, J. W. (1995). Operantly conditioned motoneuron plasticity: Possible role of sodium channels. *J. Neurophysiology*, 73(2):867–871.

Halter, J. A. and Clark, J. W. (1991). A distributed-parameter model of the myelinated nerve fiber. *J. Theo. Biol.*, 148:345–382.

Levine, D. (1995). User's guide to PGAPack parallel genetic algorithm library. Mathematics and Computer Science Division, Argonne National Laboratory, Argonne, IL.

Luba, T. (1995). Decomposition of multiple-valued functions. In *25th Intl. Symposium on Multiple-Valued Logic*, pages 256–261, Bloomigton, Indiana.

Michalski, R. S. (1986). Understanding the nature of learning: Issues and research directions. In Michalski, R., Carbonnel, J., and Michell, T., editors, *Machine Learning: An Artificial Intelligence Approach*, pages 3–25. Kaufmann, Los Atlos, CA.

Michie, D. (1995). Problem decomposition and the learning of skills. In Lavrač, N. and Wrobel, S., editors, *Machine Learning: ECML-95*, Notes in Artificial Intelligence 912, pages 17–31. Springer Verlag.

Perkowski, M. A. (1995). A survey of literature on function decomposition. Technical report, GSRP Wright Laboratories, Ohio OH.

Pfahringer, B. (1994). Controlling constructive induction in CiPF. In Bergadano, F. and Raedt, L. D., editors, *Machine Learning: ECML-94*, pages 242–256. Springer Verlag.

Phillips, M. (1994). Geomview manual. The Geometry Center, University of Minnesota.

Ragavan, H. and Rendell, L. (1993). Lookahead feature construction for learning hard concepts. In *Proc. Tenth International Machine Learning Conference*, pages 252–259. Morgan Kaufman.

Samuel, A. (1967). Some studies in machine learning using the game of checkers II: Recent progress. *IBM J. Res. Develop.*, 11:601–617.

Shapiro, A. D. (1987). *Structured Induction in Expert Systems.* Turing Institute Press in association with Addison-Wesley Publishing Company.

Stahl, I. (1991). An overview of predicate invention techniques in ILP. In *Project Report ESPRIT BRA 6020: Inductive Logic Programming.*

Zupan, B., Bohanec, M., Bratko, I., and Demšar, J. (1997). Machine learning by function decomposition. In *Proc. 14th International Conference on Machine Learning*, Nashville, TN.

Zupan, B., Halter, J. A., and Bohanec, M. (1995). Computer-assisted reasoning on principles and properties of medical physiology. In *Proc. of the Workshop on Computer-Aided Data Analysis in Medicine, CADAM-95*, pages 258–271, Bled.

16 CLASSIFICATION OF HUMAN BRAIN WAVES USING SELF-ORGANIZING MAPS

Udo Heuser,
Josef Göppert,
Wolfgang Rosenstiel,
and Andreas Stevens

Abstract: This chapter presents a method for the classification of EEG spectra by means of Kohonen's self-organizing map. We use EEG data recorded by 19 electrodes (channels), sampled at 128 Hz. Data vectors are extracted at intervals of half a second with a duration of one second each, resulting in vectors overlapping half a second. Before the training of the map, the sample vectors were compressed by either the Fast-Fourier-Transform or the Wavelet-Transform. Data preprocessed by the Fourier-Transform result in short-time power spectra. These spectra are filtered by butterworth filters that meet the EEG frequency bands of the delta-, theta-, alpha-, beta- and gamma-rhythms. Data preprocessed by the Wavelet-Transform result in wavelet coefficients that are combined and averaged. The preprocessed vectors form "clusters" on the trained self-organizing map that are related to specific EEG patterns.

16.1 INTRODUCTION

Self-organizing maps have proved to be powerful tools for the easy classification of huge amounts of data. In this chapter, we present a method for the classification and detection of specific EEG patterns that may occur in all observed test persons and at different tasks (*inter-classification*; see also [Heuser et al., 1996, Joutsiniemi et al., 1995]). First, the EEG recordings that are obtained from test persons carrying out 6 different tasks, have to be coded and packed into a sequence of vectors. Then every vector has to be preprocessed by compressing and reducing the total amount of input data. This could be obtained by the Fourier-Transform that results in power spectra. These power spectra have to be filtered again by using the butterworth filter to fit the known EEG frequency ranges or frequency rhythms. As an alternative, we use the Wavelet-Transform as preprocessing or data-compressing unit. The obtained data again have to be filtered using band-pass filters that compute averages for combined wavelet coefficients. This method detects EEG artifacts better than the Fourier-Transform.

The self-organizing map is then able to classify all major EEG patterns that may occur in every test person. Every detected class depicted as separate cluster on the map represents one major EEG pattern. The methods and tools used are explained in detail first. Next the experimental results are presented. The chapter concludes with a summary.

16.2 METHODS

16.2.1 Data coding

The experimental data used was obtained from EEG recordings that were made available by the University Clinic for Psychiatry and Psychotherapy, Tübingen. They are recorded from healthy test persons who carried out six different tasks. The tasks are described below.

The 19 electrodes (channels) are positioned according to the standard 10-20-system. We use electrodes F_{p1}, F_{p2}, F_7, F_3, F_z, F_4, F_8, T_3, C_3, C_z, C_4, T_4, T_5, P_3, P_z, P_4, T_6, O_1 and O_2. All potentials are measured against linked ears, with a resistance of < 5 kOhm. Figure 16.1 shows the positions of the electrodes. The 19 channels are drawn double-encircled.

EEG artifacts often spring from eye movements or muscle activities and lead to very high frequencies or amplitudes at the recordings. They may occur, but only artifact-free data are taken into account. This is possible, because physicians pre-analyzed the EEG spectra by visual inspection. Sequences with too many artifacts were rejected.

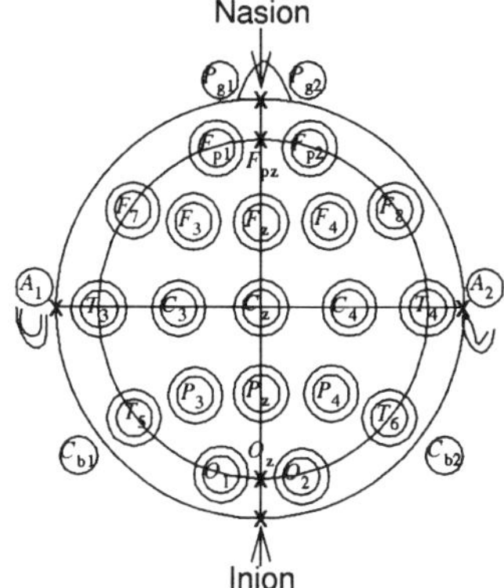

☒	F_{p1}	☒	F_{p2}	☒
F_7	F_3	F_z	F_4	F_8
T_3	C_3	C_z	C_4	T_4
T_5	P_3	P_z	P_4	T_6
☒	O_1	☒	O_2	☒

☒ not used

Figure 16.1 Left: Sample electrode positions of the 10-20-system. The 19 channels used are drawn double-encircled. Right: Visualization scheme of patterns in this chapter.

We used 10 healthy test persons who had to carry out 6 tasks. The EEG recordings contained artifact-free parts lasting at least 40 seconds per task. We used further 8 test persons, whose EEG recordings partially contained artifacts. The latter were used for the evaluation. Results of two test persons are shown in the results section. The tasks were:

- rest, eyes closed,
- rest, eyes open,
- mental calculation task,
- watch pendulum,
- figure pendulum, and
- CNV paradigm (attention task).

The EEG spectrum is digitized at the sample frequency of 128 Hz. Recordings of one second duration (128 samples) define one raw-data vector. Thus, each vector consists of 19 (channels) times 128 (samples) components. The sequence of raw-data vectors is coded every half a second and defines the input space for the Fourier-Transform and the Wavelet-Transform. Thus, the resulting vectors are overlapping in time half a second each.

16.2.2 Fourier-Transform

Each raw-data vector with 128 sample points is filtered by a *Hamming window* and Fourier-transformed. This results in a *power spectrum* that has its main

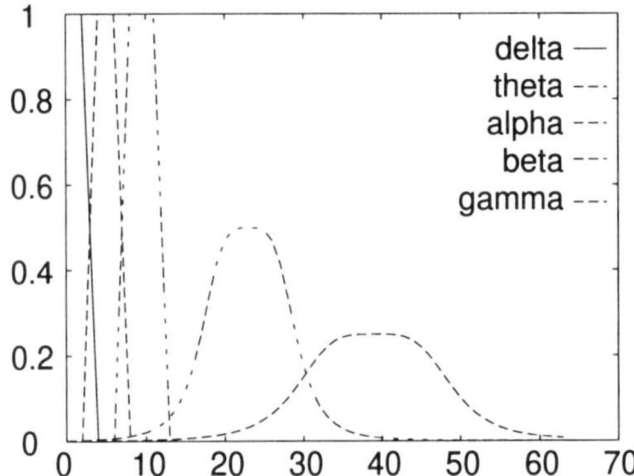

Figure 16.2 Butterworth filter covering the 5 major EEG ranges.

period from -64 Hz to 64 Hz and is symmetric to the origin. In order to avoid these redundancies, we confine the power spectrum from 0 Hz to 64 Hz. The use of Hamming windows reduces artifacts in the power spectrum that would occur if rectangular windows were used instead. Rectangular windows usually lead to high frequencies on the edges of two neighboring windows (see also [Gonzales and Wintz, 1987]).

The power spectrum of each vector is filtered with 5 *butterworth filter* covering the 5 major EEG rhythms, namely the delta-, theta-, alpha-, beta- and gamma-rhythms. According to [Cooper et al., 1974] we limit the EEG frequency ranges to fit the EEG rhythms as follows:

- delta: < 4 Hz,
- theta: $4 - 8$ Hz,
- alpha: $8 - 13$ Hz,
- beta: $13 - 30$ Hz, and
- gamma: > 30 Hz $(30 - 50$ Hz).

All five butterworth filters are plotted in Figure 16.2

We attenuate the last two frequency bands as higher frequencies often contain artifacts that we do not want to treat. For the calculation of the Fourier-Transform, the power spectra and the matrix multiplication of the power spectra with the butterworth filters we use tools of the Khoros/Cantata-v1.5 toolbox [Khoros, 1992]. The resulting vectors each have 19 (no. of channels) times 5 (no. of butterworth filters) components and serve as input to the self-organizing map.

16.2.3 Wavelet-Transform

We used the *Wavelet-Transform* as an alternative preprocessing method. In recent times, the Wavelet-Transform has more and more been used for signal processing tasks. It describes a signal in its broad shape plus its details that may vary from coarse to very fine by looking at a signal from different "levels of resolution" or different scales. It calculates the average of a signal at a given level of resolution to the next lower level of resolution. This is managed by averaging two neighboring samples at a given time and level of resolution and can be viewed as low pass filtering of the signal. In order to retrieve the original signal, the Wavelet-Transform adds some "detail coefficients" at each level of resolution. They are called the *coefficients* to the *Wavelet basic functions* and may be thought as coefficients to a frequency channel. A major property of the Wavelet-Transform is that a signal may be recovered completely by the wavelet coefficients.

The Wavelet-Transform is to a large extent analogous to the "windowed" Fourier-Transform by transforming the signal and shifting it from the time domain to the frequency domain. The main difference between Fourier- and Wavelet-Transform is that the windowed Fourier-Transform fills up the window with signals of one specific frequency, resulting in one Fourier component per frequency. This is done for all frequencies of interest. On the contrary, the Wavelet scheme transforms the signal using functions that are all derived from one mother wavelet, which is translated and dilated. High frequency portions of a signal are transformed with narrow wavelets, whereas low frequencies are transformed by broad wavelets. Thus, the Wavelet-Transform is presumed to be much more capable of detecting high frequency portions of EEG recordings such as "spikes" and "sharp waves" than the usual Fourier-Transform (for more details on Wavelet-Transforms see [Daubechies, 1992, Mallat, 1989, Stollnitz et al., 1995]). We used this preprocessing method in order to detect high frequency portions of our EEG data.

We proceed as follows: Each vector that we get from the data coding above is transformed by the 2-dimensional forward Wavelet-Transform using "bi24hd" (biorthogonal 2-dimensional high pass) as high pass filter and "bi24ld" (Daubechies 2- dimensional low pass) as low pass filter. This results in as many wavelet coefficients as sample points per second, thus 128 wavelet coefficients per vector. Mating wavelet coefficients are combined and averaged by 8 band-pass filters, thus reducing the former 128 coefficients to 8 averaged coefficients. The resulting vectors have 19 (no. of channels) times 8 (no. of band pass filter) components each.

16.2.4 Self-Organizing Map

The *Self-Organizing Map (SOM)*, also called *Kohonen's (feature) map*, is a major representative of the artificial neural networks (ANN). These are generally used to represent and generalize an input data set in an easy way [Kohonen, 1982, Kohonen, 1995].

The SOM performs an unsupervised (self-organized) adaptation scheme, no target output is needed. The learning algorithm maps the input vectors onto its two-dimensional mapping space using a neighborhood relation between adjacent neurons of the map.

SOM-Training. If an input is presented to the map, one neuron of the map "wins" this input. It is the neuron with the smallest (Euclidean) distance of its weight vector to the presented input. In the training step (weight update), the winning weight vector converges to the input vector, as well as the weight vectors of neurons in a previously defined neighborhood range around the winning neuron. It is worth mentioning that the corresponding neighboring weights do not need to have the second or third smallest distances from the input vector. It is sufficient to be adjacent to the winning neuron, according to a predefined arrangement of the neurons in a two-dimensional grid.

The training of the SOM leads to a so-called *topology preserving mapping* of the input data set to the Kohonen grid: Adjacent input vectors, that is input vectors that have small (Euclidean) distances to each other in the input space, will have neighboring coordinates on the trained grid of the map. Thus, "similar" input vectors will be mapped at the same region of the map and will form one "cluster".

Topology preservation requires an adopted dimensionality of the embedding data manifold to the map dimensionality. Note that the projection of a 3-dimensional data set on a two-dimensional map results in topological defects. Nevertheless, such a configuration may be considered because of advantageous visualization properties of two-dimensional data spaces. Kohonen recommends rectangular, not square grids, in order to avoid symmetries of the map. Distance maps may be used to show distances between neurons of the trained map and represent an important evaluation scheme. Neurons inside a cluster have slight different weight vectors, whereas neurons at the edges of different clusters show big distances. These distances are shown in distance maps, with distances between two weight vectors coded by grey-levels.

The learning process of the SOM commonly takes many steps ($10^4 - 10^6$). Therefore, the training vectors have to be presented to the map in a cyclic or randomly permutated order. The unsupervised SOM learning algorithm approximates the probability density function of the input vector space.

After the training of the map, clusters may be visualized and evaluated by prototype vectors which represent the clusters. These clusters may afterwards be identified with specific experimental conditions or patterns. Due to the unsupervised training method we do not need any information on the input EEG spectra. Another motivation of the SOM is that the user may easily identify classes of the EEG data by looking up the resulting 2-dimensional winner maps. As seen above, each EEG sample will possess a winner coordinate on the map.

16.3 RESULTS

Below, we present the classification results after the training and evaluation of the SOM. The training data is generated by the Fourier-Transform or the Wavelet-Transform.

16.3.1 Fourier-Transformation

We first concatenate 6 artifact-free tasks of 10 test persons to one huge test data set. Due to the long calculation time, we had to limit the length of each task to 5 sec (9 vectors per task, for each test person 54 vectors and for the total data set 540 vectors).

The Fourier-Transform reduces the number of components per vector from 2432 (19 channels times 128 sample points) to 95 (19 channels times 5 butterworth filters). The components are scaled between values of 0 and 1.

All 540 vectors are used to train the SOM. The map is a 2-dimensional rectangular grid with a 20x20 neuron matrix. The number of neurons is heuristically chosen to be 400. It can be seen that a lower number of neurons will collect different classes into a cluster, whereas more neurons will not yield better results. The number of training steps equals 8100. The training is repeated three times using the same number of training steps. The data is repeatedly presented in a cyclic way. The minimum and maximum initialization values are scaled to the values between 0 and 1 respectively and the initial adaptation height of 0.8 is chosen. The map is cross-evaluated by artifact-free tasks of one test person not contained in the training data (54 vectors, 95 components).

Clusters of the map are related to specific EEG patterns that consist of the spatial configuration of the power spectra of all the electrodes. The spatial configuration shows the power spectra of each electrode at the corresponding electrode position of the head. This is done for all 5 EEG frequency bands. The amplitudes of the power spectra for each of the 19 channels are normalized and visualized at different grey-levels. They are positioned according to the electrode positions of the EEG recording (see also Figure 16.1).

The maps show winner distances of one input vector to the prototype vectors arranged according to the 2-dimensional neuron grid. Black marks belong to small distances of the neuron in question and white marks to big distances.

Next we present two major results:

1. The SOM is able to differentiate between different *EEG patterns* that may occur with every test person and with every task. Some specific EEG patterns which have been detected will be presented below.

2. We are able to show the classification results for each test person in its temporal sequence. This is accomplished by using the animate-tool of the Khoros/Cantata-v1.5 toolbox [Khoros, 1992]. We use this tool in order to automatically show the winner maps for the sequence of evaluation vectors. The user is able to see the activation of the map "move" from one position of the map to the other. We may interpret each cluster as a representation of the *temporary brain function* of one test person at different time instances. A temporal sequence is visualized in a "movie"-like way and shows the sequence of the temporary brain function of the test person.

The major EEG patterns detected are presented below:

- The first typical EEG cluster consists of spectra which achieve their maximum for three anterior to posterior rows (channels F_7 to T_5, channel F_z to P_z and channel F_8 to T_6) in the delta frequency range and lasting for at least 1.5 sec (2 vectors). All other frequency ranges have low coefficients. Figure 16.3 shows at the left side the winner map trained with the complete training data set and cross-evaluated with the test person in question: the strongest activation of the map can be detected at the upper-right corner. The right side of Figure 16.3 shows the spatial configuration of spectra of all the 19 channels of the delta band that can be related to the activation of the winner map at the left side of Figure 16.3 (black marks refer to maximum spectra, white or blank marks refer to minimal spectra). This example pattern consists of the maximal spectrum at channel F_8, a submaximal spectrum at channel F_z, middle-sized spectra at T_3 and T_5 and lowest spectra at channel-rows F_{p1}, F_3, C_3, P_3 and channel- rows F_{p2}, F_4, C_4, P_4 (blank marks).

- Clusters can be detected for a second EEG pattern, consisting of maximal EEG spectra in anterior channels F_{p1} and F_{p2}, minimal spectra in all other channels, with lowest spectra in posterior electrodes (delta frequency band).

  Minimal EEG spectra may occur at channels F_{p1} and F_{p2} in the theta frequency band. Lowest spectra occur on all other frequency ranges (blink

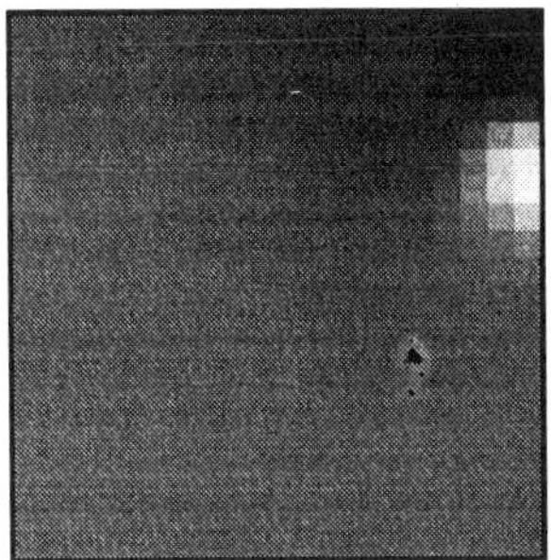

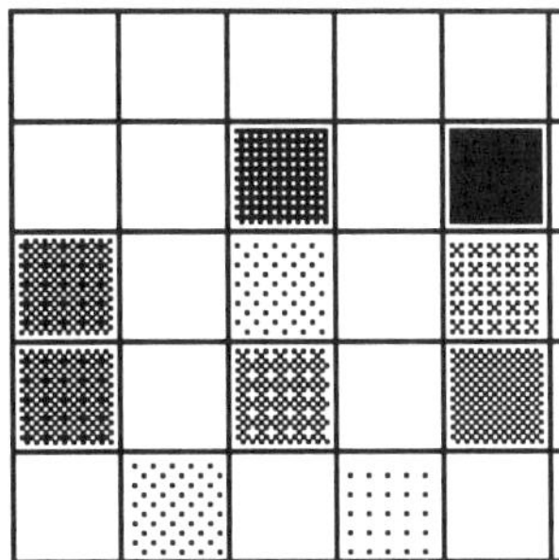

Figure 16.3 Left: Clustering results for the winner map trained with the complete training data set and evaluated with the test person (cross-evaluation of test person 1). Right: Corresponding spatial configuration (nasion on top, inion at the bottom) for the winner map of test person 1.

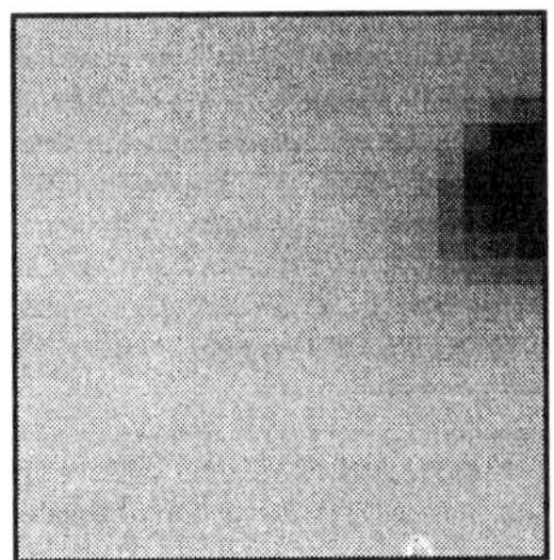

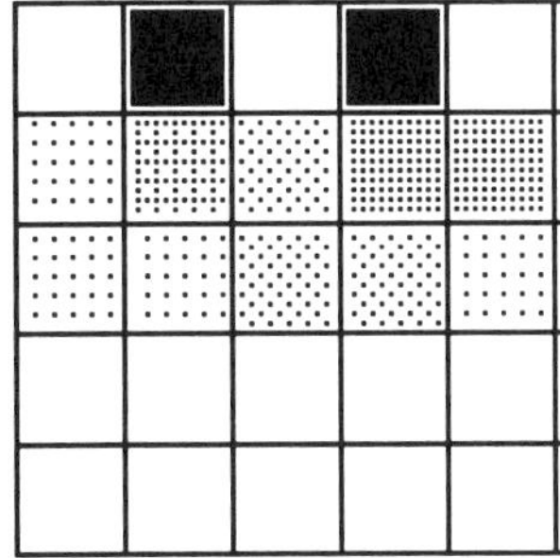

Figure 16.4 Left: Clustering results for the winner map cross-evaluated with test person 2. Right: Corresponding spatial configuration for the winner map of test person 2.

artifact). Figure 16.4 depicts the results for this second EEG pattern which are analogous to Figure 16.3.

The concrete intensities of spectra of the spatial configuration may vary.

Further EEG patterns forming clusters can be detected and these are overviewed below:

- Maximal spectrum at channel C_z and middle-sized spectra at anterior channels F_{p1} and F_{p2}, at the two channel-rows from channel F_7 through F_8 and from channel T_3 through T_4 - all in the delta range. Lowest spectra occur in all posterior channels of the delta range and in all other frequency ranges.

- Maximal spectrum in channel O_1, middle-sized spectra at "channel-rows" from channel T_5 through channel T_6 and from channel T_3 through channel T_4 - all at the delta frequency range. Lowest spectra at all other frequency ranges.

- At almost every channel sub-maximal spectra at the delta frequency range. Lowest spectra at all other frequency ranges.

- 2 channel-rows from F_{p1} through O_1 and from F_{p2} through O_2 with middle-sized spectra at all frequency ranges. All other channels have submaximal spectra at every frequency range.

An example of a time sequence of winner maps which shows the mental activations of one test person is depicted in Figure 16.5. This figure also shows the corresponding spatial EEG pattern to every Kohonen map.

The first map shows the undefined temporary brain function on the "default" rightmost-top cluster. This condition lasts from 0 to the 4th second and can not be assigned to any specific EEG pattern.

The next condition that produces an activation on the left-bottom side, which corresponds to maximal spectra at channels T_3, C_3 and C_z, middle-sized spectra at channels C_4 and T_4 and for the channel-row extending from channel F_7 through F_8, plus low-sized spectra at anterior channels F_{p1} and F_{p2} (delta range). It occurs 4.5 seconds after the beginning of the recording.

The third temporary brain function with activation at the bottom-right contains maximal spectra in channels F_{p1} and F_{p2} at the delta range and minimal spectra elsewhere and occurs five seconds after the start of the recording.

The fourth map is analogous to the first one.

The fifth map shows a cluster at the far bottom-left corner and represents the condition, when channels F_4 and F_8 have maximal spectra at the delta range and channels F_{p1} and F_{p2}, F_7 through F_z and channel-row T_3 through T_4 have submaximal spectra at the delta frequency range. All other channels have lowest spectra at delta- and all other frequency ranges. This condition is active from 7 sec to 8.5 seconds after the start of the recording.

The last but one map with an activation at the diagonal represents maximal spectra at channel C_z and middle-sized spectra at the two anterior channels F_{p1} and F_{p2}, the two channel-rows from F_7 through F_8 and from T_3 through T_4 - all at the delta range and with lowest spectra at all channels and all other frequency ranges, lasts from 8.5 sec to 13 sec after the start of the recording.

The last map again shows the default clustering for spatial configurations that can not be assigned to a specific EEG pattern.

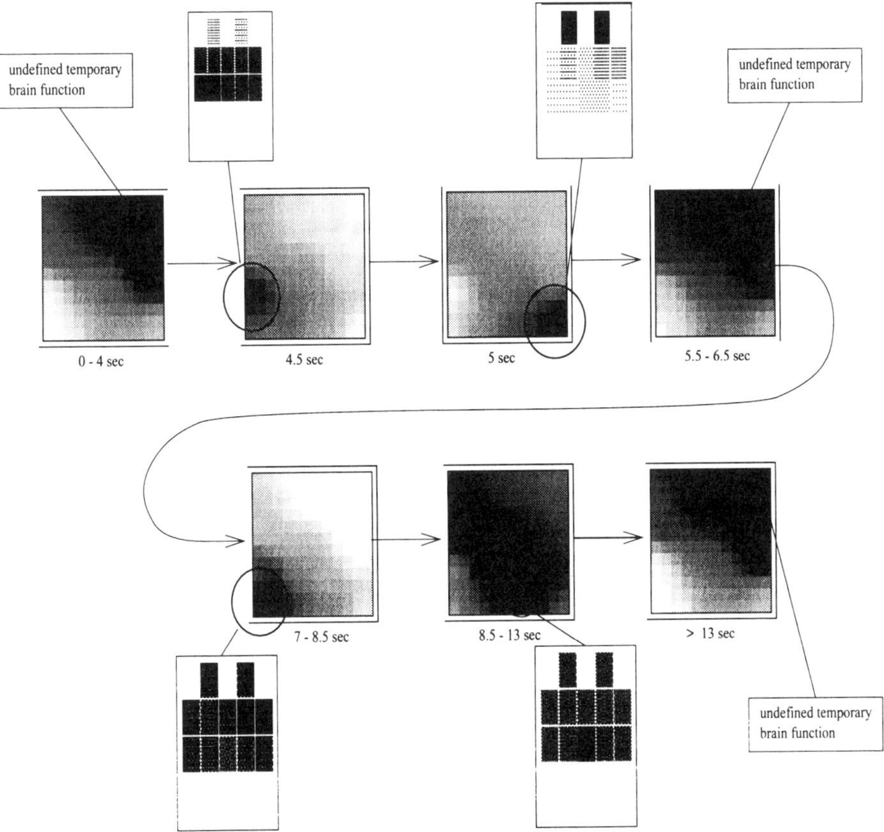

Figure 16.5 Time sequence showing the temporary brain function of an example test person evolving in time. Shown are the winner maps at different time instances with their activations or clusters plus the correlated spatial EEG patterns (all in the delta frequency range). To the first, fourth and seventh winner map can not be assigned any specific EEG pattern.

16.3.2 Wavelet-Transformation

The preprocessing unit using the Wavelet-Transform reduces the number of components per vector from 2432 (19 channels times 128 sample points) to 152 (19 channels times 8 bandpass filters). For the same reason as for the Fourier-Transform, the data have to be scaled to values between 0 and 1.

We used EEG recordings partially containing artifacts to train the SOM that is again 2-dimensional rectangular with a 20x20 neuron matrix. Analogous to the Fourier preprocessing unit, we had to limit the length of each task to 5 sec. Out of 5 test persons we obtain 270 vectors that form the test data set. The number of training steps is — like in the SOM training of the Fourier processing unit — repeated three times. For the minimum and maximum initial values and for the initial adaptation height we are using the same values as above.

The map is cross-evaluated by tasks of test persons partially containing artifacts that are not contained in the test data set (54 vectors, 152 components per test person).

According to [Clochon et al., 1993], for the detection of high frequency portions, it is sufficient to limit the data to the last bandpass filter, as the last filter represents the highest resolutions of a signal. Once again this reduces the components of each vector from 152 (19 channels times 8 bandpass filters) to 19 (19 channels times 1 bandpass filters).

Results of the cross evaluation show winner maps that consist of a specific cluster or activation. Activations of the winner map can be related to spatial configurations of filtered wavelet coefficients of all the electrodes. The spatial configurations show normalized and filtered wavelet coefficients of the last level of resolution at different grey levels. They are positioned according to the electrode positions of the EEG recording (see also Figure 16.1).

The specific "artifact activation" combines vectors that consist of highest filtered wavelet coefficients of the last level of resolution at *more than one* channel. Consequently, this activation classifies or detects potential artifacts. Furthermore, potential artifacts are projected on the same map cluster, independent of the test person in question. With that, the obtained artifact detection inter-classifies at different test persons and tasks.

Figure 16.6 shows the clustering results for the winner map cross-evaluated with example test person 3. The left side shows the specific "artifact activation" that is visible at the far left bottom of the winner map. The right side of Figure 16.6 shows a spatial configuration of the filtered and normalized wavelet coefficients of the last level of resolution that is correlated to the "artifact activation". The highest wavelet coefficients for this example are obtained at channels F_{p2} and C_4 (dark grey or black marks) 15 seconds after the start of the recording. Figure 16.7 displays the EEG recordings of the corresponding

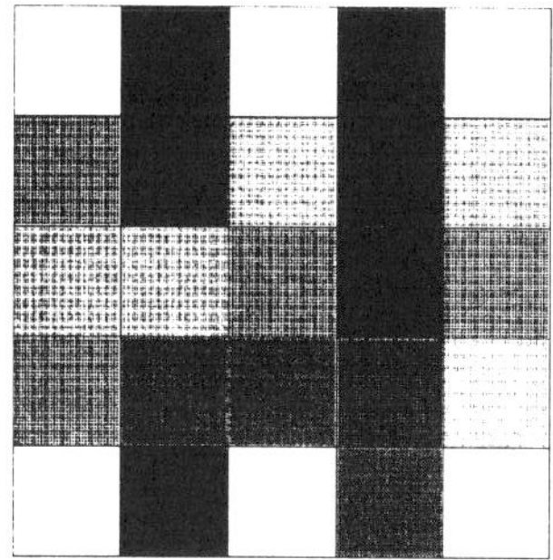

Figure 16.6 Clustering results for the winner map cross-evaluated with example test person 3. Left: "Artifact activation" visible at the far left bottom. Right: Corresponding spatial configuration of filtered wavelet coefficients.

channels (Left: channel F_{p2}, Right: channel C_4) for this example that show the highest filtered wavelet coefficients. The recordings are shown as magnifications of the total recording of test person 3 and last one second each.

Again, we are able to display the results of our artifact detection for each test person in its temporal sequence (cf. Figure 16.5). By this, the user may observe the emerging of any "artifact activation" on the winner map in time. In order to validate these results, the user may look up the corresponding "wavelet brain map" and EEG recordings of channels in question.

16.4 CONCLUSION

We have presented an easy way of detecting major EEG patterns. This is accomplished by using the SOM as a classifier and the Fourier-Transform and the Wavelet-Transform as preprocessing units.

The Fourier-Transform produces power spectra of each vector lasting one second. These vectors are filtered with masks that cover the 5 major EEG frequency bands, like delta, theta, alpha, beta and gamma. We are also able to depict the spatial configuration of the EEG spectra for all channels used and for every EEG frequency band. It is possible to correlate clusters obtained by the trained Kohonen map to specific patterns of the spatial configurations. Additionally, our map is able to evaluate unknown EEG recordings. In such a way, an inter-classification of EEG patterns that may occur with various test persons and various tasks is possible. The results can be summarized using the animate-tool: with that, the user can clearly observe the temporary brain function of any test person evolving in time. The tool automatically shows the movement of the activation on the map in a short "movie".

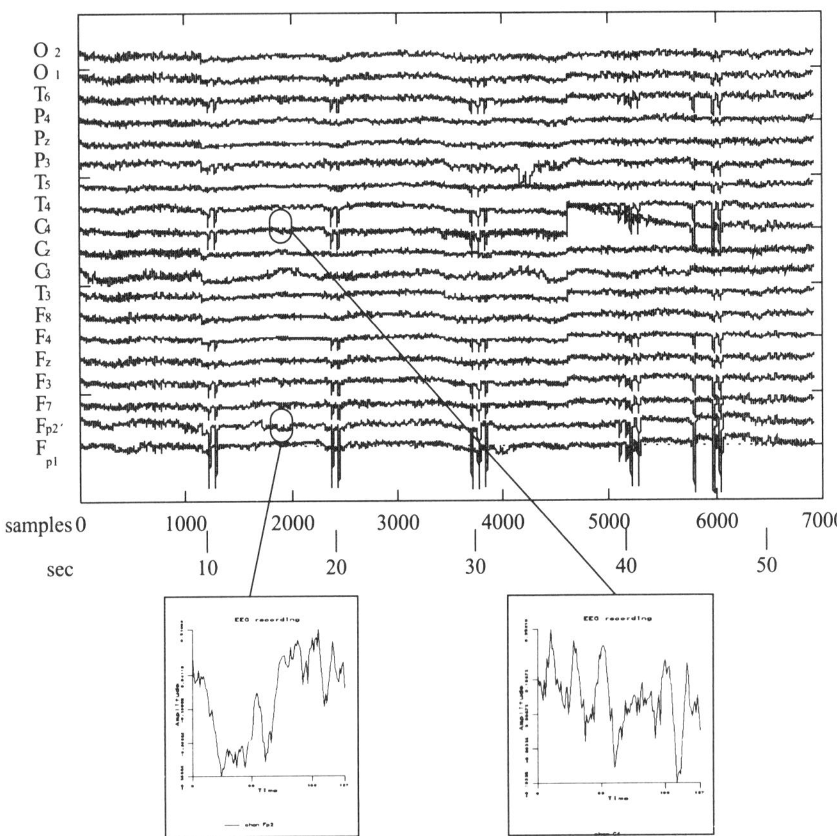

Figure 16.7 EEG recordings of corresponding channels (bottom left: F_{p2}, bottom right: C_4) showing highest wavelet coefficients. Shown are the appropriate recordings of one second duration as magnifications of the total EEG recording of test person 3.

In the second part we have presented a way of detecting potential EEG artifacts that consist of high-frequency, short time portions of the signal. Again, the SOM is used as a classifier. As the Fourier preprocessing unit is unable to detect artifacts, the Fourier-Transform is replaced by the Wavelet-Transform. The Wavelet-Transform produces Wavelet coefficients that can be divided into different levels of resolution. The input to the SOM is restricted to the filtered coefficients of the last level of resolution. The cross-evaluated winner maps show specific "artifact activations" that combine "potential artifactual EEG recordings". For the purpose of validation, EEG recordings of channels that obtain highest filtered wavelet coefficients can be displayed. Additionally, the results can be summarized using the animate-tool: the user can observe the emerging of the "artifact activation" in time.

From the medical point of view it may further be of interest to visualize pathological EEG data, like EEGs with intoxication, ischemic insult, brain tumors, epilepsy, dementia or psychiatric disease. Until now, we merely considered EEG obtained from healthy test persons. Pathological EEGs will probably deliver other map classes and spatial patterns. Especially for the epilepsy, our technique could be used for an automated evaluation of long term recordings. Other applications of our methods could be therapy monitoring and the inspection of intrapersonal changes prior to and after medication, e.g., antiepileptic medication or the ascertainment of drug effects.

References

Clochon, P., Caterini, R., Clarencon, D., Roman, V. (1993). EEG paroxystic activity detected by neural networks after wavelet transform analysis. In *Proc. ESANN'93*, Brussels, Belgium.

Cooper, R., Osselton, J. W., Shaw, J. C. (1974). *EEG-Technology*, 2nd Edition, Butterworth & Co Ltd.

Daubechies, I. (1992). Ten lectures on wavelets, Rutgers University and AT&T Bell Laboratories, *CBMS-INSF, Regional Conference Series in Applied Mathematics.*

Gonzales, R.C., Wintz, P. (1987). *Digital Image Processing*, 2nd Edition. Addison–Wesley.

Heuser, U., Göppert, J., Rosenstiel, W., Stevens, A. (1996). Classification of human brain waves using self-organizing maps. In *IDAMAP-96 Workshop Notes, ECAI'96*, Budapest, pages 37–42.

Joutsiniemi, S.-L., Kaski, S., Larsen, T.A. (1995). Self-organizing map in recognition of topographic patterns of EEG spectra. *IEEE Transactions on Biomedical Engineering*, 42(11).

Khoros manual (1992). The Khoros Group, Department of Electrical and Computer Engineering, University of New Mexico, Albuquerque, NM 87131.

Kohonen, T. (1982). Self-organized formation of topology correct feature maps. *Biological Cybernetics*, 59–69.

Kohonen, T. (1995). Adaptive-subspace SOM (ASSOM) for the implementation of wavelets and gabor filters. In *Self-Organizing Maps*, pages 161-173. Springer Verlag.

Mallat, S. (1989). A theory for multiresolution decomposition - the wavelet representation. *IEEE Transaction on Pattern Analysis and Machine Intelligence*, 2(7):674-692.

Stollnitz, E.J., DeRose, T.D., Salesin, D.H. (1995). University of Washington, Wavelets for computer graphics, Part 1 and 2. *IEEE Computer Graphics and Applications*, pages 76–83.

17 APPLYING A NEURAL NETWORK TO PROSTATE CANCER SURVIVAL DATA

Michael W. Kattan,
Haku Ishida,
Peter T. Scardino,
and J. Robert Beck

Abstract: Prediction of treatment efficacy for prostate cancer therapies has proven difficult and requires modeling of survival-type data. One reason for the difficulty may be infrequent use of flexible modeling techniques, such as artificial neural networks (ANN). The purpose of this study is to illustrate the use of an ANN to model prostate cancer survival data and compare the ANN to the traditional statistical method, Cox proportional hazards regression. Clinical data and disease follow-up for 983 men were modeled by both an ANN and a Cox model. Repeated sampling of 200 training and testing subsets were supplied to each technique. The concordance index c was calculated for each testing dataset. As further validation, ANN and Cox models were applied to a totally separate dataset. The ANN outperformed the Cox model in internal validation datasets (ANN $c = 0.76$, Cox $c = 0.74$) and on the external validation dataset (ANN $c = 0.77$, Cox $c = 0.74$). ANNs were more discriminating than Cox models for predicting cancer recurrence. Calibration of the ANN remains a problem. Once solved, it is expected that an ANN will make the most accurate predictions of prostate cancer recurrence and improve treatment decision making.

17.1 INTRODUCTION

Deciding whether to operate on patients with clinically localized prostate cancer frequently requires the urologist to classify patients into expected groups such as "remission" or "recur". When datasets containing predictor variables and the recurrence status have been collected, several statistical tools (e.g., logistic regression) are available to help form models for classification. Recently, artificial neural networks (ANNs) have become popular for medical classification decisions [Kattan and Beck, 1995]. This is largely due to their modeling flexibility since ANNs can detect certain predictor variable relationships (e.g., interactions, nonlinearities) that must be prespecified in the traditional statistical model. As a result, ANNs have frequently produced more accurate models for urological data [Kattan et al., 1996].

When predicting recurrence following surgery for prostate cancer, the endpoint of interest may take several years to occur. The reason for this is that a patient's first sign of recurrence is usually a return in his prostate specific antigen (PSA), and this may not happen for 5 years [Kattan et al., 1997a]. Thus, classification of patients into treatment successes or failures requires a lengthy follow-up, and omitting nonrecurrent patients with short follow-up will bias estimates of the probability of recurrence. The typical use of ANN models, which assume a classification decision, to predict this type of outcome is problematic.

The common statistical technique for mutivariable models which consider the time until the event is the Cox proportional hazards model [Harrell et al., 1996]. It appropriately considers the follow-up time and whether the event occurs for each patient. Although a nonparametric technique, it still makes an important assumption: that continuous predictor variables have linear relationships with the risk of the event occurring [Harrell et al., 1996]. If a priori knowledge of the variable relationships is available, the user may include nonlinear transforms of the predictors, but this is often a trial and error approach. It is usually not known a priori what specific nonlinear transform is best, or if complex variable interactions are present. The lack of flexibility of the Cox model may result in suboptimal performance for prediction purposes.

While the Cox model is well-accepted for survival analyses [Marubini and Valsecchi, 1995], the ANNs have strengths over the Cox models which may result in improved predicting ability. The ANN model is sufficiently flexible to model virtually any nonlinear relationship [Hornik et al., 1989], and rids the user of having to exactly specify the structural relationship, especially when it comes to complex interactions. As a result, it is plausible that an ANN model could outperform the Cox model in predicting prostate cancer recurrence when complex interactions or nonlinear relationships are present but not known.

However, it is not well understood how to apply an ANN to a time-until-event dataset such as this.

The purpose of this chapter is to illustrate a method of applying an ANN to radical prostatectomy follow-up data and to compare its performance with a Cox model. To do this, we adapt the suggestions of Therneau [Therneau et al., 1990] and utilize the measures of Harrell [Harrell et al., 1982] to judge predictive accuracy. An ordinary backpropagation neural network is employed with a single hidden layer and a bias neuron in both the input and hidden layers.

17.2 METHODS

The first step of our approach is the computation of the null martingale residual (NMR) [Therneau et al., 1990] using the follow-up time and the censor indicator of whether the patient recurred. As a single variable, the NMR replaces these two outcome variables (follow-up time and censor) and becomes the new outcome variable. In interpretation, the NMR is proportional to the risk of the event for the individual. Computation of the NMR is completely independent of the predictor variables and simply represents the difference between the observed and expected number of recurrences which should have been observed for that point in time (i.e., the patient's follow-up time). Thus, the adapted dataset for the ANN model contains the original predictor variables along with the NMR, which is predicted; follow-up time and censor are not used for modeling.

17.2.1 Patient data

The dataset initially consisted of records from all 1055 patients admitted to the hospital with the intent to operate on their clinically localized prostate cancer between June 1983 and December 1996. Excluded from analysis were the 55 men initially treated with radiation, and 1 treated with cryotherapy. Sixteen men whose disease status (free of disease versus cancer recurrence) was unknown were also excluded. The mean age was 63 years and 85% of the patients were Caucasian. We selected the following routinely performed clinical variables as predictors of recurrence: pretreatment serum PSA levels, primary and secondary Gleason grade in the biopsy specimen, and clinical stage (assigned using the TNM system) [Ohori, 1994]. Treatment failure was defined as either clinical evidence of cancer recurrence or a postoperative PSA (0.4 ng/ml and rising) on at least one additional evaluation. Patients who were treated with hormonal therapy (N=8) or radiotherapy (N=25) after surgery but before documented recurrence were treated as failures at the time of second therapy. Patients who had their operation aborted due to positive lymph nodes

(N=24) were considered immediate treatment failures. A separate sample was used for validation. It was composed of 168 patients from 5 surgeons at our institution.

17.2.2 Evaluating predictive accuracy - the *c* index

After training, the resulting product would be an ANN which could prospectively predict a patient's NMR, which is proportional to his risk of recurrence. For comparison, also consider a Cox statistical model that predicts the probability of the event occurring by a particular point in time (e.g., year 1). Assume both methods are used and patients are followed for a period of time. How can we tell which method predicted more accurately? Given we have two (one for each technique) predicted measures for each patient, an actual follow-up time, and an actual indicator of whether the patient recurred, we need to assess predictive accuracy. As stated previously, we cannot simply classify the patients into recur/disease-free since the patients who did not recur may not have been followed long enough. Instead, we use Harrell's c index [Harrell et al., 1982], which denotes the proportion of usable patient pairs in which the predictions are consistent with the outcome. A usable patient pair requires that at least one of the two patients recurs. If both patients recur, and the predicted disease-free time is larger for the patient who survived longer disease-free, this is a consistent pair. If one patient recurs and the other remains disease-free at least as long as the first, it is assumed that the second patient is assumed to outlasted the first, and the pair is counted as consistent pair if the recurred patient had a larger predicted probability of remaining disease-free. When predicted disease-free probabilities are identical for a patient pair, 1/2 rather than 1 is added to the count of consistent pairs in the numerator of the proportion. In this case, one is still added to the denominator of the proportion since the pair is still usable. A patient pair is not usable if both patients recur with the same follow-up or if one recurs and the other does not but with a shorter follow-up. Index c is interpreted as the probability that, given two randomly drawn patients, the patient who recurs first had a higher probability of recurrence.

17.2.3 Experimental design

As a method of internal validation, the original patient dataset is randomly divided into 2/3 training and 1/3 testing subsets. Cox and the ANN model the training subset, then predict upon the testing subset. Modeling the training subset first requires computation of the NMR for the ANN, followed by modeling of the NMR by the ANN. Predictions are then made upon the testing subset. Each technique thus has a model derived from training data, and the model is then applied to the testing dataset to obtain predictions. The testing subset predictions are then compared with actual patient results by calculating the c index. This training/testing process is repeated for a total of 200 c observations. Median and 95% confidence intervals for the c of each technique are computed. For external validation, a Cox model and an ANN were each fit on the entire dataset of 983 men and applied to the dataset of 168 men to obtain predictions. Again, c was computed. All simulations and statistical analyses are done with SPlus software (Version 3.3, Redmond WA).

17.3 RESULTS

Results from the internal validation appear in Figure 17.1. Boxplots indicate the median, surrounded by indented 95% confidence intervals, limits of second and third quartiles, and the range of observations. For the Cox model, the median c was 0.74, and for the ANN model, the median c was 0.76. Note that the confidence intervals fail to overlap suggesting a real benefit for the ANN model ($p < 0.05$). However, the benefit is very slight (a c improvement of approximately 0.02).

Figure 17.2 shows a boxplot of the paired differences between techniques as the Cox c subtracted from the ANN c for each of the 200 iterations. The paired comparisons agree with the unpaired Figure 17.1, in that the confidence interval fails to overlap 0, but the difference boxplot more precisely estimates the improvement for the ANN.

Figure 17.3 is an event chart for the Cox model predictions on the validation dataset. The y-axis is the predicted probability of remaining free from disease for each of the 168 patients, and the x-axis is the follow-up time. Open circles indicate disease-free patients, and filled triangles represent recurrences. The c index for the Cox model is 0.74. Figure 17.4 is the corresponding event chart for the ANN. The c index for this model is higher than that for Cox, with $c = 0.77$.

Figure 17.5 is a scatterplot of the validation dataset predictions for Cox and the ANN. The 45 degree line represents perfect agreement between the two techniques. Note that the predicted probabilities of remaining free from disease using the Cox model are nearly always higher than those using the ANN.

17.4 DISCUSSION

Others have developed approaches for applying ANNs to survival-type data. Some of the these involve creating multiple binary observations from each observation in the original survival dataset [De Laurentiis and Ravdin, 1994] or replacing the linear predictors of the Cox model with the nonlinear output of the neural network and maximizing the partial likelihood [Faraggi and Simon,

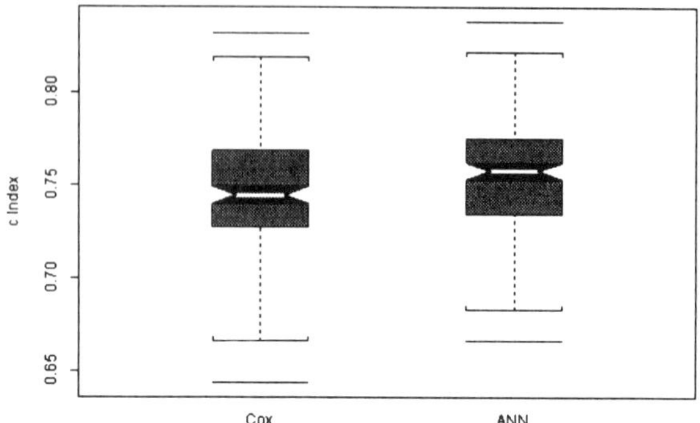

Figure 17.1 c index results from internal validation. White areas indicate medians. Indented areas are 95% confidence intervals. Dark areas outside the confidence intervals are inner quartiles. Whiskers indicate range, and horizontal lines are outliers.

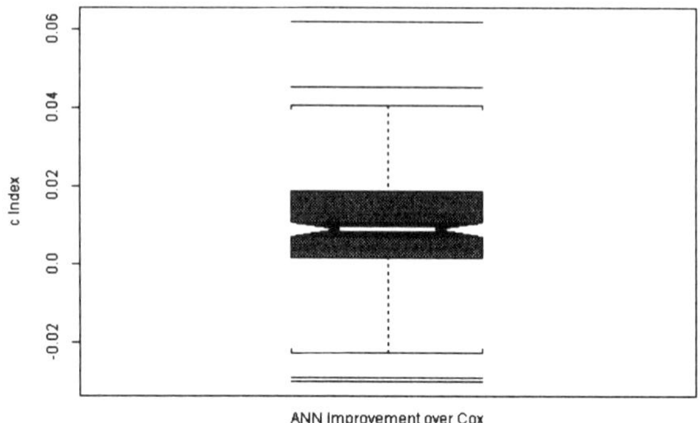

Figure 17.2 Boxplot of differences between ANN and Cox. See Figure 17.2 legend for boxplot definitions.

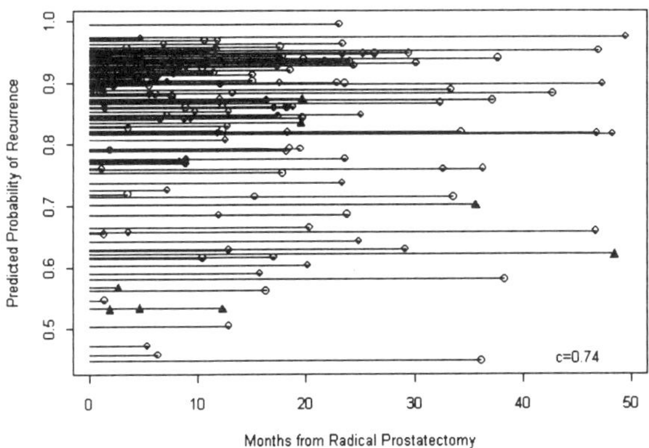

Figure 17.3 Event chart for Cox model on validation data. Open circles are disease-free patients. Closed triangles are recurrent patients.

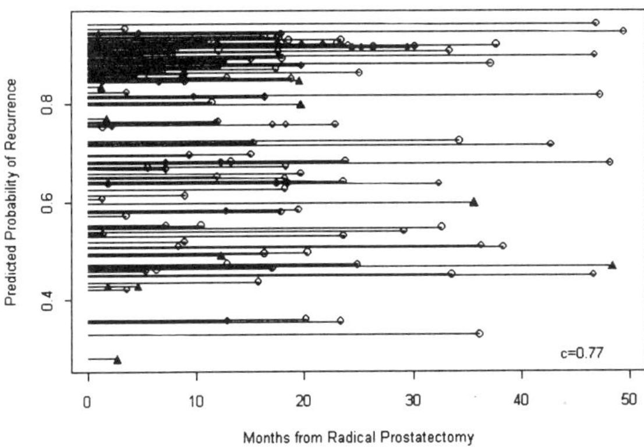

Figure 17.4 Event chart for ANN on validation data. See Figure 17.3 legend for definitions.

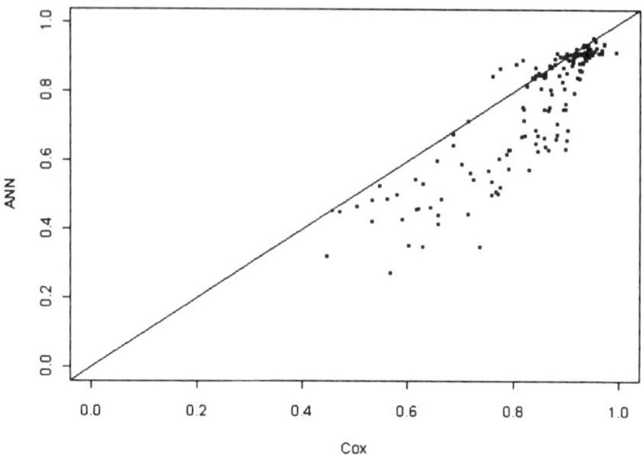

Figure 17.5 Scatterplot of the ANN and Cox predictions on the validation dataset.

1995]. We chose the NMR approach because of its simplicity. NMR calculations can be found in many biostatistical packages without having to write highly specialized code, and extensive manipulation of the original dataset is not required. Other methods for adapting ANNs to survival data may produce different results than those presented here. The simple approach we used resulted in an improvement of the ANN over the Cox model. Our approach is possible entirely within the SPlus environment with no other commercial software to obtain. This may make it easier for investigators to explore these techniques.

While there are other measures of predictive accuracy with censored data besides the c index, we believe that c is one of the easiest to conceptualize. We believe its strengths outweigh its weaknesses, such as insensitivity to slight differences, especially at the extremes of its range.

Though it remains difficult to determine a priori which technique will predict the most accurately when applied to future data, our approach suggests that ANNs should be considered for addition to the analyst's tool kit when comparing approaches. ANNs should be good at detecting nonlinear relationships or complex interactions which can be difficult to specify properly in a Cox model. Of course, a properly specified Cox model would predict at least as accurately as an ANN. However, it is not easy to explore all the interactions and nonlinearities with a Cox model. Additional research might compare the alternative models with a best subsets Cox approach that considers all possible interactions and many polynomial transforms.

While our research using the c index addresses predictive discrimination, other criteria are important to consider. In particular, ease of use for the prediction of an individual patient's outcome is a strength of the Cox model. Procedures for predicting median survival time or the probability of surviving a particular duration have been derived for the Cox model, but additional research is necessary to extend these to the ANN. For example, the ANN output could be the single, perhaps polynomial, predictor of a Cox model to facilitate these prediction estimates.

An approach for obtaining accurate predictions (i.e., calibration) for the ANN, rather than simple discrimination, appears especially important given Figure 17.5. It seems worrisome that the ANN and Cox models have such different results, given the slight discrimination improvement by the ANN. This finding suggests extreme caution before making patient decisions with the ANN until the calibration issue is resolved.

An important limitation to our approach is the assumption of proportional hazards. That is, the risk ranking of individuals does not change over time, such that if a person is expected to be at higher risk of the event by time 1, he is also assumed to be at higher risk at any later time. Relaxing this assumption does not appear easy.

A useful improvement to our methodology would be the use of bootstrapping. Bootstrapping would have important theoretical benefits and perhaps improved efficiency. Nonetheless, it would not be expected to find that bootstrapping reversed a decision of which technique is preferred. The SPlus environment should facilitate this bootstrapping improvement.

From a clinical perspective, this study has important implications. For treatment outcome following radical prostatectomy, one potential end point is the prediction of final pathologic stage, and others have used ANNs to predict stage. This particular end point, however, would be problematic in that some patients with apparently organ confined disease will later develop disease recurrence, whereas many patients with non-organ confined disease will remain disease free [Kattan et al., 1997a]. The components of pathologic stage 3 extracapsular tumor extension, seminal vesicle involvement, and positive pelvic lymph nodes 3 are adverse pathological features [Carter et al., 1989, Partin et al., 1993, Epstein et al., 1993, Stein et al., 1992]. Yet, not all patients with one or more of these findings will recur after radical prostatectomy. Partin and associates evaluated 462 men with extracapsular penetration [Partin et al., 1993]. Only 80 (17%) had evidence of disease recurrence with a mean follow-up of 53 months (range 12 to 120 months). Also, Ohori and colleagues report a PSA five year progression rate of 25% for patients with extracapsular extension in the radical prostatectomy specimen [Ohori, 1994]. Thus, using pathologic stage as an end point would limit the utility of a model to accurately predict disease recurrence following radical prostatectomy. Although final pathology has been associated with eventual treatment failure, PSA recurrence is a more appropriate measure of ultimate disease outcome [Kattan et al., 1997a] For this reason, our neural network which predicts recurrence has an advantage over the previously neural network attempts to model pathologic stage [Kattan et al., 1996].

Following radical prostatectomy designed to cure the patient of his cancer, the serum PSA should become undetectable [Stein et al., 1992]. Measurable levels of PSA after surgery suggest disease recurrence which may precede clinical detection of recurrence by several years [Partin et al., 1993]. Although an elevated serum PSA after radical prostatectomy may not be associated with death due to the cancer, it is a reasonable measure of the ability of radical prostatectomy to cure a patient with prostate cancer, provided that the follow-up is long enough.

Given that these Cox and ANN models take us closer to an accurate estimate of a patient's probability of recurrence if he chooses surgery, future research should address from the societal perspective what should be considered an acceptable probability. At levels of recurrence observed in our series, treatment appears beneficial for men under age 70, regardless of grade, and for men under 75 with moderate or poorly differentiated cancers and low comorbidity [Kattan et al., 1997b]. As the probability for recurrence increases, the morbidity of treatment may begin to outweigh the possible increase in life expectancy, resulting in a net decrease in quality-adjusted life years due to treatment. However, at the individual level, an acceptable probability of recurrence and an assessment of the risks and benefits of surgical treatment of prostate cancer remain the patient's decision.

17.5 CONCLUSION

In conclusion, this study combines the flexible modeling of an ANN adapted to survival data with the important problem of preoperatively gauging a patient's possible benefit of surgery for prostate cancer. Our results suggest that the ANN approach was better than the traditional Cox proportional hazards regression approach for ranking the patients' risk of recurrence for prostate cancer. However, additional analysis suggested that the accuracy of the ANN predictions, as measured by the difference between the predicted risk of recurrence and actual recurrence, may be a problem that future research needs to address. Upon calibration improvement for the ANN, it appears that the ANN paradigm will provide one of the most accurate and clinically useful prognostic devices currently available. Such a tool would be a welcome addition to the decision process for clinically localized prostate cancer.

Acknowledgments

Support for this work was in part provided by a Specialized Program of Research Excellence (SPORE) in prostate cancer grant (CA58204) from the National Cancer Institute and also by National Aeronautical Space Administration.

References

Carter, H. B., Partin, A. W., Oesterling, J. E., et al. (1989). The use of prostate specific antigen in the management of patients with prostate cancer: The Johns Hopkins experience. In Catalona, W.J., Coffey, D.S., Karr, J.P., editors, *Clinical aspects of prostate cancer*, pages 247–254. New York: Elsevier Science Publishing.

Epstein, J. I., Pizov, G., Walsh, P. C. (1993). Correlation of pathologic findings with progression after radical retropubic prostatectomy. *Cancer* 71:3582–3593.

Faraggi, D. and Simon, R. (1995). A neural network model for survival data. *Statistics in Medicine*, 14:73–82.

Harrell Jr., F.E., Califf, R.M., Pryor, D.B., Lee, K.L., and Rosati, R.A. (1982). Evaluating the yield of medical tests. *Journal of American Medical Association*, 247(18):2543–2546.

Harrell, F. E., Lee, K. L., Mark, D. B. (1996). Multivariable prognostic models: issues in developing models, evaluating assumptions and adequacy, and measuring and reducing errors. *Stat. Med.*, 15:361–387.

Hornik, K., Stinchcombe, M., White, H. (1989). Multilayer feedforward networks are universal approximators. *Neural Networks*, 2:359–366.

Kattan, M. W., and Beck, J. R. (1995) Artificial neural networks for medical classification decisions. *Arch. Pathol. Lab. Med.*, 119:672–677.

Kattan, M. W., Cowen, M.E., and Miles, B. J. (1996) Computer Modeling in Urology. *Urology*, 47(1):14–21.

Kattan, M. W., Stapleton, A. M. F., Wheeler, T. M., Scardino, P. T. (1997a). Evaluation of a Nomogram for Predicting Pathological Stage of Men with Clinically Localized Prostate Cancer. *Cancer*, 79(3):528–537.

Kattan, M. W., Cowen, M. E., Miles, B. J. (1997b). A decision analysis for treatment of clinically localized prostate cancer. *Journal Gen. Internal Medicine* (in press).

De Laurentiis, M., Ravdin, P. M. (1994). A technique for using neural network analysis to perform survival analysis of censored data. *Cancer Lett.*, 77:127–138.

Marubini, E., Valsecchi, M. G. (1995). *Analysing survival data from clinical trials and observational studies.* Chichester, England, Wiley & Sons Ltd.

Ohori, M., Wheeler, T. M., Scardino, P. T. (1994). The new American Joint Committee on Cancer and International Union Against Cancer TNM classification of prostate cancer: Clinicopathologic correlations. *Cancer*, 74:104–114.

Partin, A. W., Pound, C. R., Clemens, J. Q., Epstein, J. I., Walsh, P.C. (1993). Serum PSA after anatomic radical prostatectomy: The Johns Hopkins experience after 10 years. *Urol. Clin. North. Am.*, 20(4):713–725.

Stein, A., deKernion, J. B., Smith, R. B., Doug, F., Patel, H. (1992). Prostate specific antigen levels after radical prostatectomy in patients with organ confined and locally extensive prostate cancer. *Journal of Urology* 147:942.

Therneau, T.M., Grambsch, P.M., and Fleming, T.R. (1990). Martingale-based residuals for survival models. *Biometrika*, 77(1):147–160.

Index